A DOCTOR OF THEIR OWN

A DOCTOR OF
THEIR OWN

The History of
Adolescent Medicine

Heather Munro Prescott

HARVARD UNIVERSITY PRESS

Cambridge, Massachusetts
London, England   1998

Library of Congress Cataloging-in-Publication Data

Prescott, Heather Munro.
    A doctor of their own : the history of adolescent medicine /
    Heather Munro Prescott.
        p.   cm.
    Includes bibliographical references and index.
    ISBN 0-674-21461-7 (alk. paper)
    1. Adolescent medicine—United States—History.   I. Title.
RJ550.P74   1998
616'.00835—dc21
97-52222

For Wayne

Contents

Illustrations follow p. 84.

Acknowledgments

I am pleased to acknowledge the many individuals and organizations who assisted in the research and writing of this book. My greatest thanks goes to adolescent medicine's founder, Dr. J. Roswell Gallagher, whose dedication to teenagers and their problems made this work possible. Another invaluable source of support has been Joan Jacobs Brumberg, who first suggested the subject of adolescent medicine as a topic and who has carefully critiqued every draft of this project as it has evolved. I would also like to thank Margaret W. Rossiter and Bruce V. Lewenstein, who provided timely and thoughtful comments on early drafts.

Funding for research and writing came from a variety of sources. National Institutes of Health Publication Grant LM 05903-01 from the National Library of Medicine during the fall of 1995 allowed me to devote all my time to working on the book. A generous fellowship from the American College of Obstetricians and Gynecologists allowed me to spend over a month in the Washington, D.C., area conducting research at the ACOG Historical Library and other institutions. As a faculty member at Central Connecticut State University, I have been fortunate to receive financial assistance from Connecticut State University–American Association of University Professors Faculty Research Grants, which allowed me to travel to archives to conduct additional research. At Cornell University, a National Science Foundation Training Grant, a Beatrice Brown Award from the Women's Studies Program, and various fellowships from the Cornell University Graduate School provided essential sources of funding for the early stages of this project.

I am greatly indebted to the Boston Children's Hospital Medical Center for permitting me to examine patient records from the early history of the

Adolescent Unit. The unit's former director, Dr. Robert P. Masland, Jr., deserves special recognition for obtaining access to these records for me. Thanks also go to former Children's Hospital archivist Joan Krizack for helping me locate information on the broader history of this institution; to Cindy Revelle of Public Relations for helping me locate and reproduce photographs; and to former unit secretary Ruth Mersereau, former consultants Thomas Cone and Graham Blaine, and the Adolescent Unit's current director Jean Emans and physicians Esterann Grace and Elizabeth Woods for sharing their insights into the evolution of the Adolescent Unit over the years. I also acknowledge my debt to the many patients at Boston Children's Hospital. Their names have been changed to preserve their anonymity. Researchers interested in specific case records may contact me for further information.

A number of key participants in the history of adolescent medicine have helped me with this project. I am particularly grateful to Dr. Joseph L. Rauh, the official historian for the Society for Adolescent Medicine, who had the wisdom to document the history of SAM as it happened, and who has generously shared a wealth of materials and memories on the history of that organization with me. Dr. Rauh's colleague Susan L. Blumenthal offered me a place to stay while I perused the SAM records in Cincinnati. Edie Moore, executive secretary of SAM, provided additional materials on the society's history and current status. Others who have provided their insights into the development of adolescent medicine include Walter Anyan, Joseph Brenner, Robert Blum, Robert T. Brown, Michael I. Cohen, Lawrence D'Angelo, William Daniel, Robert W. Dicher, James Farrow, Marianne Felice, Dale Garell, Andrew Guthrie, Jr., Felix P. Heald, Jr., Adele Hofmann, Charles Irwin, Donald Orr, Andrew D. Rigg, Aric Schichor, S. Kenneth Schonberg, Thomas Shaffer, Tomas Silber, Victor Strasburger, Morris Wessel, and Murray Williams. Arthur J. Lesser and Vince L. Hutchins provided valuable information on the relationship between adolescent medicine and maternal and child health programs. Richard Seymour shared his recollections of the development of the Haight-Ashbury Free Clinics.

My sincere thanks also go to the librarians and archivists who have helped me with research for this book. At Cornell, librarians Robert J. Kibbee, Fred Muratori, Nancy Skipper, Carolyn Spicer, and Susan Szasz and archivist Gould Colman were particularly helpful. Julie Copenhagen, head of Interlibrary Loan at Cornell's Olin Library, patiently handled voluminous requests. At Central Connecticut State University, reference librarians Joan Packer and Emily Chasse, serials librarians Marie Kascus and Faith Merriman, and director of Interlibrary Loan June Welwood gave generous amounts of their limited time to help me find additional materials for the book. At the Francis J. Countway Library at Harvard Medical School, I was fortunate to have the able assistance of Garland Librarian Richard J. Wolfe, whose knowledge of Boston medical history was invaluable. Other librarians and archivists who deserve thanks include Thomas Rosenbaum and Gretchen Koerpel at the Rockefeller Archive Center in Sleepy Hollow, New York; Claire McCurdy, Bette Weneck, and David Ment at the Milbank Memorial Library, Teachers College, Columbia University; Patricia Cahill and Susan Young Park at the Rare Book and Manuscript Library at Columbia University; Susan Rishworth and Pamela M. Van Hine at the American College of Obstetricians and Gynecologists; and Ruth Quattlebaum, archivist for Phillips Academy, Andover, Massachusetts.

Michael Fisher, my editor at Harvard University Press, deserves my thanks for his enthusiasm about publishing the history of adolescent medicine. I would also like to thank Ann Downer-Hazell and Elizabeth Gretz for providing valuable assistance.

Completion of this project would not have been possible without the support of administrators at Central Connecticut State University who understand that research is essential for effective teaching. I would especially like to thank former Academic Vice-President Karen Beyard, former Dean of Arts and Sciences George Clarke, and Interim Dean of Arts and Sciences June Higgins for granting me reassigned time and other support necessary for completing the book. I am also grateful to Director of Sponsored Programs Dean Kleinert and Assistant Director Mimi Kaplan for helping me secure internal and external sources of funding for this project.

I have been fortunate to have had the help of faculty and students in the History Department of Central Connecticut State University. I am particularly thankful for the support of the late Charles Stephenson, who recognized the connection between the history of medicine and larger issues in recent American history. I wish he had lived to see the final product of my research. I would also like to thank former department chairs Donald Sanford, Felton Best, and Stanislaus Blejwas for helping me obtain release time from teaching to work on the book. My officemate Glen Sunshine offered moral support and his wry sense of humor at critical moments in the writing process. I am also very grateful for the research assistance of Linda Frazer, Peter Halpin, Matthew LaCrosse, Thomas Ratliff, Cynthia Riccio, Teresa Szylobryt, and John Tully, whose diligent library work was essential to the timely completion of the project.

Many individuals took time out of their busy lives to read and comment on my work. I am especially indebted to Nancy Tomes. I am also grateful to Rima Apple, Diana Long, Kathleen Jones, Steven Schlossman, and Hamilton Cravens for commenting on the portions of this book that were presented at professional meetings. Classmates in the Science and Technology Studies Department and the History Department at Cornell University, most notably Andrea Burrows, Julie Curry, John Fousek, Sergio Sismondo, and Nadine Weidman, offered their thoughts on portions of this project when it was first developing. My colleagues at Central Connecticut State University, most notably David Blitz and Cindy White, have heard me present portions of this book at faculty seminars and offered suggestions for improvement. Julia Grant, Kathleen Jones, Hans Pols, and Sarah Tracy generously shared their findings from their research in progress with me as well as offering timely and insightful comments on my own work. I would also like to thank faculty and students in the Yale University Section on the History of Medicine for offering comments on portions of the book that I have presented for their colloquium series. I am particularly grateful to John Warner for serving as my sponsor for the Yale Scholars Program, which gave me unlimited access to the resources in the Yale University Libraries and additional release time from teaching to work on this project.

Finally I would like to thank my family for supporting me throughout the years of research and writing. My aunt and uncle Carol and Bruce Perkins, my cousins Candace and Davin, and my grandmother Dorothy Rockwell Munro generously allowed me to stay in their homes during the months I spent examining materials in the greater Boston area. My parents, Sara and David Munro, and my sisters, Hope Munro Smith and Sara Munro, gave me large amounts of love and emotional support. Most of all I would like to thank my husband, Wayne, for his patience and love throughout the years it took to complete this project, and for providing valuable insights into the lives of contemporary teenagers gained through his experiences as a high school teacher.

Introduction

In May of 1965, Mr. and Mrs. Chandler brought their fifteen-year-old daughter Marnie to the Adolescent Unit at Boston Children's Hospital.[1] The unit, founded by Dr. J. Roswell Gallagher in 1951, was considered the leading facility for adolescent health care not only in the greater Boston area but worldwide. Like many parents in New England, the Chandlers learned about the clinic through the numerous articles on the clinic published in popular magazines and newspapers, and the lectures given by Gallagher and his staff to parents' groups throughout the region. Marnie's parents were concerned because their daughter appeared depressed and anxious and refused to talk to them about what was bothering her. After several months of visits at which Marnie continued to remain silent about her problems, her physician, Dr. Robert P. Masland, received a remorseful letter from Marnie disclosing the real cause of her anguish: she had spent the night drinking with a group of friends and wound up losing her virginity to a boy she did not know very well. Over the coming year, Masland successfully guided Marnie through her crisis. Toward the end of her treatment, Marnie expressed her gratitude:

> I suppose this letter is going to sound stupid but I do want to write it and thank you, for what I'm not sure, except you have really helped me and made me happy. I guess because you always listen to me and even if you knew I was wrong you did not start arguing with what I had to say at the time, it made all the difference to me in the world. I want to write you and just thank you so some day when you looked through your files you will know that your work is really worth it.[2]

Marnie's letter to her physician illuminates one of the unique features of the Adolescent Unit and similar adolescent facilities that emerged in the post–World War II period. Doctors at the unit clearly placed an emphasis on the opinions of their patients, an approach that made "all the difference in the world" to Marnie and other Boston-area teenagers.

This book will emulate this respect for the adolescent patient by demonstrating that young people themselves had a significant influence on the emergence of adolescent medicine as a distinct segment within the medical profession.[3] In particular, this book will show how this new medical field responded to broader sociocultural concerns about adolescents in mid-twentieth-century America. My interest in the social and cultural history of adolescent medicine departs somewhat from work by Sydney Halpern on the development of adolescent medicine and other behavioral areas of pediatrics. According to Halpern, "processes internal to the specialty and support from private foundations and state agencies" were the main factors behind the development of adolescent medicine.[4] Halpern's argument, however, cannot account for *why* pediatricians became interested in adolescence at the time that they did, nor can she explain why private foundations, state agencies, and the general American public supported pediatricians' movement into this area. Moreover, one cannot fully understand why laypersons bought what medicine had to offer without considering how clients viewed the emergence of adolescent medicine and how their needs shaped medical theory and practice.

Because I am interested in capturing the perspective of teenagers as well as parents, my work fits within recent scholarship on the history of childhood and youth. Rather than seeing the history of childhood solely from the perspective of adult ideas and actions, historians of childhood focus on the agency of children, the subjective experience of being a child, and the social and historical forces shaping that experience.[5]

I am also interested in examining the relationship between adolescent medicine and the emergence of an autonomous youth culture with its own unique forms of dress, style, and entertainment.[6] I argue that the development of an independent youth culture in twentieth-century American society created new strains within the family, as parents struggled to adapt to their children's increasing autonomy from parental influence and control. Adolescent medicine, among other helping professions, interceded in this growing gap between generations and tried to mediate compromises between teenagers and their parents.

In addition, this book places the emergence of adolescent medicine within the larger history and sociology of medical specialization in the United States.[7] I will show that in some ways, the rise of adolescent medicine mirrored the development of other medical specialties in the twentieth century, most notably the field's parent specialty, pediatrics.[8] Adolescent medicine, however, has encountered a unique set of professional problems that most other pediatric subspecialties have not had to face. One of the major differences between adolescent medicine and other pediatric subspecialties is that adolescent medicine is centered around an age group rather than a medical technology or organ system.[9] As a result, adolescent medicine has a low degree of what the medical sociologist Stephen M. Shortell refers to as "functional autonomy," or the degree to which a specialty infringes upon or is encroached upon by another medical specialty.[10] The field of pediatrics faced a similar dilemma in its early history. Pediatricians, however, were able to establish boundaries around the field through claims of special competency in infant feeding and the treatment of diseases unique to children.[11] The only other medical subspecialties to follow the same kind of age-group orientation are neonatology, a subspecialty of pediatrics, and geriatrics, a subspecialty of internal medicine. Yet both neonatologists and geriatric subspecialists have claims to unique technical expertise that allow them to distinguish their subspecialties from other medical disciplines.

Adolescent medicine, in contrast, does not have any technologies, diseases, or medical procedures that set it apart from other specialties. One of the cornerstones of the field throughout its history has been its insistence on looking at the "whole patient" from a variety of psychological, sociological, and physiological perspectives. Although this approach has allowed physicians who treated adolescents to assume a broad range of medical skills and problems, it has also meant that adolescent medicine has been dependent on other specialties for much of its knowledge base. Consequently, it has been difficult to find criteria that distinguished adolescent medicine from other medical segments. In fact, one of the criticisms often made by competing medical specialists is that adolescent medicine does not offer anything that is not already covered by some other medical discipline such as obstetrics and gynecology, endocrinology, or dermatology. Specialists in adolescent medicine freely admit that they do not have exclusive claims to any particular adolescent diseases or disorders. Instead, adolescent specialists argue that their approach to the teenage patient, and the relationship between practitioner and adolescent, are what set their field apart from other branches of medicine. In other words, giving teenagers a "doctor of their own" is what makes adolescent medicine unique.

Another professional problem encountered by adolescent medicine stems from its focus on the emotional, behavioral, and psychosocial problems of youth. Adolescent medicine deals with issues such as school failure, family conflicts, and more recently, substance abuse and sexually transmitted diseases. Even more straightforward medical problems such as diabetes and epilepsy frequently carry psychosocial overtones. Physicians in the organ and technology-based "bench" specialties and subspecialties tend to depict adolescent medicine, as well as other social problem–based disciplines like psychiatry and public health, as intellectually "soft" or unrigorous, much in the same way that researchers in the physical sciences tend to disparage the social sciences.[12]

The structure of this book reflects my interest in presenting a balanced portrait of the interaction between medicine and society. In Chapter 1, I explore changing perceptions about adolescence and the American medical profession's structural changes during the first half of the twentieth century that laid the foundation for adolescent medicine. I argue that adolescent medicine grew out of profound reorientations in American attitudes toward adolescents and social and ideological reform movements aimed at improving the physical and emotional well-being of this age group. These new views about American youth coincided with the professional interests of pediatricians, who were seeking new markets for their services in the 1940s and 1950s, and justified the expansion of pediatrics to include the medical care of adolescents.

Chapter 2 focuses on the career of Dr. J. Roswell Gallagher, who was school physician at Phillips Academy in Andover, Massachusetts, during the 1930s and 1940s and who served as head of the Adolescent Unit at Boston Children's Hospital Medical Center from its inception in 1951 until his retirement in 1967. Although there were other physicians who saw teenagers in their practices at this time, I have focused on Gallagher and the Adolescent Unit for three reasons. The most important is that Gallagher was the first to create a successful clinical unit devoted exclusively to adolescents. (There was an earlier, but short-lived, adolescent clinic created at Stanford University Medical School in 1916. The institutional structures necessary to support a new medical field for adolescents were not yet in place, however, and the clinic closed after two years.)[13]

A second reason for focusing on the Boston Adolescent Unit is that Gallagher's ideas on the treatment of adolescents had an impact that spread far beyond the walls of his own clinic. Through a tireless program of missionary work consisting of lectures at pediatric hospitals and medical schools around the country as well as a series of postgraduate courses offered at the Boston clinic, Gallagher eventually persuaded other institutions to create adolescent medical services modeled after his own unit. Physicians who trained at Boston went on to found clinics of their own at medical schools and hospitals throughout North America, and a few established adolescent facilities in South America, Europe, Japan, and Australia. In scarcely more than a decade after the Boston unit was founded, there were over fifty adolescent clinics in the United States and abroad.[14]

A final reason for focusing on Gallagher and Boston is a practical one: in addition to being the oldest facility of its kind, the Adolescent Unit at Boston Children's Hospital has the richest documentary record compared with other adolescent medicine services. Most other adolescent clinics have not kept primary source materials, a phenomenon that is related to adolescent medicine's tenuous position as a medical discipline. Because of their low status in relation to other pediatric services, adolescent clinics typically have had to fight for limited academic resources and hospital space. Consequently, maintenance of a documentary record has not been a high priority for directors and staff.[15]

In Chapter 3, I examine the clients' perspective, and draw on case records from the Adolescent Unit at Boston Children's Hospital to explain why parents relied on adolescent medicine rather than other professional fields for advice and treatment of their teenage children.[16] Chapter 3 also considers the Adolescent Unit from the adolescent patient's point of view and describes how young people responded to the treatment they received there. Prevailing notions of gender, race, and class were particularly important in shaping doctor-patient relationships.

Chapter 4 examines how adolescent medicine evolved beyond the Boston setting in response to the changing social needs of the 1960s and 1970s.

Physicians were forced to redefine the intellectual scope of adolescent medicine in response to dramatic changes in adolescent behavior. Young people of this period also engaged in sexual and drug-related behaviors that were increasingly at odds with parental values, and that placed them at risk for new health problems such as sexually transmitted diseases, drug addiction, and pregnancy. At the same time, adolescent medicine became enmeshed in professional problems of its own. This chapter will demonstrate that attempts to solidify adolescent medicine as a medical subspecialty were intertwined with a desire to serve all teenagers regardless of race, class, or gender. Adolescent medicine's development as a medical field was hindered by competition from other medical specialties, however, as well as by conflicts within adolescent medicine about what the proper focus of the field should be.

The Conclusion offers a historical perspective on contemporary issues in adolescent health care. I focus on one of the central paradoxes in the history of adolescent medicine: despite having a "doctor of their own," most teenagers—especially those from racial and ethnic minorities—do not receive adequate health care.[17] This chapter examines the social and cultural factors in contemporary American society that contribute to the health problems of modern teenagers.

The story outlined in the following pages not only traces the development of a new kind of medical service, but also uses the emergence of this field as a lens through which to view twentieth-century changes in American family relationships, youth culture, and the social experience of adolescence. I will demonstrate that medical ideas do not evolve independently from social needs, but instead are intimately interwoven with the views of health care consumers and the society of which they are a part. In the case of adolescent medicine, disputes about the proper place of adolescents in American society have been and continue to be at the heart of the health care problems of this age group.

1

The Professional and Social Roots
of a Medical Discipline

In 1904 the child-study pioneer and educational reformer G. Stanley Hall (1844–1924) published *Adolescence: Its Psychology and Its Relation to Physiology, Anthropology, Sociology, Sex, Crime, Religion, and Education*.[1] Although not the first work to deal with this subject, Hall's was undoubtedly one of the most widely read: the first edition alone sold over 25,000 copies in the United States, and an abridged version entitled *Youth, Its Education, Regimen, and Hygiene* (1906) became a popular textbook in teacher training institutions and normal schools.[2] Certainly no other writer of his time did more to systematize adolescence as a distinct developmental category and firmly engrave this concept on the American consciousness.[3]

Several years after *Adolescence* appeared, Hall wrote an article for the *Monthly Cyclopædia of Practical Medicine* stating that *Adolescence* had prompted a deluge of letters from "parents and relatives of young people who had given them cause for anxiety in their development." Hall wistfully added that "had I been a physician, I might have easily worked up a lucrative practice from such cases," since "children's diseases and women's diseases have become a specialty, there is now a place for another medical specialty for the treatment of adolescent troubles of mind and body."[4]

Despite Hall's insistence that his work implied the need for a field of medical practice dedicated to the care of adolescents, a new medical specialty for this age group did not appear for nearly another fifty years. The emergence of adolescent medicine in the 1950s, however, did not result from the discovery of any new "adolescent diseases" or disorders. Instead, the growth of adolescent medicine depended upon a combination of professional and social changes that provided the institutional structures necessary to support a new medical discipline for adolescents, and that placed teenagers themselves at the center of the national agenda.

"A Generalist's Specialty?": Transformations in American Pediatrics before 1950

When *Adolescence* was published, adolescent medicine's parent specialty, pediatrics, was still struggling to establish itself as a distinct medical segment. It was even more difficult to justify a special field dedicated to adolescents. One problem faced by the nascent field of pediatrics was competition from obstetricians, who were the first to take a special interest in the medical care of children. The first American textbook on the subject, *A Treatise on the Physical and Medical Treatment of Children* (1825), was written by the noted obstetrician William P. Dewees, who saw the study of child health as a logical extension of his interest in childbirth and reproduction. For much of the nineteenth century, medical schools taught pediatrics as a subset of courses on obstetric theory and practice when they addressed the subject at all. Physicians in practice seldom concentrated solely on treating children, but grouped them under the larger category of diseases of women and children. Consequently, those who tried to establish a medical specialty for children that was distinct and separate from obstetrics encountered much opposition from obstetricians who wanted to maintain exclusive control of child health care.[5]

A second obstacle to creating a specialty of pediatrics was lingering suspicions about medical specialists during the early twentieth century. According to one Milwaukee physician, the term specialist "'carried a subtle odium,' due to the 'uncontrolled reprehensible advertising of quack venereal and hernia practitioners, who invariably announced themselves to be 'specialists.'"[6] Medical specialties such as pediatrics and obstetrics and gynecology were starting to appear as distinct medical disciplines, but most medical schools and hospitals considered specialist training to be too narrow; many did not start to create departments for medical specialties until the 1930s. Consequently, the majority of American physicians in the early twentieth century (over 90 percent in 1900) were in general practice. Even those who considered themselves to be specialists in a particular field frequently spent a large portion of their practices in general medicine.[7]

In fact, many early pediatricians shared this ambivalence toward specialization, and insisted that pediatrics was a "generalist's specialty" that avoided the narrowness of organ-based fields such as ophthalmology and neurology that were also emerging at this time. For example, the pediatric pioneer Abraham Jacobi ridiculed what he considered the "exaggerated specializing tendencies of the times" and the "superficiality and wantonness displayed in the constant new formation of specialists in practice."[8]

Unfortunately, pediatricians' insistence that their field was a "generalist's specialty" centered around an age group rather than a disease or organ created a professional dilemma for the field. If pediatrics was really a "generalist's specialty," what criteria set pediatricians apart from other "generalists," namely general practitioners? How could pediatricians legitimately claim that they should have exclusive control over the health care of children, especially when other physicians were competing for the same group of patients?

To enhance the differences between themselves and other physicians, pediatricians initially focused on one specific task—artificial infant feeding. Interest in creating alternatives to breast milk began in the late nineteenth century among physicians charged with taking care of orphaned or abandoned infants in institutional settings. During the 1890s, pediatric researchers developed the "percentage method" of infant feeding, which depended upon detailed knowledge of the biochemistry of cow's milk and how to alter it to suit the delicate constitution of the infant stomach. Pediatricians argued that infant feeding was so technically complex that it required specialized medical training to understand and implement successfully. Not only was infant feeding purported to be beyond the competence of mothers and nursemaids, it was also too difficult for the general practitioner to master without specialized training. More important, the apparent efficacy of scientific methods of infant feeding in preventing death and disease helped to generate a market for pediatricians' services during the early twentieth century. Although the percentage method of infant feeding eventually fell into disrepute during the 1920s and 1930s, the scientific credibility that this technology lent to pediatrics in its early years helped to establish the field as a discrete medical discipline.[9]

The legitimacy of pediatrics as a distinct specialty was also aided by Progressive-era child welfare reform activities. Interest in protecting children began in the early 1850s, but it was only during the 1890s that this activity coalesced into a nationwide reform movement to grant children uniform protections by state and federal governments.[10] Although Progressivism encompassed a variety of political and social agendas, one of the central themes that united the various strands of the Progressive movement was protection of children from the hazards of modern industrial life. Pediatricians used this widespread concern with improving the health and welfare of American children to justify their claims to specialized knowledge in the health care of children.[11]

Pediatricians also employed new ideas about childhood as a life stage to underpin the growth of their field. By the end of the nineteenth century, most Americans recognized that childhood was a developmentally unique period of life requiring special treatment. Pediatricians went a step further and argued that there were distinct differences between the diseases of children and those of adults. "There are anomalies and diseases," wrote Jacobi in 1890, "which are met in the infant and child only." Even treatment of diseases that affected both children and adults needed to take heed of developmental differences between age groups, rather than simply reducing adult dosages to suit smaller patients. The successful medical treatment of children therefore required specialized knowledge and skill that the general physician did not possess.[12]

Between 1900 and 1940, evidence from the emerging field of child development demonstrated the specific physiological and psychological differences between children and adults, and further supported pediatricians' claims. Research on normal childhood growth and development helped to establish standardized heights, weights, and measurements for children as well as behavioral norms for each stage of development. This information was incorporated into the pediatric curriculum beginning in the 1920s, and was used as yet another way of distinguishing the knowledge base of pediatrics from other medical fields. The use of data from child development studies also justified the expansion of pediatrics into "well-child" care. Pediatricians argued that not only should they treat children when they were sick, but that they should also provide regular check-ups for apparently healthy children to ensure that they were developing on schedule.[13]

Advances in the diagnosis, treatment, and prevention of childhood diseases lent further scientific legitimacy to pediatrics. Research in nutrition and the discovery of vitamins in the 1910s allowed pediatricians to prevent or control deficiency diseases such as scurvy, rickets, and pellagra. The discovery of the sulfonamides during the 1930s and of penicillin during the 1940s gave pediatricians the ability to treat life-threatening infections such as tuberculosis, sexually transmitted diseases, and pneumonia. Finally, the development of gamma globulin in the 1940s greatly reduced the incidence and severity of childhood diseases such as measles, mumps, and rubella.[14] By the 1950s these discoveries had had a dramatic effect on the health of children. The mortality rate for infants fell from 162.4 per thousand live births in 1900 to 33 per thousand in 1950. Childhood mortality dropped from 19.8 per thousand in 1900 to 1.4 per thousand in 1950 for children ages one through four, and for children aged five through fourteen, the mortality rate fell from 3.9 per thousand to 0.6 per thousand.[15]

These therapeutic advances helped provide a favorable climate not only for the specialty of pediatrics but for medical specialization more broadly. By the time of the Second World War, advances in scientific medicine had undermined most opposition to medical specialization. Convinced that scientific research was essential to America's position as a world power, Congress approved the expansion of the National Institutes of Health in the late 1940s and the creation of the National Science Foundation in 1950.[16] Increased federal support for medical research during and after the Second World War caused a rapid growth in the number of medical specialists: in 1940, only 20 percent of American physicians were full-time medical specialists; by 1950, this percentage had doubled.[17] In particular, there was a tremendous growth in the number of specialists who identified themselves as pediatricians: in 1914, there were only 138 physicians in the United States who devoted their practices exclusively to the care of children. By the early 1950s, this number had increased to over 4,000.[18]

Yet the professional struggles of pediatricians were not over. One of the ironies of the scientific breakthroughs described above was that they threatened to undermine much of the market for pediatricians' services. Therapeutic advances in the treatment of many childhood diseases caused pediatricians to worry that demand for pediatric care would be eliminated by future medical discoveries. Although in retrospect this fear was unwarranted, it was real enough to cause pediatricians serious concern about the future of their field during the late 1940s and early 1950s.[19]

Pediatricians' professional anxieties were exacerbated by the actions of general practitioners, who were becoming more aggressive in competing for patients during the late 1940s as they saw their numbers and prestige gradually diminish as a result of growing medical specialization. The declining status of general practice was made painfully apparent during the Second World War, when specialists received higher military ranks than did general practitioners. In response, general practitioners looked for ways to revive their professional standing. One strategy was an attempt to wrest child health care away from pediatricians. In 1947, 150 general practitioners formed the American Academy of General Practitioners (AAGP), the main goal of which was to reverse the trend toward medical specialization. Promoting its members as the most logical purveyors of family health throughout the life course, the AAGP sought to provide general practitioners with better skills in pediatric care and demanded a greater emphasis on child health care in their training programs.[20]

To justify their cause, general practitioners "asserted wherever and whenever possible the special, almost mystical qualities supposedly inherent in the personal relationship of the GP with his patients."[21] General practitioners pointed to popular portrayals of medicine in novels, movies, and television shows, which depicted doctors as both heroes of modern science and exemplars of human compassion. They also drew on surveys conducted during the early 1950s that indicated that while American medical consumers were impressed with the medical discoveries of the past fifty years, they also longed for a friendly relationship with their physician reminiscent of earlier ties to the old-fashioned country doctor. Capitalizing on this nostalgia for a more humanistic approach to medical care, general practitioners projected a professional image that combined technical competence with the personal intimacy of the dedicated, traditional, family physician of the nineteenth century.[22]

In order to combat competition from general practitioners, pediatrics adopted two distinct and sometimes mutually contradictory solutions. The first strategy was the development of pediatric subspecialties such as pediatric endocrinology, cardiology, and oncology. This tactic was employed by pediatricians affiliated with large teaching hospitals and elite medical schools. Pediatricians at these institutions were especially interested in enhancing the professional status of their field relative to other medical specialties, and saw the development of science-based subspecialties as a means of enhancing the prestige and scientific content of their departments. They therefore followed the lead of surgery, radiology, and other technologically sophisticated and prestigious medical specialties by fostering the development of organ- and technology-based pediatric subspecialties.[23]

Subspecialization was fostered by the substantial increase in funding for medical research that occurred during and after the Second World War. Research grants provided by the NIH caused a tremendous expansion in the number of pediatric subspecialty programs at American medical schools. For example, in pediatric endocrinology, the number of professorships increased from twenty nationwide in 1950 to seventy-five in 1960. Thus, by the early 1960s, pediatric subspecialties were well on their way to becoming distinct, full-time, high-status academic career tracks for American doctors.[24]

A second strategy was to directly confront the rhetoric used by general practitioners by reasserting the original image of pediatrics as a "generalist's specialty." This tactic was adopted by general pediatricians in private practice and general pediatricians who ran outpatient clinics at university-affiliated children's hospitals and medical centers. In a movement variously referred to as the "new pediatrics," "ambulatory pediatrics," "comprehensive pediatrics," "developmental pediatrics," and "psychosocial" or "behavioral" pediatrics, general pediatricians argued that they were the rightful arbiters of all areas of child health and welfare. In some ways, the "new pediatrics" represented a backlash against what some general pediatricians perceived as rampant subspecialization. This criticism grew partly out of status anxiety: general pediatricians felt they were losing prestige and respect because of the increased focus on subspecialization. Advocates of the "new pediatrics" frequently criticized the fragmentation of medical care caused by subspecialization, and stressed the importance of focusing on the patient as a whole rather than on a particular disease or organ. General pediatricians claimed that because of this holistic perspective, pediatricians were uniquely qualified to treat not only the physical problems of childhood but also psychological, educational, and social issues as well. In the process, pediatricians claimed authority over psychosocial problems such as poor school performance, hyperactivity, shyness, aggressive and antisocial behavior, temper tantrums, and peer rejection.[25]

The professional outlook of the new pediatrics clashed with that of pediatric subspecialists, however, who ridiculed the movement as intellectually soft and unrigorous because it was based on social and behavioral issues rather than purely biomedical problems. Physicians in the pediatric bench subspecialties like endocrinology and cardiology were especially critical of the new pediatrics. Subspecialists claimed that by exploring areas that were not related to physical disease, the new pediatrics movement would severely damage the status of pediatrics as a whole. Charles D. May, chief of pediatrics at Columbia University, commented in 1960 that if supporters of the "new pediatrics" continued to "delude themselves by assuming they can become a priestly class of counselors on all things," then "the primary task of physical care will be diluted and dislocated beyond recognition and the pediatrician may no longer be considered a physician." By including psychosocial issues in the pediatric repertoire, claimed May, pediatrics as a whole would "slowly drift into a more pedestrian form of pediatric practice which will earn correspondingly lessened respect and fail to attract men of exceptional ability."[26]

Nevertheless, the movement to incorporate psychosocial issues into the body of pediatric knowledge met with some measure of success. The arguments used by supporters of the new pediatrics were powerful enough to convince some pediatric departments to redesign training programs to incorporate psychological and social issues into the pediatric curriculum during the 1950s and 1960s.[27] Support from a variety of public agencies and private foundations underwrote the emergence of the "new pediatrics." One of the most important financial contributors to this endeavor was the Commonwealth Fund. Originally created in the 1910s with the broad goal "to do something for the welfare of mankind," the Commonwealth Fund was one of the main funding agencies for institutions of child psychiatry and mental hygiene. By the mid-1930s the Commonwealth Fund was financing medical training programs that combined psychiatric and somatic perspectives. The fund's goal was to improve the position of psychiatry in medical training and to incorporate psychiatric principles into a broader range of medical specialties. The Commonwealth Fund was particularly interested in integrating behavioral concepts into pediatric training programs and hospital services.[28]

Medical discoveries and changing market forces were not the only factors that contributed to pediatricians' growing interest in the behavioral problems of childhood and adolescence. Instead, changing perceptions of American adolescents during the first half of the twentieth century played an equal if not more important role in justifying the idea that teenagers needed a "doctor of their own."

Adolescence: A Twentieth-Century "Invention"

Adolescence has become so firmly entrenched a category that it is difficult to imagine a time when this life stage as we know it did not exist. It is something of an exaggeration, of course, to say that adolescence was "discovered" or "invented" during the late nineteenth and early twentieth centuries: individuals between the ages of ten and twenty have undergone the biological transitions we now associate with puberty and adolescence since the beginnings of the human race. There is strong evidence, however, to suggest that even the biological aspects of adolescence have been influenced by culture. Because of improved nutrition, health care, and living conditions, the average age of physical maturity has steadily declined over the past two hundred years.[29]

More important, although historians have traced the social category of "youth" back to at least the sixteenth century, it is clear that there are fundamental differences between the early modern life stage of "youth" and the modern classification of "adolescence." As Susan M. Juster and Maris A. Vinovskis demonstrate, colonial Americans and early modern Europeans "certainly had a conceptual vocabulary that distinguished 'youth' from adulthood, but this stage of life connoted neither a fixed age span nor a uniform set of experiences." Instead, the term "youth" was applied indiscriminately to persons between the ages of seven and thirty "regardless of the nature of their activities or the degree to which they remained dependent on parental or other authorities."[30] Furthermore, the experiences of premodern youth were substantially different from those of modern adolescents: although the former certainly had an ambiguous social status that encompassed parts of both childhood and adulthood, early modern youth also enjoyed a greater flexibility of roles and larger degree of autonomy from adult supervision than do modern adolescents. Rather than being a "psychosocial moratorium" from adulthood, childhood and youth were seen as periods of gradual introduction to adult roles and responsibilities.[31]

The modern category of adolescence is a product of social and cultural changes that began in the nineteenth century and intensified during the first half of the twentieth century. One of the major factors contributing to this process was the transition to an industrial-capitalist economy, which caused dramatic changes in American class, gender, and age relationships. Although differences in status and income had existed in American society since the colonial period, industrial development and commercial expansion created clearer demarcations between "middling" farmers and businessmen; upper classes with vast sums of wealth; and a lower class of largely impoverished wage workers, tenant farmers, and sharecroppers. Class identity became associated not only with income but also with particular age and gender roles within the family. For the middle class, the family ideal corresponded to the growing geographic separation between work and home. Fathers were responsible for the public sphere of employment outside the home and were expected to be the sole breadwinners for their families. In contrast, popular advice literature depicted mothers as guardians of piety, virtue, and domesticity within the private sphere of the home, which would serve as a refuge from the cutthroat competition and social disorder of the public realm of work and commerce.[32]

Within this middle-class family ideal, children and adolescents were portrayed as innocent, immature beings who needed protection from the dangers of the adult world. Popular health writers encouraged middle-class parents to prolong their offspring's childhood for as long as possible, warning of the terrible effects on children's health should parents impose adult responsibilities and pressures at too early an age. Concerns about precocity were aimed at both genders: physicians, for example, advised parents to refrain from sending boys to school or into the work force before they had sufficient judgment to handle the temptations of the adult male world. Many physicians and asylum superintendents also claimed that premature intellectual development could induce other disturbing forms of precocious behavior, most notably masturbation. Boys who were pushed too far in their studies, these physicians warned, could become emotionally unstable and might even require hospitalization later in life.[33]

Medical warnings about precocity in girls were much more prevalent because of what Joan Jacobs Brumberg refers to as a "new timetable" in the female life course: middle-class girls were menstruating earlier but marrying later. Between 1780 and 1900, the average age of menarche declined from seventeen to thirteen or fourteen, while the average age of marriage was twenty-two or twenty-three.[34] Concerns about protecting the virtue of girls and young women were so intense that some historians of childhood and adolescence have suggested that middle-class girls were the "first adolescents," because they were the initial targets of extensive social reforms aimed at protecting them from the corrupting influence of adult society.[35]

This family ideal was not uniformly experienced by all young people aged twelve to twenty, however. The "opportunity costs" of adolescence—the loss of wages while a child attended school or resided in a protected home environment—put a prolonged period of dependency beyond the reach of most working-class, immigrant, and black families. As a result, the social experience of youth became sharply divided along class, racial, and ethnic lines. The ability to forgo a youth's wages in order to extend his or her education became a hallmark of middle-class status, one of the many ways the emerging middle classes distinguished themselves from what they considered to be the "depraved" and "vicious" habits of the immigrant and native-born working classes.[36]

Hall's work was one of the first attempts to universalize the category of adolescence by firmly linking this life stage to a specific biological process rather than social status. One of the central concepts of Hall's work was the theory of recapitulation, which stated that each stage of human development duplicated earlier periods in the biological and cultural evolution of the human race. During puberty, wrote Hall, "the floodgates of heredity seem opened and we hear from our remoter forebears." Hall further argued that this period of "savagery" was essential to both the adolescent's personal development and the survival of the race, and warned against "civilizing" adolescents too quickly by forcing them to conform to adult standards of behavior.[37]

Hall's theory of recapitulation resonated with the mood of turn-of-the-century American society. Many individuals during this era expressed a profound ambivalence about the rapid pace of social, cultural, and technological change, a sentiment that the historian Jackson Lears has termed "antimodernism."[38] Much of this attitude was rooted in the class anxieties of white, middle-class Americans, who believed that their power and prestige were being undermined by uncontrolled immigration and declining birthrates among the white, native-born middle classes. Although some admired the technological and scientific innovations of the age, others worried that poverty, crime, disease, and other social dangers fostered by urbanization, immigration, and industrialization were signs of inevitable national degeneration. Hall's image of adolescence as "the paradise of the race from which adult life is a fall," undoubtedly appealed to those who, like Hall, were haunted by fears that industrial American society was "at root morbific and sure to end in reaction and decay."[39]

Young people, particularly those from the immigrant working classes, became a focal point for much of this antimodernist anxiety about urban industrial life. Middle-class reformers had been concerned about the habits of youth from the so-called dangerous classes since the early 1830s, when a small but flourishing youth culture began to appear in large cities like New York City and Chicago. The expansion of urban youth culture was limited, however, by the kinds of employment available and the opportunities for social interaction outside the family. Most young people still worked in settings where their free time was closely scrutinized, and much of youth leisure activity still centered around the family and single-sex social groups.[40] By the late nineteenth century, the behavior of working-class youth became increasingly alarming. Rapid industrialization and urbanization created new job opportunities for young people in the cities' factories, department stores, offices, and service industries. Technological advances created dance halls, nickelodeons, amusement parks, and other new commercial centers of leisure in which urban youth could interact free from adult supervision. The most disturbing aspect of urban youth culture was the behavior of working-class girls and young women, who shirked Victorian standards of female decorum and eagerly sought the company of young men in the "cheap amusements" of the industrial city. To many middle-class observers, the behavior of working-class girls differed little from that of prostitutes, and reformers of the late nineteenth century desperately tried to find ways to contain the sexual behavior of young working-class women.[41]

Hall's theories on adolescence provided a scientific explanation for the new behavior of urban youth. Hall observed that much of the apparent depravity of working-class adolescents was due to society's failure to provide them with a wholesome environment in which to play out their "primal hereditary impulses." Although youth from middle-class families had ready access to the simple, premodern environment prescribed by Hall, urban youth were "especially divorced in city life from the steadying laws of recapitulation which insure emergence in due season into a higher state, and so [are] all the more plastic, helpless, disoriented, and in need of succor." In order to counteract the debilitating effects of urban industrial life, Hall suggested helping working-class youth "by devising more wholesome and natural expressions for the instincts" than those available in most urban slums.[42]

Hall's recapitulation theory justified a variety of Progressive-era reforms for adolescents. These included laws mandating school attendance, legislation against child labor, and the creation of adult-sponsored youth organizations such as the Boys' Clubs of America and the Association of Working Girls' Clubs. Like other Progressive reforms, those created for youth were based on a white, middle-class model to which all adolescents and their families were expected to aspire. Progressive reformers advised working-class and immigrant parents to adopt the same attitudes toward child nurture as their middle-class, native-born counterparts, and keep their offspring within the sheltered environments of home and school until they were adequately prepared for the adult world. Parents who could not or would not control wayward adolescents frequently found themselves the target of social workers and juvenile justice officials. Some Progressive reformers did make concessions to the economic realities of working-class families, and originally the maximum age for compulsory schooling was set as low as age fourteen in some cities. The preference, however, was to encourage students to stay in school. To facilitate compulsory schooling, many Progressives campaigned for a family wage for male workers that would make it unnecessary for children and adolescents, as well as wives and mothers, to work outside the home to help support the family.[43]

As a result of Progressive reforms, school attendance for adolescents grew dramatically. In 1890, only 6.7 percent of fourteen- to seventeen-year-olds were enrolled in high school. By 1920 this figure had risen to 32.3 percent, and by 1930 over 50 percent of the high-school-aged population was enrolled in school. The Great Depression would accelerate this trend even further: unemployment combined with New Deal incentives to stay in school pushed high school attendance rates to 75 percent and graduation rates to 50 percent. Although inequalities in educational opportunities persisted, high school attendance was starting to become the rule rather than the exception for most adolescents.[44]

Progressives were less successful in redirecting the behavior of urban working-class and immigrant youth. Despite reformers' efforts to provide alternatives, youth continued to flock to dance halls, movie theaters, and other leisure activities of the industrial city. Settlement house workers and organizers of youth clubs were eventually forced to compromise on the issue of youth culture, and cautiously allowed mixed-sex dances and social activities among club members.[45]

Not only did Progressive reforms fail to eliminate urban, working-class youth culture, during the late 1910s, a new alarming trend appeared: middle-class youth were beginning to engage in the same activities. Kathy Peiss observes that during the years surrounding the First World War, urban middle-class youth "increasingly embraced new 'manners and morals' . . . associating it with a sense of twentieth century modernity."[46] By the 1920s hundreds of books and articles were decrying the behavior of middle-class, "flaming" youth: their disregard for parental values, their odd clothing and hairstyles, their bizarre slang-filled language, their wild dances, and "lewd" activities such as "petting parties" and drinking binges. Commentators were particularly concerned about the appearance and behavior of young women. During the First World War, social workers and vice officials noted with alarm the growing problem of "khaki fever" among middle-class girls who "succumbed to the emotional conditions produced by the war" and eagerly pursued romantic relationships with young men in uniform.[47] By the 1920s, the behavior of middle-class girls appeared to degenerate even further, as young "flappers" shortened their hair and skirts, and smoked, drank, danced, swore, and adopted the same "loose" attitudes toward sex as men.[48]

Ironically, the spread of youth culture to middle-class adolescents was fostered by the very reforms that were designed to shelter working-class adolescents from the hazards of urban industrial life. Compulsory education laws and growing rates of high school attendance isolated adolescents from adult roles and responsibilities, but also brought together youth of different socioeconomic classes in settings that were exclusively theirs. To be sure, youth culture was by no means monolithic, and many high schools contained a variety of subcultures based on race, ethnicity, and class. High schools did, however, help create an unprecedented, national peer-group consciousness that frequently transcended racial and economic boundaries. Although schools tried to homogenize the behavior of all students into middle-class standards of dress and conduct, middle-class youth nevertheless admired and emulated some aspects of working-class and minority subcultures.[49]

The new centers of commercialized leisure also helped to feed the growth of a cross-class youth culture. Although dance halls, movie theaters, and amusement parks were initially the province of working-class youth, by the late 1910s and 1920s affluent urban and suburban youth were also flocking to these entertainments. Commercialized forms of leisure eventually crossed ethnic and class boundaries, forming a "common cultural currency" for youth from a variety of ethnic and socioeconomic backgrounds.[50]

Hall's attempts to universalize the experience of adolescence therefore had unintended consequences. On the one hand, Progressive reforms did extend some of the benefits enjoyed by middle class adolescents to working-class youth, and made an extended period of segregation from the adult world a normative experience for all adolescents. On the other hand, reformers who adopted Hall's theories on adolescence not only failed to contain working-class youth culture, but created conditions that unintentionally allowed youth culture to spread to middle-class adolescents as well. By the 1920s, Hall's vision of adolescence as a means of containing the unstable forces of modern life seemed increasingly inappropriate. Instead, experts on adolescence would try to come to terms with modernity by creating a model of development that could accommodate rather than condemn the radical changes in youthful behavior.

"A Strategic Group for Social Change": The Normalization of Adolescent Rebellion

Initially, the antics of middle-class youth prompted the same antimodernist anxiety that had been directed at the behavior of working-class adolescents two decades earlier. For example, Judge William McAdoo, city magistrate of New York City, attributed the "frightful" behavior of modern youth to a kind of "moral bolshevism" that signaled the imminent collapse of American civilization. McAdoo and other juvenile justice authorities warned middle-class parents that their children were headed down the same "road to destruction" as their less-fortunate counterparts, and would ultimately wind up in jail unless parents took timely action to change their children's errant ways. Some communities, particularly those in the South and Midwest, treated youth culture as a form of criminal behavior and passed laws that forbid "lewd" forms of dancing, smoking by women, and flapper fashions. The growing popularity of the Ku Klux Klan during this period grew partly out of its claims that "immoral youth" were as much a threat to traditional American values as were immigrants, blacks, Catholics, and Jews.[51]

During the Great Depression and the Second World War, as adolescent behavior seemed to be getting worse rather than better, adult anxieties about the problem of youth culture intensified. Statistics on juvenile delinquency collected during the Depression and the war underscored these fears: court cases and the FBI annual compendium of police arrests demonstrated an almost 100 percent increase in juvenile cases handled between 1940 and 1945.[52] By the late 1940s, "42 percent of the adult respondents were convinced that teenagers behaved worse than their parents' generation; only 9 percent thought that youthful behavior had improved."[53]

The involvement of adolescents in totalitarian movements in Europe contributed to the sense of social danger posed by American youth. During the 1920s and 1930s, Germany, Italy, and the Soviet Union had all created organizations and work camps for unemployed young people, and used these institutions to cultivate party loyalty from an early age.[54] Some made a direct link between the ominous characteristics of American youth culture and the involvement of adolescents in totalitarian movements overseas. The noted child psychologist Erik Erikson argued that Hitler capitalized on the phenomenon of adolescent rebellion, and "tried to replace the complicated conflict of adolescence . . . with simple patterns of hypnotic action and freedom from thought." Employing the motto "Youth shapes its own destiny," the Hitler youth movement encouraged German teenagers to free themselves from the preconceived ideas of their parents and ally themselves with the new social and moral order of National Socialism.[55]

The language used to describe the threats posed by youth culture employed many of the same metaphors used to depict the threat to American democracy posed by authoritarian movements overseas. In 1936 FBI director J. Edgar Hoover drew an analogy between delinquency and communism, describing the delinquent as "the traitor, the vile enemy in our political family which seeks to disrupt our institutions of government; who knifes from within; who has only selfish purposes; who is the antagonist of everything that is honorable in our present-day form of government."[56] President Franklin Delano Roosevelt used less inflammatory language, yet still drew upon metaphors of disease and contagion to describe the problem of Depression-era youth, arguing that "any neglected group . . . can infect our whole national life and produce widespread misery."[57] In some critics' minds, therefore, juvenile delinquency and youth culture represented pathologies that needed to be contained and controlled before they infected the rest of the American body politic.

Most middle-class parents, however, were reluctant to believe that their children were incipient criminals. Instead, parents turned to the emerging field of mental hygiene for help with their errant offspring. Founded in 1909 by Clifford Beers, a former mental patient, the mental hygiene movement was based on a "dynamic" approach to mental illness that emphasized the role of early childhood experiences and family and social environment in psychological development. According to the medical historian Sol Cohen, although the dynamic approach is usually associated with the work of Freud and other psychoanalysts, in the United States the term "dynamic psychiatry" was used to refer to a variety of approaches that focused on life history and personality development, rather than neurological injury or heredity, as the causes of mental illness. These included Adolf Meyer's "psychobiological" approach, which tried to find a psychiatry of the "whole person" and John B. Watson's behaviorist psychology, as well as the psychoanalytic approach advocated by Freud and his followers. Although Freudian theories eventually came to dominate, American mental hygienists tended to take a more optimistic view of human nature than did Freud. Mental hygienists, like Freud, downplayed the role of heredity in mental illness, and placed a greater emphasis on environmental causes, particularly the influence of parenting practices on children and adolescents. Mental hygienists also claimed that the majority of mental problems could be prevented entirely through timely psychiatric intervention.[59]

Because many mental problems had their roots in childhood experiences, the mental hygiene movement directed much of its preventive efforts at children and adolescents. In the words of one leader in the field, childhood was the "period par excellence for prophylaxis." Much of the movement's work therefore focused on incorporating principles of mental hygiene into institutions affecting children and adolescents.[59]

One accomplishment of the mental hygiene movement was its reconceptualization of theories about the causes of juvenile delinquency: mental hygienists argued that juvenile delinquency was a sign of deep-rooted personality disorders, not the product of innate mental depravity. Juvenile offenders deserved psychiatric treatment rather than incarceration in reformatories. This new view of juvenile delinquency fostered the creation of child guidance clinics, which were aimed primarily at treating children and adolescents who had already gone astray, but also helped identify "predelinquent" children who could be rescued through timely intervention. At first these clinics were used mainly as arms of the juvenile justice system, and were viewed as humane alternatives to incarceration for working-class youngsters. During the 1920s and 1930s, growing numbers of middle-class parents consulted child guidance clinics for help with the distressing behavior of their "modern" sons and daughters. Child guidance personnel in turn adapted their institutions to suit the needs of an increasingly middle-class clientele, and created new services to give advice to these perplexed parents.[60]

To further meet this demand for mental hygiene advice, the National Committee for Mental Hygiene (NCMH), in collaboration with private philanthropies like the Rockefeller Foundation and the Commonwealth Fund, encouraged the formation of parent education groups that would help disseminate information on child rearing and mental hygiene to anxious parents. One of the largest projects in this area was the Laura Spelman Rockefeller Memorial (LSRM), a branch of the Rockefeller Foundation. The LSRM funded research projects on child and adolescent development at several major universities around the country, as well as a nationwide system of parent education that disseminated child development research to concerned mothers and (to a lesser extent) fathers who wanted assistance in raising their children.[61]

The most prominent figure in the parent education movement was Lawrence K. Frank, who directed the LSRM during the 1920s and 1930s and had a widespread influence on ideas about youth and society during the interwar years.[62] In some ways, Frank echoed Hall's antimodernist fears about the future of American society. In a classic essay entitled "Society as the Patient" (1936), Frank argued that the rise of totalitarian regimes overseas and massive socioeconomic problems at home were evidence that Western civilization was "sick, mentally disordered, and in need of treatment." Unlike Hall, however, Frank believed that the solution to the problems facing American society was not to abandon modernity, but to embrace it. Borrowing from the language of mental hygiene, Frank claimed that many social and political problems arose out of "frantic efforts" of maladjusted, mentally unstable individuals to adapt to a rapidly changing society "being remade by scientific research and technology." The best way to prevent cultural disintegration, argued Frank, was to treat all of society as a "patient" whose personality needed to be "adjusted" to the social, political, and technological changes of the early twentieth century.[63]

Like Hall, adolescents were at the center of Frank's concern about the "sickness" facing modern American society. Frank recognized the potentially destructive consequences of adolescent rebellion, claiming that the appeal dictators held for European youth was "a warning of what neglect of this group may entail." Yet Frank also argued that if rebellion could be channeled into productive and acceptable channels, youth could become "a strategic group for social change."[64]

Frank's ideas about the relationship between adolescence and social change drew upon the work of the sociologist William Fielding Ogburn and the cultural anthropologist Margaret Mead. According to Ogburn's theory of "cultural lag" articulated in his book *Social Change: With Respect to Culture and Original Nature* (1922), there was a widening gap between the material changes in American life caused by rapid advances in science and technology and the ability of traditional institutions like the family to deal with such changes.[65] Mead elaborated upon this idea during the 1930s and 1940s, arguing that American society was gradually being transformed from a "postfigurative" culture to a "prefigurative" culture. In postfigurative cultures, claimed Mead, cultural change was slow, and the values and social roles of parents were no different from the roles and responsibilities that children would occupy when they reached adulthood. In contrast, Mead argued, prefigurative cultures like the United States were characterized by rapid change that was so great that the past was no longer an adequate guide for the future. Therefore, children could no longer look to their parents for guidance about adult roles.[66]

Likewise, Frank argued that youngsters who had "escaped the older formulations and the prevalent distortions of today" were the ones best able to "assimilate these startling new ideas and beliefs coming from scientific research . . . and thus begin not only to build the society that is to come, but to reconstruct our culture."[67] In order to give adolescents the skills to renew American society, adults must abandon Hall's recapitulation theory: although such a model was fine for "a static, tradition-bound society," it was unsuited to the rapid social and political upheavals of twentieth-century America. "If society is to change and continually adapt itself to new knowledge and novel practices," wrote Frank, "children must to some extent relinquish parental beliefs and practices and learn the ideas, techniques, and the patterns of conduct of their own generation." In short, Frank claimed that parents must encourage rather than discourage adolescent rebellion, and help adolescents adapt to the future rather than forcing them to recapitulate the moribund traditions of the past.[68]

Frank's ideas on the relationship between youth and society were shared by child development specialists, educators, mental hygienists, and other professionals who worked with adolescents during the 1930s and 1940s. One of the leading proponents of Frank's interpretation of modern adolescence was Erik Erikson. Although Erikson recognized the potential dangers of youth rebellion, he also claimed that rejection of parental values and allegiance with the views of the peer group were vital components of adolescents' progress toward adulthood. Moreover, noted Erikson, the ability to move beyond the values and ideas of one's parents and adapt to rapidly changing social and political conditions was essential to the progress of American society. Rather than viewing teenage rebellion as a sign of deeper emotional pathology, Erikson insisted that defiance of adult authority was a sign that the adolescent was successfully on the road to maturity. According to Erikson, juvenile delinquency and the involvement of adolescents in totalitarian youth organizations were simply exaggerated versions of normal adolescent development.[69]

Frank and Erikson thus offered a theory of adolescent development that normalized rebellion by making identification with the peer group more important than compliance with parental wishes. Within this model, adolescents who did not fit in with their age cohort were considered more of a problem than those who rebelled against parental authority, since it was they, not the teen rebels, who inhibited cultural progress.

Frank did not, however, abandon adult control entirely: he did believe that lack of discipline and disregard for group values were responsible for nearly as much social chaos as overly restrictive parenting styles. As a middle ground, Frank proposed a variation on what the historian William Graebner refers to as "democratic social engineering," which combined a more permissive attitude toward child rearing with timely yet benevolent adult intervention should children's behavior become out of control.[70] According to Frank, cooperation with group ideals "to be really effective, must function, not in physical coercion and police supervision, but within the individual himself." The pressure to win approval from peers, rather than overt forms of coercion by adults, argued Frank, would force adolescents to internalize and conform to group standards.[71]

Frank therefore had a tremendous faith in the ability of the peer group to keep most adolescents in line. Frank argued that the desire to "be like everyone else" and avoid social ostracism by friends and classmates would prevent most adolescents from crossing the line into antisocial and delinquent behavior. When peer culture itself bordered on the delinquent, Frank and adolescent development experts who shared his views recommended prompt yet gentle intervention from parents, teachers, psychologists, and other adult advisors.

The Tyranny of the Norm

Frank recognized that the conformist tendencies of youth culture came at a price: those who failed to fit in with their peers could develop irrevocable personality disorders and mental problems. To support his ideas, Frank drew upon the ideas of the Viennese psychoanalyst Alfred Adler, whose idea of the inferiority complex received increasing attention in the United States during the 1920s and 1930s. Although Adler's therapeutic approach was eventually abandoned in favor of Freud's, the concept of the inferiority complex remained an important organizing principle in American psychiatry.[72] Elaborating on Adler, Frank observed that adolescents as a group were "especially anxious about their normality" and constantly worried about how they compared to others their age. Frank claimed that most adolescents were vulnerable to this kind of "stress and strain" about their body image, but those who were different from their peers because of illness, disability, or some other physical or emotional problem were particularly likely to develop intense feelings of inferiority. Although some adolescents reacted to their distress by becoming passive and withdrawn, others could overcompensate for their perceived inadequacies by acting out in socially unacceptable ways.[73]

Frank argued that adolescents' anxiety about their normality was exacerbated by parents' confusion over the parameters of normal human growth and development. The idea that children and adolescents developed according to distinct stages was first suggested by Hall's recapitulation theory and elaborated by the pediatrician and child development specialist Arnold

Gesell, director of the Yale Child Development Clinic. Gesell popularized this "stage theory" of development in a series of advice manuals for parents, which detailed what physical and mental characteristics parents could expect at particular stages in their child's growth. Although Gesell insisted that his stages were meant to be guidelines and not rigid developmental categories, there is substantial evidence that parents tended to interpret Gesell's advice too literally and panicked when their children did not develop "on schedule."[74]

Frank observed that "confusion and misunderstanding" about normal adolescent development could lead to poor medical care of teenagers. Usually, physicians would attempt to bring apparently abnormal adolescents into line with average height and weight charts through diet and exercise.[75] The discovery of hormones affecting growth and development during the 1920s and 1930s made hormonal therapy an increasingly popular option for treating adolescents who appeared to be ahead of or behind their peers developmentally. Physicians were especially apt to use hormone treatment for sex-inappropriate developmental characteristics that they believed originated from hormonal imbalances. For example, obese boys with underdeveloped genitalia and sluggish behavior were believed to have a pituitary disturbance called Frölich's syndrome, which required treatment with pituitary gland extract. Likewise, girls who were considered tall for their age would often be given estrogen therapy to prevent further growth.[76]

Frank did not disregard the possibility that there was a hormonal basis for some growth disorders. Some late-bloomers, for example, could have hormonal imbalances that inhibited their growth and development. Early maturers—particularly those who entered puberty at extremely young ages (less than eight or nine) could have pituitary tumors that could turn malignant without medical attention. Frank also argued, however, that the vast majority of adolescents would eventually "fall into step" with their peers without medical intervention. Frank liked to use the analogy of 100 boys and 100 girls traveling from New York to Chicago: some youngsters would reach their destination "by airplane, some by Twentieth Century Limited, others by bus, some by water, some by hitch-hiking, and others trudging along on foot. Those who get to Chicago will arrive at different times and in different conditions, depending upon their mode of travel."[77]

Rather than subject adolescents to the "tyranny of the norm," Frank believed that physicians should take a "psychocultural" approach that acknowledged the "patient as a personality" whose growth, development, and response to health and disease were unique to that individual. To be sure, Frank did not trivialize the psychological trauma that resulted from an adolescent's failure to measure up to his or her peers. Frank insisted, however, that surgical or endocrinological manipulation of the body simply escalated the anxiety felt by an adolescent who was already psychologically disturbed by being different. Instead Frank recommended that parents, pediatricians, teachers, and others who worked with adolescents should find ways for a young person to find acceptance within his or her peer group.[78]

Frank made a clear link between this "psychocultural approach" and the preservation of the American way of life. According to Frank, enforced conformity presented the "gravest danger to democracy" because it created "distorted, immature, unhappy personalities" who would "sacrifice freedom and follow demagogues and dictators." By becoming increasingly aware of individual differences and protecting children and adolescents from "unnecessary traumas" caused by forced adherence to group standards, physicians and social scientists would go a long way toward "reaffirming our democratic goals and values."[79]

Frank's ideas on body image and personality development were supported by longitudinal studies of adolescent growth and development that were conducted at Harvard, Yale, Antioch, Case Western Reserve, Catholic University, the University of Iowa, the University of Chicago, the University of California, and other child development centers during the 1930s and 1940s. Many of these programs were funded by the Laura Spellman Rockefeller Memorial, the Macy Foundation, and other philanthropic organizations administered by Frank over the course of his career, and shared his concerns about the relationship between adolescent mental hygiene and cultural progress. Under Frank's guidance, much of the research conducted at the Rockefeller-funded child development institutes was aimed at uncovering the normal range of individual variation in growth and development. All of these programs were interdisciplinary and examined the relationship between physical and psychological development as well as the impact of environmental factors such as the family, the school, and socioeconomic class on adolescent development.[80]

Although the adolescent development studies directed by Frank did offer an expanded notion of what it meant to be "normal," they carried some unexamined assumptions about race and class. The majority of subjects chosen for these studies were from white, middle-class families, although some studies did include small numbers of African Americans, Asian Americans, and Native Americans. Developmental researchers justified their choice of subjects by claiming that they wanted to exclude "contaminating" factors such as race and class from their study of "normal" adolescent development, but seemed unconcerned by the fact that their definition of normal was based largely on a white, middle-class model.[81]

Furthermore, many of these adolescent development studies reflected anxieties about changes in American gender roles caused by the Depression and the Second World War. During the Depression, gender roles in many families were reversed as men lost their jobs and women were forced to find work to support their families. Even in families where the father remained employed, the need to economize and supplement the family's income gave women greater control over economic decisions than they had enjoyed before.[82] The war upset gender roles even further, as women assumed jobs that had previously been limited to men and as mothers assumed the authority vacated by fathers who left to fight overseas. Historians have demonstrated that Americans did not accept these challenges to traditional gender roles willingly, and constantly looked for ways to underscore traditional notions of masculinity and femininity.[83]

Frank and other experts on adolescent development expressed many of the same concerns about the effect of the Depression and war on American gender roles. Developmental researchers observed that unemployment reversed the "natural" pattern of gender relations in the family by diminishing the authority of fathers, while elevating the position of mothers who went out to work or were responsible for family purchases. Developmental researchers warned of the dire consequences of "emasculated fathers" and "domineering mothers" for adolescent psychological development. The presence of a weak father and a strong mother could cause "effeminate" behavior and even lead to homosexual tendencies in some young men. Others might overcompensate by becoming hypermasculine and attempt to prove their manhood through reckless and even delinquent behavior. Girls could also be led astray by inappropriate role models in the home: they could become "masculinized" by emulating a domineering mother's behavior; or the presence of a weak father could lead girls to seek surrogate father figures outside the home and engage in sexual relationships with older men.

For both boys and girls, the financial pressures of the Depression inhibited their participation in the peer culture and interfered with their gender role identity. Boys were often forced to take jobs, and were unable to participate in sports and other activities that won them approval from male peers and admiring female fans. Economic problems could also prevent boys from taking girls on dates, and thereby inhibit development of normal heterosexual desires. Increased responsibilities in the home and chronic shortages of cash had the same effect on girls: they could not purchase cosmetics and other beauty aids to make them attractive to the opposite sex, they frequently did not have time to go out on dates because of domestic chores, and they were often rejected by boys in favor of girls with more promising economic prospects. Like boys, girls who were barred from the dating culture because of economic circumstances could also fail to develop proper heterosexual attitudes.[84]

Concerns about gender-appropriate behavior are also apparent in studies of physical growth. Although researchers examined a variety of problems that stemmed from an adolescent's failure to develop at the same rate as his or her peers, they were especially concerned about youngsters who had sex-inappropriate physical characteristics: girls who were too tall, lacked breasts or other secondary sexual characteristics, or had masculine facial characteristics and physiques; and boys who were too short, had underdeveloped genitals, high-pitched voices, and/or flabby, "feminine" body types characterized by wide hips, short waists, and fatty, breastlike deposits on their chests.[85]

Adolescent development researchers found that all adolescents who fell outside the average for the age group had some kind of problem with peer adjustment. Early and late maturity had different meanings, however, for boys and girls. Researchers recognized that for boys, athletic ability and a "manly" physical appearance (that is, facial hair, a muscular physique, well-developed genitals, and so forth) ensured popularity. Boys who matured early tended to fit in better with their peers and even excel as leaders within their peer group. Late maturing boys were usually less popular, since they had difficulty competing with other boys in sports and felt embarrassed about their infantile secondary sexual characteristics. These boys were believed to be at risk for developing homosexual tendencies, since their lack of popularity prevented them from winning dates with girls and developing heterosexual interests. Mothers also tended to overprotect late-maturing boys, making the development of effeminate behavior even more likely.[86]

For girls, early maturity often posed the biggest problem. Although developmental researchers found that all girls were upset if they failed to develop a feminine figure by the age of sixteen or seventeen, those who "blossomed" at a very early age (between ten and fourteen) were embarrassed by their appearance and by unwanted male attention. Early maturing girls presented another social problem as well, particularly if accompanied by early onset of menses: researchers worried that girls who matured too early would be more likely to be "sexual delinquents," that is, engage in sexual intercourse, acquire venereal diseases, and become pregnant.[87]

Even adolescents who developed according to standardized height and weight charts could experience problems with body image and gender role identification. Researchers argued that the adolescent's natural self-consciousness and desire for peer approval could wreak emotional havoc even in those adolescents who developed normally, but were unprepared for the changes in their developing bodies. Developmental scientists blamed this lack of preparation on parents who failed to teach their children about impending sexual development out of fear that such knowledge would lead to sexual activity. Experts warned that adolescents who were not prepared for the physical changes of puberty could experience severe emotional distress when their bodies began developing in strange and unexpected ways. Researchers warned that without timely therapeutic intervention, an adolescent might become so disgusted with his or her body that he or she would reject sexuality altogether or, worse, identify with the wrong gender role. Girls, for example, might adopt tomboyish attire and behavior in order to hide their developing breasts; boys might become overly passive or feminine.[88]

Although development researchers admitted that all adolescents had difficulty adjusting to their developing bodies, they pointed out that adolescents with sex-inappropriate characteristics had the most difficult time fitting in with their peer group, and consequently exhibited a greater degree of psychopathology and antisocial behavior than those who developed normally.[89] Sometimes the burden of being different could result in severe mental disorder. Nancy Bayley and Read D. Tuddenbaum of the Child Welfare Institute at Berkeley observed that "a tendency toward the morphological characteristics of the opposite sex, were conspicuously more common among three thousand young schizophrenics than among the general population."[90]

Like Frank, developmental researchers resisted labeling these adolescents as "abnormal" and instead advised parents and professionals on how to help adolescents "fit in" with their peers. Once again, advice fell along marked gender lines. Boys, for example, could win peer approval by excelling in sports (if they were large for their age) or artistic and intellectual pursuits (if they were smaller or frailer than other boys their age). Herbert Stolz of Berkeley presented the case study of "Ben," an overweight boy who made up for his feminine appearance through success on the football field. Athletic success not only improved Ben's self-confidence and popularity, observed Stolz, but eventually eliminated the excess fat that had been the source of ridicule for many years.[91] Girls, however, were advised to compensate for physical shortcomings by developing a "friendly, outgoing personality" or by focusing on some other aspect of their appearance such as their face, hairstyle, or clothing.[92]

During the Second World War, concerns about the impact of physical difference on adolescent emotional health were heightened by studies of military recruits that showed the substantial toll that the Great Depression had taken on the physical health of the nation's youth. According to a Selective Service report, approximately 25 percent of the eighteen- and nineteen-year-old registrants were rejected for military service because of physical and mental defects.[93] These findings prompted Frank to call the adolescent "the forgotten child" whose health had been neglected by medical experts.[94]

Physicians and mental hygiene experts worried not only about the physical consequences of poor nutrition and inadequate health care but about the emotional consequences of disease as well. Infectious diseases such as tuberculosis and polio, to which adolescents were particularly susceptible because of their lifestyles and rapid growth, not only could cripple a young person physically, but could cause deep-rooted psychological scars if physical disability prevented successful integration into the youth culture. Likewise, chronic diseases like diabetes, enteric disorders, heart problems, scoliosis, epilepsy, or asthma, which required a special diet, medication, braces, or periodic hospitalization that marked a young person as different, could have devastating psychological consequences.[95]

Concerns about the consequences of physical illnesses, however, differed according to gender. For boys, the main concern was how illness affected athletic ability, scholastic performance, and masculine role identity. Physicians worried that parents—particularly mothers—would "coddle" boys with chronic illnesses like diabetes or asthma and prevent them from participating in sports and other activities that were crucial to their acceptance by male peers and popularity with girls. Although physicians recognized that boys had to accept some physical limitations imposed by their illnesses, too many restrictions would inhibit peer approval and keep boys from turning into "real men."[96]

For girls, physicians were mainly interested in how illness might affect physical appearance, feminine role identification, and marriageability. Physicians recognized that some infectious and chronic diseases—particularly tuberculosis and diabetes—could inhibit menstruation and the development of breasts and other secondary sexual characteristics. Although some parents undoubtedly considered delayed puberty in their daughters to be a blessing, physicians warned that such girls might become so discouraged by their lack of "feminine" features that they would reject their gender role altogether and adopt "tomboyish" and even lesbian behaviors.[97]

After the Second World War, disclosures about the poor mental and physical condition of American youth prompted a number of medical experts to begin focusing more attention on the health needs of adolescents. Dermatology benefited from adolescent anxiety about pimples and the psychological consequences of having a flawed complexion.[98] Fields like plastic surgery, orthodontics, endocrinology, and orthopedics capitalized on new ideas about the relationship between physical appearance and adolescent peer adjustment. Even experts in serious chronic and acute diseases in adolescents became concerned with not just the physical affects of illness but the psychological consequences of diseases that made an adolescent different from his or her peers.

Anxieties about the impact of adolescents and their problems on national security thus served to justify a more aggressive professional response to adolescent physical and mental health. Experts interested in adolescent mental hygiene worried about the potentially destructive force of adolescent youth culture. Yet they also argued that encouraging the development of "healthy personalities" could contain the disruptive tendencies of youth, and instead employ youthful exuberance as a means of carrying American society forward into the atomic age.

Experts in adolescent development also argued that parents could not always ensure the growth of healthy personalities without expert intervention, for too many things could go wrong on the way to adulthood: teenagers with disabilities and illnesses not only suffered physically, but could also become psychologically warped if their disorders prevented them from fitting in with their peers. Experts also pointed out that differentiating between normal variations in growth and development and genuine hormonal or physiological disorders required extensive technical expertise that laypersons did not possess. At the very least, adolescents who differed from their peers needed extra attention from mental health experts to prevent inferiority complexes or other psychological difficulties related to their physical appearance. If adolescents did not receive proper attention to their emotional and physical well-being, these experts argued, then social chaos would result.

These new ideas about American adolescents meshed nicely with the professional interests of pediatricians, who were seeking to expand their therapeutic mandate during this period. Until the mid-twentieth century, pediatricians seldom included adolescents in their practices. By the 1950s, however, pediatricians in the United States had entered into a period of crisis and retrenchment that resulted in the redefinition of the professional boundaries and intellectual scope of the field. These intraprofessional concerns, combined with larger social anxieties about American youth, gradually legitimized pediatricians' movement into the medical care of adolescents.

It was in this climate of heightened concern about young people and the need to find new markets for pediatrics that adolescent medicine emerged. Among the numerous projects in psychosocial pediatrics financed by the Commonwealth Fund was the Adolescent Unit at Boston Children's Hospital. Those who supported this clinic would draw upon the rhetoric of the new pediatrics to justify the establishment of a new field for adolescents, claiming that specialization and subspecialization had fragmented medical care for this age group. Like pediatricians before them, physicians in adolescent medicine would argue that their field was a "generalist's specialty" that treated the patient as a whole rather than a single organ system or medical problem. Consequently, adolescent medicine would experience some of the same professional struggles as had pediatrics over a half century earlier.

J. Roswell Gallagher and the
Origins of Adolescent Medicine

The origins of adolescent medicine are commonly credited to J. Roswell Gallagher, founder of the first service for adolescents in the United States at Boston Children's Hospital. Gallagher himself was rather modest about his accomplishments, and once remarked that "had it not been for the Great Depression, I would have become a cardiologist" instead of creating a new field of medicine devoted to teenagers. Gallagher received his medical degree from Yale University in 1929, and did his residency training in internal medicine and cardiology during the early years of the Depression. Full-time positions for cardiologists were scarce even for Ivy League graduates, however, and the only job Gallagher could find was as a school physician. Gallagher served as an assistant physician at the Hill School in Pottstown, Pennsylvania, for two years (1932–1934) and then became the director of health services at Phillips Academy in Andover, Massachusetts, where he worked for the next fourteen years.[1]

Although Gallagher's early employment was driven primarily by economic circumstances, it formed the foundation for his long and distinguished career in the field of adolescent medicine. Unlike most school physicians of the time, Gallagher maintained an interest in medical research that he had developed during his cardiology residency. Within a few years of his arrival at Phillips Academy, Gallagher set up a research unit to study adolescent growth and development. This work allowed Gallagher to establish professional contacts with leaders in the field of child development, particularly Lawrence Frank. The close proximity of Phillips Academy to Boston also permitted Gallagher to form close professional relationships with physicians at Boston Children's Hospital, Harvard Medical School, and the Harvard School of Public Health. By the late 1940s

Gallagher was widely recognized as *the* major authority on adolescent health issues in the Boston area, a reputation that made him the natural choice to head the Adolescent Unit at Boston Children's Hospital in 1951.

Gallagher also observed that the Adolescent Unit would never have come about without the support of physicians and administrators at Children's Hospital and Harvard. In an acceptance speech for the C. Anderson Aldrich Award, which was given to Gallagher by the American Academy of Pediatrics in recognition of his work in the developmental and behavioral aspects of pediatrics, Gallagher noted that "a large share of the award belongs to the trustees and staff of the Children's Hospital," most notably Charles Alderson Janeway, who was physician-in-chief at Children's Hospital when the Adolescent Unit was founded. According to Gallagher, Janeway and many other physicians at Children's Hospital and Harvard Medical School "wanted to establish a medical service for adolescents, and they supported it enthusiastically."[2]

Gallagher was not simply being humble when he said that other individuals and circumstances contributed to his success: his interest in adolescent health care was clearly shaped by larger developments within society and medicine during the 1930s and 1940s. Like his close friend Lawrence Frank, Gallagher was disturbed by the social and political turmoil of the era, and believed that emotional maladjustments were responsible for many of the problems of the day. As a school physician, Gallagher found high rates of emotional problems and physical illness among his young patients, despite their relatively privileged socioeconomic circumstances. Gallagher blamed many of these problems on faulty methods of child nurture, which forced adolescents to conform to the "tyranny" of fixed standards of growth and development. Gallagher's empathy for young people who were different grew out of his own experiences as a teenager: he suffered from severe acne and tuberculosis, the latter of which forced him to leave high school and be tutored at home.[3] Gallagher's observation of similar kinds of emotional turmoil among Phillips Academy students was a major factor in his decision to start a research unit on adolescence at the private school, and later shaped his work at Boston Children's Hospital.

Gallagher's clinic for adolescents also emerged at a critical time in both the history of American pediatrics and the evolution of Boston Children's Hospital as a major center for pediatric education and practice. Like their contemporaries at other medical facilities around the country, members of the pediatric staff at Children's Hospital and Harvard Medical School were engaged in an intense debate about the future of pediatric care in the United States. As Janeway recalled, "we wanted to redefine pediatrics—in its broadest sense—as the field of health and medical care for boys and girls throughout the period of growth."[4] One of the strategies used to "redefine pediatrics" was to expand the field to include the physical and emotional problems of adolescents.

"A Mistaken Spartan Air": Reforming Health Services and Education at Phillips Academy

When Gallagher arrived at Phillips Academy in 1934, he discovered the health services to be primitive compared with the state-of-the-art facilities he had been accustomed to as a medical student and resident. Although the academy had appointed Dr. Peirson S. Page as its first full-time school physician and director of athletics in 1902, and built an infirmary in 1912, the academy's headmaster, Claude Moore Fuess, considered the health service "obsolescent" because it lacked even the most basic diagnostic equipment.[5] More important, in Fuess's opinion, Page's abilities as a physician "left a good deal to be desired." Page was able to deal with relatively simple ailments such as sprained ankles, colds, and upset stomachs, but had to turn to Boston area specialists for more serious complaints. When he did treat illnesses and injuries himself, Page tended to be haphazard in his use of medication, earning the nickname "paint it with iodine" because of his indiscriminate use of this remedy for nearly every ailment.[6]

Gallagher attributed the state of the academy's health services to the mistaken assumption that the students, the majority of whom came from middle- and upper-middle class backgrounds, did not have serious health problems, and therefore did not need a highly sophisticated medical service on campus. Gallagher soon discovered that despite their privileged upbringing, many of the first-year students were in poor physical health upon their arrival at the academy. During his first year as school physician, Gallagher found more than ninety preventable defects among an entering class of approximately 250 students.[7] Although most of these cases involved relatively minor and easily correctable problems such as acne, poor posture, and nearsightedness, Gallagher also discovered a remarkably high incidence of potentially life-threatening disease among the students he examined. For example, in a survey of 910 students conducted between 1935 and 1943, Gallagher found that over a quarter of these boys tested positive for tuberculosis, an unusually high rate for upper-middle-class individuals at this time.[8]

Gallagher put some of the blame for these problems on parents—particularly mothers—who did not ensure that their sons received proper medical care during childhood. In one of his earliest reports on the health service, Gallagher noted that while few students had serious medical problems, it was "surprising" how many students had never had a proper physical examination. Gallagher suggested that perhaps mothers assumed that since their sons lived in privileged circumstances, they did not need as diligent attention to health as did children from more modest socioeconomic backgrounds.[9]

An even greater danger, claimed Gallagher, were mothers who succumbed to medical "fads" and "quacks" rather than consulting trained medical professionals. Like other highly trained medical professionals at this time, Gallagher distrusted the ability of mothers to raise their own children without professional assistance, and believed that scientific experts like himself should make up for maternal shortcomings. In *Understanding Your Son's Adolescence,* an advice manual for parents based on his experiences at Phillips Academy, Gallagher lamented the disastrous results of mothers' misapplication of medical information. For example, Gallagher described the case of "Ralph," who had come to the infirmary with a cold. When given the simple instructions to stay in bed and rest until his symptoms subsided, Ralph anxiously asked Gallagher, "Gee, Doc, aren't you going to do anything for my cold? My mother always gives me a laxative, paints my throat, gives me aspirin, fills me up with hot lemonade, makes me drink lots of water and gives me nose drops." Gallagher claimed the mother's "random self-medication" and distrust of doctors had given Ralph an "irrational" and neurotic approach to illness. Cases like Ralph's, Gallagher believed, demonstrated the need to convince adolescents and their parents to cease the indiscriminate use of home remedies, and allow trained experts with "patience, prestige and knowledge" to decide the proper course of medical treatment.[10]

A side effect of this "maternal incompetence," observed Gallagher, was that many students he encountered were, in his opinion, remarkably ignorant about the causes of illness. Gallagher found this situation disgraceful, arguing that "a preparatory school training is not complete" if it "does not develop by example and teaching those habits of living which are essential to good health and the enjoyment of one's education." To achieve this goal, Gallagher began a program in health education that would provide students with "individual instruction" and "the distribution of reliable information free of fads and fancy regarding the causes of illness."[11]

Although parents received the most blame for the ill health of students, Gallagher also argued that many physical diseases and injuries were exacerbated by the physical and social environment at the academy. Like other elite private schools in the United States, Phillips Academy grew out of fears about the "feminizing" influences of "lady teachers" and overprotective mothers on adolescent male development. By providing boys with an appropriately masculine environment dominated by athletics, rigid discipline, moral and religious training, and strenuous living in rural settings, schoolmasters at these boarding schools hoped to turn "overcivilized" boys into virile young men. Those who "made the grade" and excelled in this austere atmosphere would go on to assume privileged places in politics, business, and the professions. Those who failed to "measure up" were systematically expelled from further study.[12]

Gallagher argued that this "mistaken Spartan air" encouraged students to endure illnesses and injuries manfully rather than seeking prompt medical attention. Although Gallagher admitted that there were some "malingerers" who possessed an "unnatural" concern with their health and a "morbid interest in disease," they were far less of a problem than boys who failed to consult the school physician for their ailments. Not only did such boys put themselves at risk for more serious complications, but those with infectious diseases jeopardized the health of the entire student population. Rather than allowing boys to suffer in silence, Gallagher encouraged students and faculty to report all illnesses and injuries, no matter how minor.[13]

At the same time Gallagher began a drastic overhaul of the academy's health services. A generous donation from Fannie R. Dennis funded the construction of a large addition to the infirmary and the purchase of an X-ray machine and other diagnostic equipment. Funds from the Dennis bequest also allowed Gallagher to hire five resident nurses, a dietitian, a secretary, and several other assistants to help run the infirmary. By the late 1930s the health services more closely resembled a small hospital of the period than a typical private school infirmary.

Gallagher also improved preventive health procedures at the academy. At the request of the Massachusetts Department of Public Health, Gallagher required all students to obtain thorough medical examinations and immunization against smallpox and diphtheria before attendance at school, had his staff examine food handlers for communicable diseases, investigated the bacteriological content of the swimming pool, and revised the school schedule so that students would be absent from the campus during the worst cold and flu seasons.[14]

Gallagher soon discovered that he needed to do more than improve the quality of health services available to adolescents: studies on adolescence were just beginning in the early 1930s, and there simply was not enough knowledge about normal adolescent growth and development to serve as an adequate guide to medical treatment of this age group. He felt particularly overwhelmed in the area of adolescent mental hygiene: although he had been trained by leading psychiatric experts during his years at Yale Medical School, he felt unprepared to deal with the everyday emotional turmoil of adolescent boys. Gallagher recalled, "My hospital training had given me an acquaintance with the care of severe, and often terminal, disorders . . . [but] I found myself woefully deficient in the care of an adolescent troubled with delayed growth, a Sprinter's fracture, homesickness, acne, epilepsy, obesity, an anxiety state, diabetes, a sprained knee or school failure, to confess only a few."[15]

Gallagher was not the only school physician who felt his knowledge of adolescent development was inadequate: he noted that many of his colleagues at other boarding schools "were almost equally frustrated and often could offer little more than a concerned 'someone really ought to look into that.'"[16] Yet Gallagher possessed a combination of intellectual curiosity and professional ambition that set him apart from other school physicians at the time, and in 1937 he decided to start his own study of adolescent growth and development.[17]

Gallagher's reasons for proposing an adolescent study unit were partly professional: he wanted to improve his own professional standing as a medical researcher. In a grant proposal to the Carnegie Corporation, Gallagher wrote that the value of a research project on adolescent development "lies not only in the data obtained and the conclusions drawn, but also in the salutary effect upon the department's morale and standards; such a department without research tends to deteriorate because of its limitations in the fields of medical care and prophylaxis."[18] Elsewhere, he noted that school and college health programs that do not conduct medical research "lose their vitality, fail to command student respect, and gradually acquire a less alert, less progressive, and less efficient staff."[19] As a medical student at Yale University, he was exposed to an academic system that made original research and publication critical to tenure and promotion. Gallagher may have felt that his position at Phillips Academy was something of an intellectual backwater, and that by conducting research he could enhance his standing in a medical community that was placing greater emphasis on research. He may also have wanted to cultivate connections outside of Andover in case his position at the academy was eliminated because of budgetary constraints.

Professional status was not Gallagher's only motivation: he also argued that developing an adolescent research institute could be used as a marketing tool for Phillips Academy. In several letters to Headmaster Fuess, Gallagher noted the "prestige" that a medical research department lent to the academy, and claimed that by offering students a quality of medical care that equaled or surpassed "that which their parents would seek at times of illness," Phillips Academy would have a distinct marketing edge over other elite preparatory schools.[20]

Finally, Gallagher's interest in improving knowledge about adolescent growth and development was influenced by contemporary concerns about the relationship between adolescent mental hygiene and social stability. Like Frank, Gallagher believed that personality disorders were at the root of fascism, crime, juvenile delinquency, and other social problems facing Western society. Gallagher was particularly worried about eliminating emotional problems in the kinds of boys who attended Phillips Academy, most of whom went on to assume prominent positions in American business, the professions, and government.[21] "Nothing is more futile and wasteful than to equip a student with an Phillips Academy education and leave uncorrected his anarchistic attitudes or psychopathic trends," wrote Gallagher. If Phillips Academy was to do its part in drawing the nation out of the Depression and preventing a totalitarian regime from emerging on American soil, then it needed to do a better job of preparing elite young men for leadership roles in American society. According to Gallagher, this entailed more than providing a superior education: it also meant studying each "students' characteristics and attempt to remedy those which presage one or another type of individual or social disaster" similar to the ones seen among the dictators and their followers in Europe.[22]

Gallagher claimed that the competitive academic environment at the academy exacerbated adolescent emotional problems, and was dismayed that faculty and administrators did not take emotional problems into account when they considered academic dismissals. In fact, Gallagher often interceded on behalf of boys who were in danger of being expelled. The home he shared with his wife, Constance Dann Gallagher, became a haven for students who were homesick and/or having trouble adjusting to the rigorous academic and behavioral expectations at the school.[23]

During the fall of 1937 Gallagher met with Headmaster Fuess and the academy's registrar, Dr. Willet L. Eccles, to discuss the possibility of studying a group of adolescent boys at the school that would "better the physical and scholastic and social adjustment of the individual student" as well as improve medical care and education for this age group more broadly.[24] Fuess greeted Gallagher's proposal for an adolescent study unit enthusiastically, because it fit perfectly with the headmaster's approach to educating adolescent boys. As a faculty member during the 1920s, Fuess became disillusioned with what he saw as a rigid, authoritarian system, which allowed the schoolmaster to be a "legalized tyrant" and which dealt with students "as if they were units in an army platoon to be handled in the same way, without attention to individual differences or abnormalities."[25] Fuess argued that such a policy was particularly unfair on the "less conspicuous" boys of modest ability, who while intellectually capable of meeting the academy's academic standards, lacked the "Olympian" qualities of the "big men on campus."[26]

Fuess's description of tyrannical schoolmasters echoed contemporary anxieties about the rise of totalitarian movements in Europe: rather than turning out independent-minded, self-reliant, responsible citizens and leaders, Fuess argued, authoritarian teachers could produce young men whose only skill was blind obedience to authority. In contrast, Fuess wanted Phillips Academy to produce young men who were "tolerant, open-minded, and liberal in their attitude toward current problems," and who would "become good citizens, interested in the welfare of mankind."[27]

Fuess's interest in transforming the educational philosophy at Phillips Academy was further shaped by larger developments in public and private secondary education, particularly the progressive educational movement that was inspired by the work of G. Stanley Hall. According to Hall's recapitulation theory, education should be fitted to each developmental stage, rather than forcing students to study subjects that were beyond their capabilities. Proponents of progressive education carried this notion further and suggested that education should be fitted to each individual student. To be sure, the goals and outcome of progressive education were often just as elitist as the systems they were supposed to replace: indeed, some historians have argued that one of the motivations behind progressive education was to protect native-born, middle-class students from the "bad influences" of working-class immigrant and minority students by tracking the latter into less rigorous academic programs and excluding them from elite private schools. One of the methods used to sort students by ability were the new intelligence quotient (IQ) and aptitude tests developed by researchers in applied psychology. Although psychologists claimed that these tests were based on an objective "meritocracy of the mind" that transcended traditional sources of social privilege based on ethnicity and class, critics argued that these tests were culturally biased and tended to favor children from white, native-born, upper- and middle-class backgrounds. Despite this elitist slant, progressive education did for the first time attempt to demonstrate that education needed to be tailored to the abilities of individual students.[28]

By the early 1930s the progressive approach to education had been expanded to include an interest in the emotional needs of school-age children and adolescents. According to this "mental hygiene point of view," not only did inflexible academic programs doom some students to failure, they also thwarted healthy personality development by breeding feelings of inferiority in students who were forced into academic programs that did not fit their unique needs and interests.[29]

Although Fuess remained skeptical about some aspects of progressive education, he nevertheless shared the progressive belief that each boy was "an individual" with unique talents and abilities.[30] Rather than forcing boys into an inflexible educational program, argued Fuess, the goal of a private school should be to test each boy's individual aptitude, "to advise him wisely, and to help him adjust himself to the society of which he was a unit."[31]

Fuess's interest in progressive educational principles was part of a broader attempt to make Phillips Academy more meritocratic. During the late nineteenth and early twentieth centuries, the academy increasingly based its admissions decisions on ability rather than social connections, and in the 1920s instituted a system of entrance exams and aptitude tests designed to select the best and brightest students regardless of social background. These revised admissions policies significantly increased the diversity of the students at Phillips Academy: by 1930 nearly one-third of the students were on some form of financial aid. This figure grew partly out of the increased economic pressures on middle- and upper-class families at this time, but also reflected a sincere effort by admissions personnel to attract students from lower socioeconomic backgrounds. In terms of religion and ethnicity, Fuess liked to brag that "in a school established by rather bigoted Calvinistic Congregationalists, we had nearly 10 percent of Jews and about the same proportion of Roman Catholics" during his term as headmaster, a significant increase from previous administrations. Fuess also noted that the academy "usually had two or three Negroes and would have accepted more if they could have met the stiff entrance requirements." [32]

There were limits to Fuess's tolerance of racial and ethnic minorities, however: like most private schools and colleges and universities at this time, Phillips Academy had strict quotas governing the admission of Jews and blacks. In his private correspondence, Fuess admitted that he and the admissions personnel tried to keep the academy "as predominantly Aryan as possible," adding that if Jews were admitted on the same basis as Gentiles he would soon be "overwhelmed" by applications. In the case of blacks, Fuess did not mind admitting one or two per year, but felt that having more than a few blacks on campus would "make trouble." [33] Despite Fuess's claims to meritocracy, therefore, the majority of Phillips Academy students were still white, Anglo-Saxon, Protestant, and relatively wealthy. [34] Nevertheless, the socioeconomic and ethnic composition of the student body was becoming sufficiently diverse to convince Fuess that an educational philosophy that treated students as interchangeable units was no longer appropriate.

Fuess' interest in tailoring education to the individual boy made him receptive to Gallagher's plan for a research program that would improve understanding of the physical and mental hygiene of adolescent boys. Fuess gained the support of the trustees for the Adolescent Study Unit and helped Gallagher obtain a five-year research grant from the Carnegie Corporation, which allowed Gallagher to enlarge the infirmary facilities and to hire sufficient additional staff to accommodate the new research project.[35]

"There Is No Average Boy": The Adolescent Study Unit at Phillips Academy

Gallagher's research on adolescent development soon brought him into contact with the leading adolescent development researchers in the United States. William Greulich of the Yale Child Study Department was a frequent visitor at Phillips Academy, and helped Gallagher collect data on the relationship between skeletal development and sexual maturation.[36] Gallagher in return participated in several of Greulich's research projects at Yale, and a major portion of the research subjects for Greulich's landmark studies of somatic development in adolescent boys were students at Phillips Academy.[37] Other frequent collaborators in Gallagher's research projects were Lawrence Frank; Harold Coe Stuart, who conducted research on children and adolescents at the Harvard School of Public Health; and Arlie Bock, director of the Health Services Department at Harvard University, and his associates Dana Farnsworth and Clark Wright Heath.[38]

Gallagher's association with the Harvard Health Department was particularly significant since it drew him into a major study of "normal" adolescence and young adulthood that was conducted by Bock and his associates. Commonly referred to as the "Grant Study" because it was the first research project funded by the William T. Grant Foundation, this study grew out of Bock's observation that many of the students under his care were not physically ill, but rather were "unhappy and badly adjusted to their environment." Like Gallagher, Bock suggested that these emotional problems were due to an inadequate understanding of the normal individual, that is, one who is free from gross physical and mental disease, and how to help him adjust to college and professional life. Believing that the purpose of higher education was "to build a man and aid him in the expression of the capacities he has within him," Bock decided to start an interdisciplinary study of "normal" young men that would be used to improve medical, psychological, and vocational guidance services for this age group.[39] Grant, a former patient in Bock's private practice, agreed to fund the study because it fit with his foundation's goal to help "people or peoples to live more contentedly and peacefully and well in body and mind."[40] Grant was also puzzled by psychological troubles and career failures of "normal, at times even highly promising persons" who worked for him, and wanted a fool-proof method of selecting successful managers and salesmen for his company.[41] After several meetings with Bock during the summer and fall of 1937, Grant agreed to give the Harvard Hygiene Department $60,000 per year for five years to fund his project.[42]

The selection of Harvard undergraduates and Phillips Academy students as research subjects was done partly for convenience, but also demon-strated that Grant researchers equated "normal" with privileged, white, native-born males. Earnest A. Hooton, one of the physical anthropologists involved in the study, described the reasoning behind the choice of research subjects in "Young Man, You Are Normal" (1945), a popular book on the Grant Study.[43] Although Hooton was a close associate of the physical an-thropologist Franz Boas and helped Boas lead a campaign against Nazi racial policies during the 1930s, Hooton's views on racial issues were incon-sistent.[44] On the one hand, Hooton frequently argued that abnormality knew no racial, ethnic, or class boundaries, claiming that "every tree that bears bad fruit" regardless of background, "should be cut down and cast into the fire." Indeed, Hooton claimed that the Nazis were misguided in targeting Jews for extermination, because centuries of persecution had made Jews superior to other races by "weeding out" the weaker individu-als.[45] Hooton even suggested that the rise of fascism in Europe was due to a prevalence of "morons" and other deviants among the Gentiles, a situation that allowed "men like Hitler and Mussolini [to] impose their evil wills upon stupid and suggestible masses."[46] On the other hand, Hooton be-lieved that race, class, and gender were "complicating variables" and that the white middle classes should be used as the "baseline" for the study of society. Hooton therefore claimed that "it would be foolish to include Negro babies and inmates of a home for old men, with Radcliffe seniors" in a study of normal human development.[47]

Consequently, despite efforts to ensure a broad range of geographic, socioeconomic, and ethnic backgrounds, 61 percent of the Harvard sample came from New England or New York State, 64 percent came from families that made more than $5,000 per year, nearly 50 percent of the participants were educated exclusively at private schools, the majority were affiliated with Protestant denominations, all of them were white, and all but eight were born in the United States.[48] This roughly approximated the undergraduate population at Harvard at the time, although researchers were quick to point out that the Grantees were taller, heavier, more muscular, had better posture, and came from better families than the "average" Harvard man.[49] The Phillips Academy sample closely mirrored that at Harvard: all of them were white, most were native-born of native parentage, over half were from New England and other northeastern states, and all but 5% came from families with annual incomes of $1,500 or more.[50]

Gallagher seems to have been more tolerant of racial diversity than the other Grant researchers: during the early 1940s, for example, he proposed using some of his funds from the Carnegie Corporation to do comparative studies of Indian boys in the Southwest and Negro boys in inner-city Cleveland in order to discern whether "the standards and norms of skeletal development derived from white populations can be applied to other races as well."[51] The Carnegie Corporation turned down his request, however, stating that it needed information on "normal groups" that had "a more or less direct relationship to the national emergency." The Carnegie Corporation clearly did not believe that Native and African Americans would play an important role in leading the country out of the Depression, nor could they serve as a guideline for "normal" adolescent growth and development.[52]

Nevertheless, Gallagher did share some of the other Grant researchers' ideas about class and gender. In his original proposal for the research project, Gallagher pointed out the benefits of studying the "normal adolescent who has the hereditary and nutritional background of the upper and middle class social level," and believed that by discerning the developmental factors that contributed to academic success among elite boys, he and the admissions officers would be able to eliminate potentially unsuccessful candidates before they came to the academy.[53] Gallagher also did not seem particularly concerned with the developmental factors that contributed to young women's academic success, possibly because he did not have much contact with female adolescents during his career at Phillips Academy. Gallagher did publish an article on female development during this time, but stated that studies of female adolescence should be used to help girls perform their future roles as wives and mothers.[54]

Once they were selected for the study, each student spent about twenty hours undergoing various physical and psychological tests, including urinalysis, blood count, lung X-rays, hearing tests, measurement of basal metabolic rate, and psychological and intelligence examinations such as the Rorschach test and Wechsler-Bellevue intelligence test that would determine the students' mental state and aptitude for college work. A social worker also interviewed each young man and his family regarding their socioeconomic status and family background.[55]

A major preoccupation of the Grant Study was the relationship between somatotype or body composition and personality. All subjects were photographed in the nude from the front, side, and rear. The physical anthropologist involved in the study—Carl Seltzer—used these photographs to assign body types to each subject using a scale developed by William T. Sheldon of the psychology department at Harvard. According to Sheldon's scale, there were three primary components of physique: endomorphy, a tendency toward a round, soft appearance; mesomorphy, a hard, muscular, athletic appearance; and ectomorphy, a linear, thin, fragile appearance.[56] Seltzer also assigned each body type a rating on a "scale of masculinity," with highly muscular, mesomorphic individuals receiving the highest masculinity rating, and plump, flabby men or extremely thin men with little or no muscular development receiving the lowest masculinity ratings. In general, Seltzer found that men with highly masculine physiques tended to be "well integrated," "vital" in affect, emotionally stable, friendly in their social relations, interested in "practical" fields like physical science and engineering, "with strongly pragmatic, humanistic, and political attitudes." Men with weakly masculine physiques, in contrast, tended to be "less well integrated" in personality, to be "sensitive" in affect, emotionally unstable, shy and asocial, interested in "creative" and "ideational" fields like art, literature, and music, and were more often "self-conscious and inhibited and perhaps more likely to drive themselves by an exercise of will power against their natural tendencies."[57] In short, "highly masculine" men were more like what American society at the time expected men to be, while "weakly masculine" men fit popular stereotypes about women and their abilities.

There were some similarities between the Grant Study and research on homosexuality during this time period. During the 1930s and 1940s, researchers in gynecology, psychology, physical anthropology, and the emerging field of sexology attempted to determine if homosexuality was caused by psychogenic factors, as suggested by the work of Sigmund Freud, or whether it arose out of innate biological characteristics such as endocrine dysfunction or brain abnormalities. Sex researchers examined every aspect of the body—including hair texture, skin complexion, body type, and the size and shape of the genitals—as well as personality characteristics that set homosexuals apart from heterosexuals.[58] Although the Grant Study borrowed some techniques from research on homosexuals, the Grant Study staff was rather vague on the exact relationship between a "weak masculine component" and homosexuality. Bock noted that those with low masculinity had "mincing expressive movements, soft voice, delicacy, grace, or mannerisms usually thought of under this category," but also claimed that a man who had such characteristics was not necessarily homosexual.[59] Conversely, Grant researchers noted that homosexuals did not always possess a "pathological" deviation toward femininity, and could even have a thoroughly "normal" masculine physique. This latter observation could have been an attempt to explain away the fact that despite the Grant researchers' supposedly meticulous selection procedure, several students in the study were discharged from military service during World War II for homosexuality. Therefore, in order to underscore the "normality" of their sample, Grant researchers claimed that even the homosexuals in their sample had the same bodily characteristics as "normal" young men.[60] Grant researchers insisted, however, that large deviations from the "highly masculine" ideal were definitely "abnormal," and they were quick to note that 90 percent of their sample fell into the "strongly masculine" category.[61] Thus they clearly associated a highly masculine body type with "normality."

Although one would think that flabby and "feminine" appearing men could become more masculine through body building or dieting, most Grant researchers insisted that the somatotype and the personality that went with it were immutable and could not be altered through environmental changes. The Harvard researchers were careful to distinguish between men who were masculine but "out of shape," and men who were inherently "feminine" in their body type. They were also adamant that once a young man was characterized as "weakly masculine," no amount of physical training could make him "highly masculine," although it might make him healthier and slightly more physically fit.[62]

Rather than engaging in futile attempts to change a young man's natural endowments, Grant researchers suggested that private schools, colleges, and universities should focus on guiding young men into careers suited to their individual characteristics. Highly masculine men, for example, should go into "manly" professions such as business, law, and medicine. In contrast, "less masculine" men should pursue careers in "feminine" fields in the arts and humanities. Grant researchers underscored this association between masculinity and traditionally "male" careers through a study of fifty-two of the most successful salesmen and managers from Grant's five-and-ten store chain. The researchers found that the managers "showed an essentially characteristic 'male physique'" that was "similar to the physical type found in undergraduates intending to go into business."[63]

Gallagher was less pessimistic about the somatotypes of Phillips Academy students. In fact, there is some evidence in Gallagher's correspondence with the Carnegie Corporation that he felt uneasy about some of the implications of Seltzer's work, and collaborated with Seltzer only because he valued his advisor Hooton's advice and support.[64] Gallagher argued that because adolescent boys were still growing, it was more difficult to determine whether the somatotype they were assigned as freshmen would be "permanent" or whether they would "outgrow" it as they progressed through adolescence. Gallagher was aware of growth studies at Berkeley that indicated a "fat period" was common during male puberty, and that some boys classified as "weakly masculine" would eventually appear more masculine as they matured and their "baby fat" turned to muscle. To compensate for the fluctuations in size during adolescence and young adulthood, Gallagher and Seltzer worked out a special somatotype scale for the adolescent group. An accurate estimate of the degree to which adolescent somatotypes were permanent, Gallagher observed, would have to wait until he could compare the somatotypes of his students in early adolescence with those of the same individuals in early adulthood.[65]

Furthermore, Gallagher's contact with other researchers in adolescent development made him cautious about the rigid use of standards of adolescent growth. Gallagher shared Frank's criticism of the "tyranny of the norm" and its negative impact on adolescent mental hygiene. Gallagher was particularly concerned about the emotional problems that resulted from delayed physical development. Boys who were "late bloomers," noted Gallagher, constantly wondered whether they would "ever be a man." Since the dormitory conditions at Phillips Academy were notorious for their lack of privacy, Gallagher observed, boys who appeared "unmanly" in any way had trouble gaining acceptance from their classmates. Gallagher noticed the same problems with peer adjustment in boys who had some sort of chronic illness such as heart disease or diabetes that prevented them from participating in sports or other extracurricular activities that were the main routes to popularity at the academy.[66]

A typical example of the kinds of emotional problems Gallagher observed at Phillips Academy was the case of "Billy," whom Gallagher described in a faculty seminar on growth and development and later published in an *Atlantic Monthly* article entitled "There is No Average Boy." [67] Although Billy was sixteen, he weighed only 115 pounds, was only five feet four inches tall, and "although a little fuzz had begun to appear on his cheeks, he had no real excuse for shaving." Up until his third year of school, Billy had been a "model boy": his grades were excellent and his behavior faultless. During his junior year, Billy's grades dropped dramatically, he became uncommunicative when at home, and was unwilling to participate in school and family gatherings. Billy's mother was frantic about his physical immaturity, and asked Gallagher whether the boy had a problem with his glands and needed to take "thyroid" or some other "tonic" to help stimulate his growth.

Rather than to succumbing to the mother's demands for a biomedical solution to Billy's problems, Gallagher convinced her that the boy simply demonstrated "that adolescents vary tremendously in the rate and manner of their growth and development." "No one ever did adolescents a greater disservice," observed Gallagher, "than the person who initiated the idea that there is an 'average' weight, or height." "The fact is," said Gallagher, "that wide ranges exist in all these matters in perfectly normal boys . . . Height tables, weight tables, charts and growth graphs all have their uses," said Gallagher, "but to evaluate a youngster's growth or health solely on the basis of these devices, to regard a number on a chart or a dot on a graph as a diagnosis instead of a fact, is to develop anxiety both in boys already fearful lest they be 'different' and in mothers who are always comparing Tom with Cousin Kate's invariably perfect son." Parents who insisted that their sons conform to average height and weight charts, warned Gallagher, "should remember that by suggesting treatment they can be fostering in the boy the idea that he is abnormal." Instead, Gallagher advised parents to recognize that a wide variation from the average was still within normal range.[68]

Gallagher added that the pressure to conform to parental expectations was not confined to physical growth, but could include unreasonable academic demands. The case of "Jerry" typifies the kind of emotional problems that could arise out of the intense academic pressure experienced by many boys at Phillips Academy. Jerry had been a good student during his first two years at school, and his family "expected great things of him." Jerry's father was a "highly respected and wealthy citizen," who wanted Jerry to pursue his own unfulfilled dream of becoming a doctor. During his third year at school, Jerry's grades began to go downhill, and Jerry became increasingly sullen and withdrawn. After weeks of conflict with parents and teachers, Jerry was finally referred to Gallagher, who was not surprised to find that Jerry's problems were rooted in his father's high expectations and his refusal to allow Jerry to choose his own career.[69]

Cases like those of Billy and Jerry convinced Gallagher that many of the "anxieties and fears and somatic complaints" that he saw in his office were due to "the inhibitions, frustrations, traditions and prejudices to which the adolescent is subjected from birth." If parents learned to be more flexible, said Gallagher, then many of the emotional problems of adolescence could be avoided, but "on the other hand, should the individual be subjected to further frustrations, defeats, and persecutions, as may easily occur in our highly competitive society, we may soon have on our hands a person of mental unbalance: a fanatic seeking revenge, a hypochondriac seeking physicians, a recluse seeking solitude."[70]

Gallagher did not put all of the blame on parents: he argued that the competitive academic environment at the academy was as much at fault for adolescent emotional problems as were unreasonable parental expectations. To prevent such emotional difficulties, Gallagher believed that the faculty should view every boy "as an individual whose growth pattern, attitudes, capabilities, personality, constitutional type and psychological needs should be considered by an educator who is attempting to foster his development. The futility and inefficiency of any system which does not recognize the incongruities and variations within members of this age group," said Gallagher, was evident in the intense emotional turmoil experienced by boys who sought refuge at Gallagher's home and office.[71]

In order to improve educational opportunities for the students, Gallagher disseminated information on the relationship between adolescent development and academic success to the Phillips Academy faculty through faculty seminars and lectures delivered periodically throughout his career at the school. In these talks, Gallagher pleaded with faculty to recognize the "great variety which exists in any given class at Phillips Academy." Using the case of Billy described earlier, Gallagher argued that faculty needed to take a more individualized approach to education, which took into account the various features of each adolescent's unique physical and psychological development. "Any program of character building, studies, athletics or health improvement which does not take into account all the information it can gather about the product to be educated starts off at a tremendous handicap." Gallagher hoped that by educating the faculty in the principles of adolescent development, they would learn to "judge the adolescent on his potentialities rather than on his present state or past achievement," and tailor the individual boy's education to suit his own developmental needs and interests.[72]

Gallagher was careful to point out that by individualizing education to meet the needs of the boy, he did not mean that students should be given unlimited freedom at the school. Like Frank, Gallagher believed that "benevolent" forms of control would help adolescents internalize rules and restrictions without causing emotional difficulties. In one of his faculty seminars, Gallagher argued that while the "development of independence and responsibility is very desirable," the imposition of "reasonable restrictions" on adolescent behavior was "in itself a valuable method of educating adolescents in the true principles of democracy, and furnishes an excellent opportunity to acquaint them with the fact that democracy is a system in which the individual and common good are so fully recognized and appreciated that reasonable restrictions are inevitable."[73]

The most striking example of Gallagher's desire to structure education to match the needs of each individual boy was his program in language training, which was designed to help boys who had what Gallagher called "specific language disability" (SLD) or what is now referred to as dyslexia. The idea for the language training program began when Headmaster Fuess asked Gallagher to assist with the remedial reading program in the Department of English, a program designed to "salvage" boys who showed academic promise but whose reading skills were below average. In the course of working with these students, Gallagher found a fair number of boys who had above-average or even superior intelligence, but had perceptual difficulties in handling written language.

The case of "Ben" illustrates the kind of student Gallagher treated for

SLD. Before his sophomore year in school, Ben had always excelled in mathematics, but had just barely passed in English and Latin. During his sophomore year, Ben began to have more and more trouble with his schoolwork, and failed all his subjects except mathematics. Although Ben's parents were "disgusted with him" and blamed his scholastic problems on laziness and carelessness, they reluctantly agreed to have him examined to see what was causing his problems. A series of tests administered at the academy's health department indicated a great discrepancy between Ben's reading ability and his intelligence quotient: although only able to read at a fifth-grade level, Ben's Wechsler-Bellevue IQ score was 126, placing him in the top 3 percent of the general population.[74] Believing that these kinds of students deserved to be given a second chance, Gallagher enlisted the help of the Boston neuropsychologist Edwin Cole, who ran a clinic for special language disability at the Massachusetts General Hospital, to assist him in diagnosing and treating students with SLD.[75]

Fuess supported Gallagher's work on SLD, but faculty members proved harder to persuade. Many believed that allowing students with obviously poor academic records to remain in school would undercut the prestige of Phillips Academy and its ability to compete with other elite boarding schools.[76] Gallagher tried to quiet these objections by appealing to the same elitist language used by his opponents. He argued that while Phillips Academy should "provide adequate facilities for those boys who come to us with such handicaps and who have demonstrated themselves to be reasonably intelligent and desirable citizens," the school should not go out of its way to recruit such students and thus court the image of being a school for educationally handicapped students.[77] Furthermore, observed Gallagher, only boys who had an intelligence quotient indicating their aptitude for the educational environment at Phillips Academy should be permitted into the program. "Other handicapped students," said Gallagher, "should go to schools where the standards are less high."[78]

The faculty's fears that Phillips Academy would become a school for students with SLD were eventually eliminated when other preparatory schools began to recognize the value of language training for certain individuals. In his health department report for spring 1949, Gallagher observed that most faculty had accepted the Language Training Program because other schools were implementing similar programs, "and the old argument 'Why does Phillips Academy need such work if Exeter doesn't have to have it' has died a natural death."[79] It is unclear exactly why other schools instituted language training programs during this time, but it could be related to the fact that upper-class parents found a diagnosis of SLD more favorable than alternative explanations of school failure, which blamed poor academic performance on emotional conflicts, bad parenting, and low intelligence. Perhaps Phillips Academy's competitors imitated Gallagher's work because they realized that doing so would attract parents who were eager to accept the possibility that their son's academic career could be "saved" through special language training programs.[80]

Despite his interest in recognizing individual differences, Gallagher's work did tend to reinforce accepted notions about gender and sexuality. Like the other Grant researchers, Gallagher found that boys with masculine physiques were more likely to have "sound personalities" and were better able to adjust to the highly competitive academic environment than were those with weak masculine somatotypes. Although Gallagher insisted that even boys with low masculinity ratings should not be labeled "abnormal," he did share the Harvard researchers' opinion that body type and personality were genetically linked. Rather than attempting to change an adolescent's body type, Gallagher recommended that masculinity ratings be used to advise students on academic majors and what sport to select.[81]

Gallagher and the other Grant Study researchers did sympathize with their subjects, and realized that even elite institutions should be more tolerant of individual differences in personality, development, and somatotype. Researchers were careful to point out that a wide variety of body types—including "feminine" ones—could be considered within the spectrum of "normal" masculinity. The findings of the study, however, were essentially conservative: although the Grant researchers found that more than one kind of masculinity was "normal," they also found that only certain kinds of masculine traits were suited to academic success at elite institutions and in traditionally masculine fields. Rather than changing these institutions to make them more accommodating to individuals who did not have the ideal masculine characteristics, the goal of the Grant Study was to help boys and young men accept their limitations gracefully and adjust to their predetermined place in society.

This connection between "masculine" characteristics and career choice intensified during the Second World War, as members of the Grant Study staff become involved in the examination of young men who were joining the armed services. Grant researchers were aware of the high rate of rejection and discharge for psychiatric reasons, and wanted to find a reliable means of determining who would succeed in particular areas of the service.[82] Moreover, military officials were interested in finding a way of identifying and eliminating potential homosexuals before they entered the service, and saw the work of the Grant Study as an ideal method for accomplishing this goal.[83]

Once again, notions about the relationship between masculinity and success were paramount. Grant researchers found that men with the strongest masculine component were the most successful in combat duty, while those with medium or weak masculinity were more suited to noncombat positions. Grant researchers argued that strongly masculine men were also more successful as officers. In contrast, "leadership qualities of the nature required of combat officers were noticeably lacking in individuals with weakness of the masculine component." Therefore, those with low masculinity ratings tended to be in enlisted positions, regardless of socioeconomic status before joining the military.[84]

Despite this determinism about body type and military rank, researchers at both Harvard and Phillips Academy did increase their emphasis on physical fitness training, in the hopes that they could help all young men achieve their full physical potential. Gallagher found that many of his students, even those with highly masculine somatotypes, did not have the physical stamina required for an officer's position in the armed services. Gallagher blamed this fact partly on the physical education department's preoccupation with creating a winning football team rather than with developing a high level of individual fitness in all students. Arguing that the physical education program needed to be redesigned to suit the needs of "a private school whose graduates are likely to see military service soon after graduation," Gallagher convinced Headmaster Fuess to allow him to assume control over the physical education department. During the early 1940s, Gallagher created a new program that provided each student with an individualized exercise regimen geared at improving his overall cardiovascular fitness and physical strength.[85]

Gallagher and his colleagues at the Adolescent Study Unit also developed methods for testing the fitness level, eyesight, and color vision of adolescents. In his report to the Carnegie Corporation, Gallagher noted that these tests attracted the attention of "various individuals and organizations connected with the war effort: The Royal Air Force and the Bureau of Medicine and Surgery of the United States Navy have been particularly interested in our color vision studies; the Children's Bureau of the U.S. Department of Labor are in touch with our methods of testing vision; and the Massachusetts Department of Public Health, the Health Council of the Boy Scouts of America, and many schools have been interested in our studies of dynamic physical fitness."[86] For example, Colonel Leonard G. Rowntree of the United States Army Medical Reserve Corps wrote Gallagher "to commend the splendid work you are doing at Phillips Academy . . . In my opinion the work that you are doing is most desirable—not only will the students become fit for military service but for the full responsibilities of their life's work." Rowntree concluded that "such efforts should be carried on in all the schools and colleges of the country. I believe you are creating a model which should prove exceedingly valuable in this connection."[87] Arthur H. Steinhaus, chief of the Health Education and Physical Fitness Department of the U.S. Office of Education, added that Gallagher's program was a great way for American boys to develop the same level of fitness that German youth gained through programs of "Ausgeleichende Ubungen" or complementary exercises, and believed that Gallagher's work would make an excellent contribution toward beating the Axis powers.[88]

By the late 1940s, Gallagher's work at the Adolescent Study Unit had earned him a strong reputation as an expert in developmental research and adolescent health care that extended well beyond the Phillips Academy community. Gallagher published dozens of articles on his research during this period and received numerous requests for reprints from other physicians, who were particularly interested in Gallagher's work on language training. The response to Gallagher's paper on "Specific Language Disabilities" published in the *New England Journal of Medicine* in 1950 was particularly overwhelming: he received over three thousand reprint requests from other physicians by the end of the year.[89] Another major sign that Gallagher had won the admiration of his medical colleagues was an invitation made by the president of the American Academy of Pediatrics, Borden S. Veeder, to help organize a symposium on adolescence at the AAP's annual meeting in 1941. Other contributors to the symposium included Lawrence Frank and William Greulich, a fact that no doubt assured Gallagher that the Academy of Pediatrics regarded his work as equal in caliber to that of these eminent adolescent development researchers.[90]

Gallagher actively promoted his image as a scientific expert on adolescence among the American public at large. During the late 1940s and early 1950s, Gallagher published a series of articles in the *Atlantic Monthly* on adolescent growth and development, learning disabilities, teenage rebellion, and various other topics related to adolescent health.[91] Gallagher recalled that he received "hundreds" of "pathetically favorable" letters from parents, thanking him for his advice on adolescent health problems.[92] During the late 1940s Gallagher even began offering limited consultation services on language disabilities for adolescents who were not Phillips Academy students.[93] As a result of all these activities, Gallagher established himself as one of the leading authorities on adolescent health and development in the United States. Other developmental scientists willingly collaborated with him on research projects. Pediatricians asked for his recommendations regarding adolescent health topics. Finally, parents and other nonscientists eagerly began to seek his advice on how to raise their teenagers in a healthy manner.

Despite Gallagher's growing national reputation, administrative support for his work at Phillips Academy ran out soon after Headmaster Fuess retired in 1948. Fuess was replaced by John M. Kemper, a retired army colonel whose managerial style departed little from his former career as a company commander. During Fuess's tenure as headmaster, Gallagher had complete control over the running of the health service. Fuess never interfered with Gallagher's operation of the health department and the Adolescent Study Unit, and seldom refused Gallagher's request for improvements and financial assistance. Although Kemper eagerly supported the research at the Adolescent Study Unit and believed it improved Phillips Academy's competitive edge in the educational marketplace, he was unwilling to allow Gallagher the professional freedom he enjoyed under Fuess.

Kemper resented the degree of control Gallagher had over decisions about which boys should be expelled from school and who should be permitted to stay. During the Fuess administration, Gallagher was allowed to intercede on the behalf of a boy threatened with expulsion if he felt that exceptions should be made for the boy's health, emotional problems, or other extenuating circumstances. Although Fuess felt this was an acceptable practice, Kemper did not agree.

Gallagher soon found the conditions of Kemper's headmastership intolerable, because Kemper seemed to undo all the work he and Fuess had done to improve the educational climate at the academy, particularly in the area of student mental health. When Gallagher was offered a position as college physician at Wesleyan University in 1950, he saw it as a chance to move to a more hospitable professional climate. He left Phillips Academy that year, bringing most of the staff from the Adolescent Study Unit with him.[94]

By this point Gallagher's intellectual interests were beginning to move beyond Phillips Academy as well. Gallagher knew that the surprisingly high incidence of physical and emotional ill-health among Phillips Academy students was a bad sign for adolescent health more broadly: if this many problems could be found among a relatively privileged group, then the situation of less fortunate adolescents who had lived through the past decade of economic and social turmoil must be even more dire. Thus Gallagher's experiences with the boys of Phillips Academy eventually convinced him of the need for adequate care for all adolescents.[95] At the same time, developments were under way at Boston Children's Hospital that made this institution more interested in the medical care of adolescents.

"A Spirit of Friendly Cooperation": The New Pediatrics at Boston Children's Hospital

The history of the Children's Hospital of Boston provides an excellent case study of some of the tensions within pediatrics during the years following the Second World War. Boston Children's Hospital was the main teaching facility for the Harvard Medical School Department of Pediatrics, and was an exemplar of highly specialized medical care and education. As with other pediatric hospitals, the pace of subspecialization at the Children's Hospital accelerated dramatically during the late 1940s and early 1950s. The hospital's Department of Medicine alone added nineteen subspecialty divisions, including pediatric cardiology, gastroenterology, endocrinology, and neonatology.[96]

The expansion of pediatric subspecialties at Children's Hospital was part of a larger movement to transform the institution into a major medical center for child health care for the New England region. One of the most enthusiastic advocates of this endeavor was the president of the Hospital board of trustees, John Wells Farley. Soon after his appointment as president in 1944, Farley proposed that if the Children's Hospital was to become a major center for child health care, it must cover "all phases of pediatrics," including prevention, mental hygiene, and well-child care. "The function of this Center," argued Farley, "would not only be hospital treatment but preventive pediatrics." It was only by expanding into all branches of child health care, concluded Farley, that the Children's Hospital could "make the greatest possible contribution to the health and well-being of our children."[97]

To accomplish Farley's goals, the Children's Hospital merged with local child welfare organizations that had originated out of Progressive-era child-saving efforts, and that until the mid-1940s were responsible for the bulk of services in preventive medicine and mental hygiene. Beginning in the late 1940s, the Children's Hospital incorporated ten local institutions, including the Infants' Hospital, the Hospital and Convalescent Home for Children, and the Judge Baker Guidance Center, into a new institution called the Children's Hospital Medical Center (CHMC), which provided a full spectrum of pediatric care, education, and research for the New England area.[98]

Some members of the pediatric faculty at Harvard Medical School and the School of Public Health worried that the growing emphasis on developing pediatric subspecialties was isolating medical training from everyday pediatric practice. Janeway, as physician-in-chief, was particularly concerned about the impact of subspecialization on the training and practice of pediatricians. Although Janeway enthusiastically endorsed the expansion of medical research and subspecialty services at the hospital, he feared that the predominance of subspecialists on the pediatric faculty was fragmenting pediatric education and causing pediatricians to lose the humanistic touch he believed was so vital to successful medical care. In his annual report for 1950, Janeway warned that "no matter what the size and complexity of the institution, it is essential that not only the professional skill, but the friendly personal touch, the humane concern for the welfare of the individual patient . . . which has been characteristic of the Children's Hospital for its 80 years, should remain . . . They are more important than size, and we must constantly cherish them." Although Janeway admitted that "no technical advances are possible without specialization," he insisted that in order to correct the fragmentation of medical care, the hospital administration must foster a "friendly spirit of cooperation" among the various divisions of the hospital. Indeed, noted Janeway, the main purpose of a medical center was to provide "the opportunity for collaboration in the care of patients and in research." It was only through this kind of "friendly cooperation" that the hospital could counteract "the centrifugal tendency of the trend toward specialization."[99]

Janeway was particularly concerned about the lack of training in the psychological aspects of childhood health and disease in most pediatric residency programs. In a conference on Pediatrics and the Emotional Needs of the Child, Janeway claimed that by overlooking the total needs of the child, particularly psychological needs, pediatrics was slowly losing ground to the general practitioner who dealt with the patient and his or her family as a whole. Janeway warned that if pediatric education continued to focus on increasingly rare pediatric medical problems, rather than training general pediatricians to care for the patient as a whole, pediatrics would soon become a "luxury" limited to a few elite researchers in the subspecialties. Eventually, said Janeway, the bulk of child health care would be taken over by general practitioners and most pediatricians would be driven out of business.[100]

For Janeway, more was at stake than the professional status of pediatrics: his interest in the psychological aspects of pediatric care also stemmed from his concern about the relationship between the emotional problems of children and adolescents and the stability of American society. Janeway was familiar with the high rate of psychiatric casualties among combatants in the Second World War, and shared Frank's belief that fostering good mental hygiene in American youth was at the heart of preserving the nation's democratic institutions.[101] In recognition of his expertise in both pediatrics and mental hygiene, Janeway was appointed by President Truman to the national committee in charge of planning the Mid-Century White House Conference on Children and Youth, which adopted as its major goal the development of a "healthy personality" in all of the nation's children.[102]

Janeway's experience during the war indicated that there were not enough professionals trained in psychiatry and psychology to deal with the multitude of emotional problems witnessed among combatants and civilians. Moreover, Janeway believed that if pediatricians were adequately trained in the psychiatric aspects of child health, they could stem emotional problems before they blossomed into full-blown mental illness. Indeed, Janeway believed that pediatricians were in some ways better equipped to deal with mental hygiene issues in childhood than were child psychiatrists: according to Janeway, child psychiatrists "only deal with a portion of the individual, and by and large may tend to neglect the physical side, which is as important as the psychological and which is indissolubly linked with it." Pediatricians, in contrast, were much more likely to see how physical and psychological factors interacted in the causation of mental disease. Janeway argued that the best way to prevent mental illness was to train pediatricians in the behavioral sciences.[103]

One of Janeway's starting points for the reform of pediatric residencies at the Children's Hospital was the creation of a division of psychiatry within the hospital's Department of Medicine, which would serve to train pediatric residents in psychiatric aspects of pediatric care. In 1948 Janeway appointed Dane Prugh, a former resident at the Children's Hospital, to head this new service.[104] Prugh soon found himself overwhelmed by requests for his services from other areas of the hospital. It is unclear whether this increased demand for psychiatric services was the result of growing consumer interest or simply a reflection of the fact that many of the Children's Hospital staff were not trained or interested in the treatment of children's emotional problems. In 1950 the nearby Judge Baker Child Guidance Clinic agreed to "lend" Prugh some of its personnel to help ease his patient load. Demand for child psychiatry services at the hospital continued to grow over the next several years, compelling Janeway to formalize the hospital's affiliation with the Judge Baker by creating a Department of Psychiatry with George Edward Gardner, director of the Judge Baker, as psychiatrist-in-chief.[105]

The creation of the psychiatric service was only a preliminary step in Janeway's larger plan to thoroughly revise medical services at the hospital with regard to the total health needs of the patient. Janeway soon found what he was looking for at Gallagher's Adolescent Study Unit at Phillips Academy. To Janeway, Gallagher's efforts to study the adolescent from a variety of disciplinary perspectives was the perfect embodiment of integrated health care and clinical instruction that Janeway wanted to create at Children's Hospital.

Resolving the Tug of War between Generalist and Specialist

At first Janeway only proposed to use Gallagher as a consultant for a long-term collaborative research program on adolescence involving the Adolescent Study Unit at Phillips Academy, the Children's Hospital, and the Department of Pediatrics at Harvard Medical School.[106] When Gallagher left Phillips Academy in 1950, Janeway's plans became more ambitious. In early 1951 Gallagher and Janeway submitted a proposal for a new Adolescent Unit at the Children's Hospital to the hospital's board of trustees.[107]

In his personal correspondence and published writings, Janeway claimed that most of the trustees and staff at Children's Hospital were enthusiastic about the plans for an Adolescent Unit. Indeed, efforts to get rid of the twelve-year age limit at the hospital had been under way for almost a decade. According to Janeway, before 1940 "twelve to thirteen came to be the terminal age for much of our research and treatment" at Children's Hospital, partly "because at that age you must separate the sexes and provide facilities for each."[108] Collaborative research projects between the staff of the Children's Hospital and those in adult medical departments in the other Harvard-affiliated hospitals were signs that physicians at the Children's Hospital were willing to explore the health problems of children older than the age of twelve. For example, joint research projects between Sidney Farber, head of the pathology department at Children's Hospital, and George Thorn, at the Peter Bent Brigham Hospital, were described in the Medical Department annual report for 1942 as "but one more sign of the eradication of the 'twelve year line' which once tended to create separation of scientific interests of this hospital and those of neighboring hospitals."[109]

Board of trustees president John Wells Farley was particularly enthusiastic about incorporating adolescent health services into the Children's Hospital because he saw it as an excellent way to expand the hospital's clientele. Farley predicted that the postwar rise in the American birthrate would eventually result in a sizable population of teenagers in the greater Boston area, and he wanted Children's Hospital to be the first to tap into this new market. Moreover, Farley was keenly aware of the emotional problems precipitated by the Great Depression and the war, and believed that "nothing else [could] . . . be more important for the future of our Country" than to improve the emotional well-being of the nation's children and youth. As early as 1945 Farley had included an Adolescent Unit as part of his general plan to update the services offered at Children's Hospital, and he was thus receptive to Janeway and Gallagher's proposal to start an Adolescent Unit in 1951.[110]

Another enthusiastic supporter of the Adolescent Unit was George Packer Berry, dean of Harvard Medical School. Like Janeway, Berry was concerned that medical education had become too focused on specific diseases and scientific specialties rather than giving students an understanding of the patient as a whole. When Janeway and Gallagher proposed creating an adolescent facility that would train pediatricians in patient-centered care, Berry saw it as an excellent way to reform clinical training at the medical school.[111]

Despite the support from the dean of Harvard Medical School and the Children's Hospital board of trustees, there is ample evidence that Janeway and Gallagher encountered resistance from members of the pediatric faculty at Harvard Medical School and the Children's Hospital. These conflicts are particularly apparent in Gallagher's correspondence with the Commonwealth Fund, one of the main financial supporters of the Adolescent Unit during its early years. Gallagher first approached the Commonwealth Fund for financial support in 1952: his fellowship with the Grant Foundation was about to expire, and he was uncertain whether Grant would continue supporting his research in the future.[112] In his proposal to the Commonwealth Fund, Gallagher argued that the Adolescent Unit fit perfectly with the fund's attempts to promote a comprehensive approach to medical care that incorporated principles of mental hygiene as well as knowledge of physical illness. Although Gallagher acknowledged that a clinic focused exclusively on the treatment of adolescents might fragment medical education and practice even further, he also argued that "a Unit which focuses its attention upon an age group and which seeks specialists' help for the individuals under its care (but which avoids sending its problems to specialists) is in a position to offer training to medical students and physicians which emphasizes the importance of fulfilling an individual's psychological and social as well as his medical needs." More important, argued Gallagher, a unit for adolescents was needed because "at present no institution is devoting a major portion of its effort to a comprehensive service-research-teaching program aimed at the care and study of the adolescent." Gallagher claimed that adolescence "has correctly but for too long been spoken of as the neglected age group; no longer boy or girl and not yet man or woman, they are not regarded as the special responsibility of either the pediatrician or the internist." In order to more fully serve teenagers, a new medical service that was aware of adolescents' special needs was required.[113]

Some members of the Commonwealth Fund staff were skeptical about whether Gallagher could fulfill his goals given the setting in which he was trying to work. For example, the fund's medical director, Lester Evans, observed that "pediatrics is fragmented to a considerable extent" at both the Medical School and the Children's Hospital, and doubted that Gallagher's hopes could "ever be fully achieved in such a highly structured and compartmentalized a set-up as the Boston Children's Hospital or the Harvard Medical School setting."[114] The fund's social work consultant, Mildred Scoville, suggested that a clinic devoted exclusively to adolescents would actually be counterproductive. Although she admitted that adolescents had been slighted by the medical profession, she believed that knowledge about adolescent health and development "should be part of the understanding of all physicians." Rather than providing a model of holistic patient care, Scoville argued, "an elaborate institute such as the one proposed [by Gallagher] with emphasis on pathology and age period sounds almost like equating adolescence with a disease entity."[115] In the end, the Commonwealth Fund staff decided to adopt a "wait and see" attitude, and held off funding the Adolescent Unit until it could more firmly establish itself within the Children's Hospital and the Medical School.[116]

During the next few years Gallagher slowly carved a niche for himself and the Adolescent Unit within the Harvard-Longwood hospital complex. The new clinic filled a void for adolescent medical care in the greater Boston area: the number of clinic visits grew by 300 percent in the first year alone, and by 1954 the clinic was handling over five thousand visits per year.[117] The growing demand for services prompted the hospital administration to allot more resources to the Adolescent Unit. In October of 1952, the unit received its own office space within the hospital, and these quarters were expanded gradually during the following years. The Children's Hospital administration also substantially increased Gallagher's budget, raising it from a initial allocation of $25,000 in 1951 to almost $45,000 by the end of

1953. The increased budget allowed Gallagher to bring in more consultants and to hire two full-time associates, Felix P. Heald and Robert P. Masland, to assist him in coordinating patient care at the unit.[118] Heald graduated from the University of Pennsylvania School of Medicine in 1946. During the early 1950s, he started a fellowship in pediatric oncology under Sidney Farber at the Children's Hospital. The strain of seeing young patients die of cancer proved too much for Heald to handle, however, and he requested a transfer to another service in the hospital. Farber told him that the Children's Hospital was going to start an adolescent clinic and that it would fit perfectly with Heald's budding interests in the psychological features of childhood illness. Heald agreed, and in 1952 became the Adolescent Unit's first trainee.

Masland received his medical degree from Columbia in 1946 and completed a residency in internal medicine at Northwestern University in 1949. In order to avoid military service in the Korean War, Masland volunteered as a physician in rural South Dakota. After a year, Masland found he did not like either the professional isolation of a rural medical practice or the long winters in South Dakota, and he sent letters to college health services all over the East Coast in search of a job. In early 1954 Masland received an encouraging letter from Dana Farnsworth, head of the college health service at the Massachusetts Institute of Technology, who told Masland of Gallagher's work and suggested that there might be a position available at Children's Hospital. Masland immediately contacted Gallagher, arranged an interview during one of Gallagher's workshops in Kansas City, and was appointed an assistant to the unit in 1954.

Like Gallagher, Heald and Masland both had medical histories that made them sympathetic to the anxieties faced by adolescent patients. Heald had contracted tuberculosis while in medical school and was sensitive to the restrictions that a debilitating disease could impose on a young person. As a youth, Masland had spent a good deal of his time laid up in the hospital with various sports-related injuries. It was an experience during his undergraduate years at Yale University, however, that formed the basis for Masland's therapeutic style with adolescents: during his senior year, Masland was admitted to the college infirmary with severe abdominal pain. The attending physician was "not very nice" and assumed that Masland was drunk or hungover when in fact he was suffering from a ruptured appendix. Masland's close brush with death and the insensitivity of the attending physician convinced him of the need to listen carefully to young patients.[119]

The arrival of Heald and Masland helped Gallagher further the goal of "friendly cooperation" and patient-centered care that Janeway was trying to foster throughout the Children's Hospital. Although Gallagher drew on a variety of specialists within the hospital as consultants in particular cases, he was careful to keep the focus of treatment on the "patient as a whole" rather than on a particular disease or disorder. Each patient was assigned to either Gallagher, Heald, or Masland, who would then serve as the main care-giver, and who was responsible for orchestrating a team of medical consultants, social workers, guidance counselors, and other experts who would attend to a particular patient's total needs.

Gallagher's research projects were also designed to encourage collaboration among members of the various departments in the Harvard Medical School, the School of Public Health, and the Longwood Avenue hospitals. For example, in 1952 Gallagher began a collaborative research project on dysmenorrhea with Somers Sturgis of the Peter Bent Brigham Hospital. Gallagher also relied regularly on Prugh from the Children's Hospital psychiatric service for consultation on psychological and emotional problems of adolescents. Other collaborative projects included research on the differential diagnosis of hypothyroidism in adolescence, conducted with George W. Thorn of the Brigham Hospital; a multidisciplinary approach to the etiology of specific language disability with hematologists from the Children's Hospital's Blood Grouping Laboratory and geneticists at the Children's Cancer Research Foundation; a joint study with the Judge Baker Guidance Center on "school phobia"; and a longitudinal study of adolescent growth and development performed in conjunction with the Department of Anthropology at Harvard University and the Department of Maternal and Child Health at the Harvard School of Public Health.[120]

Despite the addition of Heald to the staff in 1952 and the arrival of Masland in 1954, the unit was chronically understaffed during the early years of its existence, and almost all of the staff's time was devoted to seeing patients rather than to its original goal of training medical students and residents in comprehensive approaches to health care. Once again, Gallagher turned to the Commonwealth Fund for financial assistance. Arguing that "in order to establish our Unit as a training center we first need to train those physicians who will form the basis of our teaching staff," Gallagher asked the Commonwealth Fund for a three-year grant to pay the salaries of those individuals who would become the core medical personnel for the Adolescent Unit.[121]

The Commonwealth Fund was still reluctant to provide funding for the Adolescent Unit, however. Although fund staff members were encouraged by Dean Berry's enthusiastic support, they still worried that the Adolescent Unit was too isolated from the Harvard Medical School to truly serve as an instrument of educational reform. The fund's main concern was that Gallagher and his colleagues would not be considered qualified to serve on the Harvard faculty, a fear that was borne out during the early years of the unit. One of the chief difficulties Gallagher encountered was his lack of specialty training and academic experience in pediatrics: Gallagher's residency training was in internal medicine, and he was not board certified in either pediatrics or a pediatric subspecialty. Janeway also was trained as an internist, but had won the respect of the pediatric faculty by his reputation as an outstanding "bench" researcher in pediatric immunology. In Gallagher's case, most of the pediatric faculty viewed his work at Phillips Academy as somewhat old-fashioned, and doubted whether his training and background could meet the high academic standards required for tenure at Harvard Medical School. It was only at the insistence of Dean Berry that Gallagher was finally given an appointment as assistant professor of pediatrics in March of 1953.[122]

The Commonwealth Fund staff also believed that the psychiatric component of the unit was rather weak, especially considering the fact that at least two-thirds of the patients seen at the clinic needed some form of psychological care or child guidance. The clinic employed only one psychiatrist, Herbert Harris, and even he was present at the clinic for only two and half days per week.[123] Fund staff members were alerted to the problems in the unit by the newly appointed chief of psychiatry, George Gardner. Soon after his appointment to the Children's Hospital in April of 1953, Gardner began to complain that Gallagher was paying insufficient attention to the psychiatric needs of patients, despite his claims that the clinic was intended to address the needs of the "whole patient." Gallagher refused Gardner's suggestion that he employ more psychiatrists and psychiatric social workers at the unit. Gallagher argued that he did not want to traumatize patients by sending them to a mental health specialist for what he considered to be relatively minor psychological problems. He also claimed that by too hastily sending youngsters to psychiatrists, their total health needs would be overlooked.[124] According to a report made by the Commonwealth Fund's social work consultant, Mildred Scoville, "Dr. Gallagher seems so convinced of the soundness of his own approach to problems of adolescents that he does not think too clearly regarding some of the psychiatric aspects." Scoville was trained as a psychiatric social worker, and was skeptical about whether Gallagher had sufficient training in mental hygiene to adequately address the psychological needs of adolescent patients.[125] It was only at the insistence of the Commonwealth Fund's Lester Evans that Gallagher finally yielded to Gardner's suggestions and agreed to add two more psychiatrists to the clinic's staff.[126]

Despite the shortage of psychiatric staff at the Adolescent Unit, Evans found that the clinic's interdisciplinary approach to adolescent health problems had great potential for reforming clinical instruction at Harvard. When he visited the clinic in September of 1953, he agreed with Janeway's claims that the Adolescent Unit was "the best example they now have of what integrated service might become . . . with principal emphasis on the patient's problem and not on the technique of treatment."[127] Evans was further persuaded by Janeway's observation that the Adolescent Unit provided an excellent model for resolving the "tug of war" between "the general practitioner who knows his patient and the specialist who knows his disease."[128] Hoping that the Adolescent Unit would serve as a model of reform in pediatric education for the rest of the country, the Commonwealth Fund agreed to provide the Children's Hospital with a $70,000 grant to further develop Gallagher's unit.[129]

The fortunes of the Adolescent Unit improved considerably under the Commonwealth Fund's support. The grant allowed Gallagher to appoint more full-time staff for the unit, to hire additional psychiatric consultants, to greatly expand and renovate the unit's physical quarters, to purchase more sophisticated research equipment, and to finance more elaborate research activities.[130] These improvements allowed the Adolescent Unit to more fully attain its objective of integrating medical training at Harvard. According to Janeway's report to the Commonwealth Fund in 1957, the Adolescent Unit "helped to break down interdepartmental and interhospital barriers, as a place where pediatricians, internists, and psychiatrists, and representatives of many specialties from various teaching hospitals have worked closely together in the interests of teaching and of study of the medical peculiarities and needs of this age group." More important, said Janeway, expansion of the Adolescent Unit allowed more residents to receive instruction in the model of patient care provided at the unit. In 1955 the Harvard Medical School added an elective course in adolescence to its catalog, and by 1956 all out-patient residents spent part of their rotations on the Adolescent Unit.[131]

Support from the Commonwealth Fund also enabled the Adolescent Unit to become a nationally recognized training center for the medical care of adolescents. As early as 1952, physicians from other medical institutions turned to Gallagher for advice in the care of adolescents. By the mid-fifties, the Adolescent Unit had formalized its postgraduate training program, and offered as many as twelve fellowships per year to postgraduate physicians who were interested in receiving instruction in adolescent health care.[132]

The comprehensive model of patient care embodied in the Adolescent Unit never really caught on either at Harvard or among the medical profession as a whole. A. McGehee Harvey and Susan Abrams note in their history of the Commonwealth Fund that Evans and his staff were "swimming against the tide" by trying to develop patient-centered programs "just when many medical schools were turning their backs on comprehensive care, family medicine, and health-care research. More glamorous areas, such as cardiology, were competing for students' interest, and medical faculties were seduced by federal research training grants in medical specialties." Consequently, despite much early enthusiasm for the comprehensive care movement in medical education in the 1950s, few medical schools sustained these programs for very long.[133]

Fortunately, this fate did not befall the Adolescent Unit at the Boston Children's Hospital. Support from local benefactors, various private foundations, and a tremendous demand for services made the unit relatively self-sufficient by the mid-1950s. Yet there is also ample evidence from the Commonwealth Fund records that the unit had little effect on the overall teaching program at Harvard Medical School, despite support from Dean Berry.[134]

Thus one of the ironies of the history of the Adolescent Unit at Children's Hospital was that it emerged at an institution that was rapidly moving away from Gallagher's generalist outlook on adolescent health care. The Harvard Medical School and its affiliated hospitals were exemplars of the highly specialized and technically sophisticated medicine that dominated postwar medical practice. Although the pediatric specialists at the Children's Hospital and Harvard Medical School were somewhat willing to expand the age limit of the hospital beyond the traditional "twelve year line," they were less enthusiastic about the comprehensive approach to pediatrics advocated by Gallagher and Janeway. As a result, the establishment of the Adolescent Unit encountered many obstacles because its philosophy on medical research and patient care came in direct conflict with the professional ethos of the mainstream of the postwar American medical profession. This "tug of war" between the generalist approach of adolescent medicine and the drive toward specialization in the rest of the medical profession would be a major obstacle for adolescent medicine for many years to come.

Gallagher and Janeway had an easier time persuading Boston area parents and adolescents of the value of the Adolescent Unit. For parents, the unit became a way to deal with the more troubling aspects of postwar youth culture. For adolescents, Gallagher was the first to seriously consider the idea that young people needed a "doctor of their own."

The Adolescent Unit at Boston Children's Hospital

In March of 1960 an article by Gallagher entitled "Why We Feel Sick" appeared in *Seventeen* magazine. The article described "a noted clinic, The Adolescent Unit of the Children's Hospital in Boston," which was "devoted exclusively to the treatment of the physical illnesses and worries of boys and girls from twelve to twenty-one." The bulk of the article consisted of four "actual case histories" that demonstrated the range of problems treated at the Adolescent Unit, and showed the "powerful link" between emotional upheaval and physical ailments in the teen years, "when rapid body growth goes hand in hand with rapidly changing emotions." The article made it clear that patients were seen separately from their parents, and that doctors took their opinions seriously.[1]

The *Seventeen* article was only one of many efforts made by Gallagher and his staff to promote the clinic directly to teenagers and their parents both in the greater Boston area and nationwide. Soon after his appointment to the staff at Children's Hospital, Gallagher publicized the clinic's services through articles in *Parents' Magazine,* the *Saturday Evening Post,* and other nationally published periodicals.[2] Gallagher and his staff advertised the clinic's services through countless lectures and demonstrations for parent groups and youth organizations, as well as numerous appearances on both local and national television and radio programs, including NBC's "Today Show."[3]

Gallagher was especially concerned with distinguishing his service from other medical specialists who treated adolescents. According to Gallagher, other specialists who saw adolescents in their practices, such as child psychiatrists, endocrinologists, orthodontists, and dermatologists, offered a one-sided approach to adolescent health care because they focused on only one problem rather than addressing the total health needs of the teenage patient. Gallagher claimed that because the staff members at the Adolescent Unit looked at the "patient as a whole" they were better able to diagnose and treat adolescent medical complaints than other medical specialists.

Although Gallagher aimed his public relations campaigns at both parents and their adolescent children, he was particularly interested in making his message appealing to teenagers. Even articles that appeared in adult-oriented magazines created an image of the clinic that would appeal to teenage tastes. For example, an article in the July 1954 issue of the *Saturday Evening Post* entitled "The Adolescents Get a Doctor of Their Own" pointed out that despite the location of the Adolescent Unit in a pediatric medical center, every attempt was made to create "an atmosphere that is certainly not 'children's' and only part 'hospital.' It has its own entrance from the street to a corridor and reception room, where the furniture and the magazines depart from the general pattern in the Children's Medical Center in being completely adult."[4]

Gallagher's attempts to "sell" his services to Boston-area teenagers was part of a larger movement to "normalize" adolescent rebellion. Developmental psychologists during the 1940s and 1950s argued that adolescent rebellion, within certain boundaries, was a healthy sign of progress toward adulthood. Within this model, adolescents who did not achieve independence from their parents and identify with their peers were seen as more problematic than teen rebels who challenged adult authority. To be sure, these developmental experts recognized that some adolescent rebellion could cross the line into juvenile delinquency. However, they argued that true delinquency was relatively rare and that for most adolescents, rebellion took on innocuous forms such as dress, hairstyle, and tastes in popular music.

Similarly, Gallagher believed that attaining independence from parents and identifying with the peer culture were essential to normal psychological development. Indeed, Gallagher was more worried about young people who were overly compliant with adults and did not socialize with their peers. Drawing on his own painful experiences with acne and tuberculosis as an adolescent, Gallagher focused much of his attention on physical disorders and psychological conflicts that interfered with successful peer integration. Gallagher argued that physicians who treated this age group should not only recognize the adolescent's natural need for independence, but should use the doctor-patient relationship as a way of facilitating adolescent individuation. In the process, Gallagher created a new role for physicians. Not only would doctors provide adolescents with good health care, they would also serve as guides on the arduous path toward adulthood.

Publicity campaigns and salesmanship are not the only factors that attracted Boston-area parents and their children to the Adolescent Unit: clients would not have come to this facility unless they were convinced it offered a service that met their needs and that no other facility in the Boston area was prepared to give. To help elucidate what made the Adolescent Unit appealing to Boston-area parents, I randomly sampled 430 case records of private patients treated at the unit between 1952 and 1973. Of this sample, 191 were from the 1950s, 202 were from the 1960s, and the remainder were from the early 1970s.[5] From its inception, the unit treated patients from a variety of socioeconomic backgrounds and classified them into two categories: "clinic" cases, which tended to come from low-income backgrounds, and "private" patients, who came from middle-class or upper-class families who were able to afford the full cost of medical treatment.[6] Physicians at the unit also provided low-cost medical care for local child welfare organizations, such as the Hayden Goodwill Inn for delinquent boys, the Industrial School for Crippled Children, and the Boys' and Girls' Clubs of Boston. The condition of the documentary record, however, made it impossible for me to obtain samples of non-private patient records.[7]

Nevertheless, an examination of private patient records gives tremendous insight into the inner workings of the Adolescent Unit. Before the advent of Medicaid during the mid-1960s, private patients were the ones who literally kept the unit in business. Although Gallagher was able to obtain some money from private foundations, most of the unit's funds came from private patient fees and donations from grateful parents and personal friends of Gallagher. Therefore, in assessing how the concept of adolescent medicine was "sold" to local medical consumers, one needs to understand what attracted private patients to the Adolescent Unit and how they viewed the medical care that physicians offered.

Teen Markets and Teen Doctors

Gallagher and his staff were not the first ones to recognize the importance of aiming their public relations efforts directly at teenagers. Advertisements and products designed specifically for children and youth began to appear as early as the 1860s, and market analyses of purchases made by children and youth date back to at least the 1920s.[8] What was new about youth marketing of the post–Second World War period was its use of theories about adolescent development. Drawing on the work of Erikson and others on adolescent psychology, advertisers argued that independence from adult authority and identification with the peer group was a normal part of adolescent development, and that advertising copy directed at this age group should reflect this fact. In the words of the youth marketing guru Eugene Gilbert, advertisers needed to keep in mind that "young people are in the process of growing up" and should be treated differently from both younger children and adults.[9] The term "teenager," first coined in the early 1940s, was a recognition that the adolescent age group was a distinct market segment with its own tastes and opinions. The fact that there were more adolescents in the American population (over 9 million in 1940) than at any other time in U.S. history also made this age group attractive to advertisers and merchandisers.[10]

Gallagher was influenced by the same concepts about adolescent development, and was the first to apply the idea of "niche marketing" to the medical care of adolescents. Like youth marketers of this period, Gallagher believed that respect for the patients' point of view was a crucial component of successful medical care for adolescents. Gallagher noted in his textbook on adolescent medical care:

> Adolescents are very quick to reject anyone who tries to impose his will or ideas upon them, whose interest is feigned, or who seems to have little regard for what they are, do, think, or say. In short, they literally demand that you pay as much attention to them as you do their symptoms. When you fail to do so, you may expect monosyllabic replies, broken appointments, [and] discarded advice."[11]

Gallagher's therapeutic style differed markedly from earlier interactions between teenage patients and physicians. Joan Jacobs Brumberg argues in her history of anorexia nervosa that during the nineteenth century, adolescent girls were not given the chance to tell their own story in the doctor's office. Physicians examined the patient and solicited the opinions of her parents, but they did not ask the girl herself for an explanation of her food refusal. Instead, says Brumberg, the relationship between doctor and adolescent was a product of Victorian social conventions and views on child rearing. Just as the child was supposed to be "seen and not heard" in the bourgeois home, so too was she expected to be silent in the doctor's office.[12]

Kathleen Jones's history of child psychiatry demonstrates that the first half of the twentieth century saw little change in the relationship between doctors and young patients. Rather than allowing children and adolescents to "tell their own story in their own words," Jones observes, child psychiatrists were interested mainly in manipulating factors in the child's environment—usually maladjusted mothers and occasionally fathers—that contributed to the child's emotional and behavioral problems. Thus the parents, not children, were the "real" clients of child psychiatry services.[13]

Gallagher realized the importance of respecting the patient's perspective by observing the behavior of young people who, while unable to consent to or pay for their own medical care, were nevertheless able to subvert medical intervention by refusing to take their medication, neglecting to keep appointments, ignoring medical advice, or refusing to see a doctor altogether. The case of Betty Algers illustrates the degree of control that patients could exert in the doctor's office. Betty's parents had taken her to a variety of specialists in a futile attempt to get her to lose weight. Betty's doctor described her as a "fiercely independent girl," who insisted that she was "happy the way I am" and would "lose weight when I am good and ready." Betty resisted all of her parents' pressure by refusing to diet or even to come in for a second visit to the unit.[14]

Conversely, Gallagher realized that adolescents could persuade their parents to take them to the Adolescent Unit, even when the parents were somewhat apathetic about seeking treatment for a particular condition. For example, Steve Ellis's parents brushed off his recurring episodes of anxiety as typical teenage moodiness, and did not think it serious enough to seek a doctor's advice. Steve eventually convinced his parents that he needed help for his problems and specifically requested that his parents take him to the Adolescent Unit for treatment.[15] Cases like Steve's were rare, however, and the unit's staff soon realized that if they were going to gain their young patients' cooperation, they needed to make their services appealing to teen-agers as well as to parents.

One of the most obvious concessions that Gallagher made to teenage tastes was in the physical environment of the unit. Because the entrance to the Adolescent Unit was separate from the rest of Children's Hospital, patients did not have to see younger children as they entered the Unit. The waiting area was free of toys or childish furniture, and was stocked with a plentiful supply of teen magazines and comic books. The walls of the waiting room were decorated with pictures of teen idols and original art-work created by patients and other local teens. Gallagher justified the physi-cal appearance of the clinic by arguing that the "major value" of an office designed according to youthful tastes was "to lure the reluctant adolescent, and to offer tangible evidence to all [teenagers] that this clinic . . . has a special interest in them."[16]

Efforts to gain adolescents' approval were also evident in the clinical demeanor of the unit's physicians and support staff. If doctors wanted to avoid being rejected by adolescents, Gallagher wrote, then a teenager's "visit to a physician's office should be different from that of a child. They [adoles-cents] are no longer little people, their hand in Mother's, being taken to the doctor to whom Mother will tell the story and be given the explanations and advice."[17] In marked contrast to a typical pediatric office visit, Gal-lagher ensured that from the moment a teenager entered the Adolescent Unit, he or she was treated with the same level of respect and dignity as an adult patient. Gallagher insisted that patients be seen separately from their parents so that they would feel that the doctor was truly interested in them rather than in their parents. Although parents were the only ones allowed to set up the first appointment, Gallagher recommended that patients themselves be allowed to make all further appointments so that they would not feel they were being forced to come to the clinic. The receptionist would introduce patients to their doctors as "Miss" or "Mr." Gallagher advised his physicians to avoid a patronizing tone when dealing with pa-tients. "It is important to do everything possible to avoid an authoritarian atmosphere," wrote Gallagher, for adolescents "quickly recognize, and re-spond well to a physician who is slow to suggest, more eager to listen than to talk, and who usually listens without apparent approval or disapproval of what he is told." Gallagher recommended that doctors avoid lecturing patients from behind a desk and instead conduct their interview from a chair placed next to or in front of the patient so that patients would feel that doctors were treating them as equals rather than as subordinates.[18]

Yet Gallagher warned that pandering too shamelessly to teenagers would turn a patient off just as surely as being too dictatorial. "Adolescents want someone interested in them, someone they can trust and respect," Gallagher wrote, "but they are suspicious of and not comfortable with adults who are too friendly, whom they cannot respect, and who, when asked for an opinion, agree with everything they say." Although it was important for physicians to "recognize that these people neither like to be nor should be pushed around," Gallagher said, "it is equally important to remember that they respect an adult who knows what he is doing." Physicians should therefore find a balance between being "overbearing, officious, and authoritarian" and trying to be "pals" with their patients.[19]

Gallagher was particularly careful to warn against using the interviewing style employed by psychiatrists, which involved sitting and waiting for the patient to express his or her thoughts. This approach, Gallagher claimed, would only increase the adolescent's anxiety, "and because of this, although it is very useful psychiatric technique in the treatment of adults, it is usually less than helpful in interviewing adolescents."[20] Gallagher's advice on this subject appears to have been a way of making his service more appealing to adolescents by distinguishing it from psychiatry. In his textbook on adolescent health care, he observed that nonpsychiatrists were in a "favorable position" when it came to "adolescents who have some personality, emotional, or behavioral problem and yet who refuse to see a psychiatrist." "However, these same young people," Gallagher observed, "will often be willing to see their family doctor or some other physician whom he suggests." By providing a therapeutic setting that these youngsters found appealing, Gallagher argued, the physician could attract patients who would ordinarily have been sent to a mental health professional or not have received medical treatment at all.[21]

Another important component of Gallagher's approach was to make sure adolescents were adequately informed about the nature of their problem and the course of treatment. Drawing on the work of the child psychologist Jean Piaget, who suggested that adolescents possessed the capacity for rational thought and decision making, Gallagher believed that adolescents had sufficient cognitive maturity to understand and contribute to their own health care.[22] This meant that physicians should tell patients about all diagnoses and treatment decisions, rather than simply relaying this information to their parents. "An adolescent wants to know, and should know, what ails him," wrote Gallagher in a promotional brochure on the unit: physicians should not simply assume that adolescents were "too young to understand" what was happening to them. Gallagher argued that if physicians were completely sincere about a patient's condition, adolescents would in turn be more honest with their physicians and more willing to comply with medical advice. "The more adolescents know about their ailments," claimed Gallagher, "the better the chances that they'll do what is best for their own health."[23]

Failing to fully inform adolescents about their illnesses, Gallagher warned, not only would decrease the likelihood that a teenager would comply with medical advice, but could also lead to unnecessary panic in the young person, and possibly cause unacceptable and self-destructive forms of behavior. In his various publications on adolescent medical care, Gallagher recounted the disastrous consequences that resulted from patients' ignorance about their own medical problems. For example, in an article for *Parents' Magazine,* Gallagher presented the case of thirteen-year-old Ralph, who had been told by previous physicians that he had "heart trouble" but had not been told what this entailed. As a result, Ralph was terrified that he would jeopardize his life if he engaged in even the slightest physical exertion. Ralph's doctor at the Adolescent Unit, however, carefully explained that his problem was relatively minor and easy to take care of. When Ralph left the clinic, "his heart condition was no longer a complete mystery, a matter for fear and for shame: it was beginning to be a matter of fact that he could comprehend." Most important, "because someone had considered him mature enough to 'talk straight' to him, Ralph was more willing to assume some responsibility for his health than he had been before."[24]

Gallagher insistence that adolescents be given the opportunity to develop an independent and confidential relationship with their doctors was perhaps the most revolutionary aspect of his treatment philosophy. One of the main reasons for seeing patients without their parents was to ensure that patients would take responsibility for their own recovery. Gallagher also believed that fostering a confidential relationship between adolescents and physicians would contribute to the adolescents' progress toward adulthood. Gallagher pointed out that adolescents "have reached the stage of development where they can profit from, and may badly need, the benefits of a confidential relationship which a doctor of their own offers . . . They are now old enough to have their own doctor, tell their own story, listen to his explanation, ask questions, to be given advice, and in short, to begin themselves to take the responsibility for their own health." The more that doctors allow adolescents to "tell their own story" independently of parental control or influence, concluded Gallagher, "the greater will be their doctor's contribution both to their well-being and to their acquisition of maturity." [25] Giving adolescents a "doctor of their own" involved more than providing them with adequate medical care: it also entailed helping young people prepare for adulthood by giving them responsibility for their own health. By providing adolescents with a clinical setting that contained familiar icons of teenage popular culture and allowing patients to "tell their own story," doctors hoped that their young patients would be more willing to come to the unit for treatment and accept medical advice.

"Selling" to adolescents was one thing, but getting teenagers to "buy" what doctors were offering was another. Although there is no way to quantify the impact of the unit's public relations strategies, some adolescent patients who came in for treatment specifically mentioned seeing or hearing publications and programs about the clinic. Robert Black, for example, told his parents he wanted to visit the unit after seeing Gallagher on a local television program. [26] Mike Gilman, a seventeen-year-old with ulcerative colitis, an autoimmune disease of the colon, convinced his parents to travel all the way from the Midwest to Boston because he was so impressed by an article on the Adolescent Unit in the *Saturday Evening Post.* [27]

There is also some evidence that information about the clinic was spread among Boston-area teenagers by word of mouth. Typically, a youngster who had a positive experience at the clinic would recommend it to a friend or relative who was having similar problems. [28]

Although it is difficult to say exactly how many adolescents were attracted to the clinic because of publicity or recommendations by friends and relatives, the teen-centered environment and the sympathetic style of the clinic's staff made a positive impression on many young patients. Ellen Jacobs, for example, mentioned to her parents that she was eager to see Dr. Masland after her return from school because she had found him to be "such a nice guy" during her last visit. [29] Johnny Hurtz expressed similar feelings about his sessions at the unit, telling his father after one visit that "I feel good now for the first time" since leaving an unpleasant school environment. Johnny's father added that his son found Masland to be "most kind and understanding, which is a situation which has been somewhat unfamiliar to him in recent months."[30]

The unit's therapeutic style had a positive effect on many other patients who did not put their feelings into words. The patient case records contain numerous instances of patients who improved markedly after visiting the clinic. Howard Dailey's mother, for instance, told Masland that "Howie is very happy when he arrives home after his visit with you."[31] Patients such as Daniel Burg and Eddie Knight, who came in for headaches or stomach aches, reported that their symptoms disappeared after being given a chance to express their feelings to one of the doctors at the clinic.[32] One patient, Roseanne Bloom, noted that her stress headaches disappeared after just a single visit to the unit.[33]

According to physicians' reports, adolescents became more cooperative if their doctor demonstrated an interest in the young person's point of view. Laura Chase was an especially recalcitrant patient who was eventually won over by the unit's nonthreatening approach. During her first visits to the clinic, Laura would frequently refuse to talk or would leave a session early, saying, "This isn't doing me any good, and I don't want to come in anymore. I have nothing to talk about." After a few years of sporadic visits to the clinic, however, Laura's relationship gradually improved. In a letter written to Masland after one of her last visits to the unit, Laura wrote: "I was really glad to have been able to see you over vacation. Not just because I wanted to tell you how I've been, but also just to . . . have a conversation like an old friend would want to have with someone they hadn't seen in awhile."[34]

Adolescent patients were particularly impressed with the difference between the clinical style at the Adolescent Unit and that of child psychiatry. Adolescent patients frequently worried that being sent to a psychiatrist meant that they were seriously mentally ill. Kathy Barton, for example, associated psychiatrists with her father's stay in a mental institution. She refused to go to a psychiatrist despite her mother's request, insisting, "I'm not crazy." Kathy in fact was so suspicious of psychiatric methods that she refused to cooperate with doctors at the Adolescent Unit, terminating treatment after only a few sessions.[35] Many more patients, however, mentioned that they found the Adolescent Unit to be a less threatening therapeutic environment than most psychiatric offices. Mike Gilman was typical of many young patients who had unpleasant experiences with psychiatrists:

> There would be these, what seemed like, long pauses where he'd be watching you as if you were supposed to go on talking when actually there was nothing to say. Two eyes peering at you beneath a blue haze of cigarette smoke . . . It seemed as if he were trying to classify me in a category where I didn't belong. Maybe we got spoiled when we came to Boston and saw you. But frankly, he wasn't anything at all like you and I found it rather hard to talk to him.[36]

The opportunity to tell their own story without threat of parental knowledge or interference and without the clinical stance typical of psychiatry was effective with many young people. Teenagers who visited the Adolescent Unit were undoubtedly attracted to the youth-oriented environment at the CHMC and to physicians who treated them as responsible young people rather than as children. In the words of one patient: "I wouldn't go anywhere else for medical care. They respect my confidences; they treat me like a person instead of a mama's boy; they understand my problems. As far as I'm concerned, that's the name of the game."[37]

"The Greatest Sin in Adolescence Is to Be Different"

Among those who received the most comfort from the clinical approach at the Adolescent Unit were patients who had some sort of physical disease or flaw that prevented them from being accepted by other teenagers. Looking back to his own youthful experience, Gallagher was painfully aware of the psychological trauma caused by having a disease or problem that set a teenager apart from his or her peers. In both his popular and his scientific publications, Gallagher continually remarked on adolescents' intense self-consciousness and obsession with being part of the group, noting that the "greatest sin" an adolescent could commit was to be "different" from other teenagers. Although many of the problems facing adolescents were not life-threatening, and frequently seemed trivial to adults, they could be devastating to the emotional well-being of an adolescent. Therefore, Gallagher insisted that his staff take an adolescent's concerns about his or her

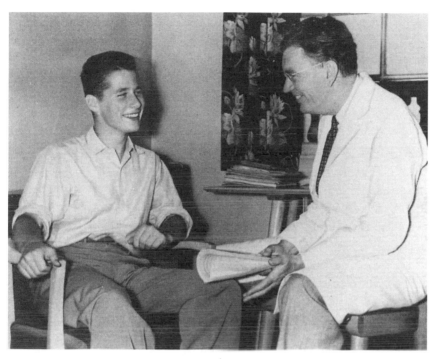

Dr. Gallagher and patient. In order to provide a friendly, nonthreatening environment for patients, Gallagher recommended that physicians avoid lecturing their patients from behind a desk. Instead, he advised sitting next to or across from a patient to give the impression that the doctor regarded the patient as an equal, rather than as a subordinate. *Courtesy of Children's Hospital Archives, Boston, Massachusetts.*

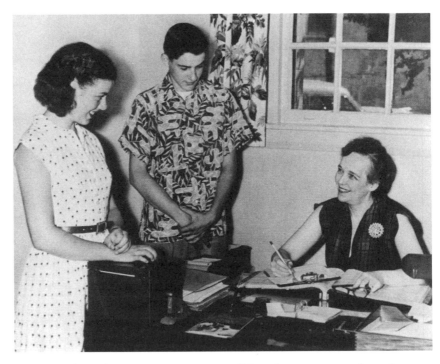

Patients making their own appointments. Although parents were the only ones allowed to set up the first appointment, Gallagher recommended that patients themselves be allowed to make all further appointments so that they would not feel that they were being forced to come to the clinic. *Courtesy of Children's Hospital Archives, Boston, Massachusetts.*

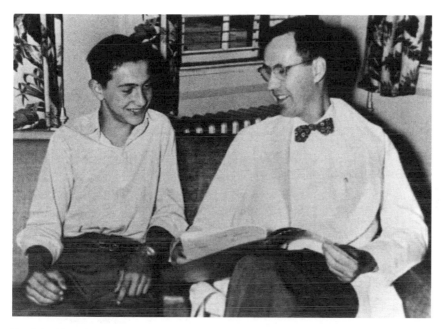

Dr. Heald and patient. Gallagher believed that adolescents possessed sufficient cognitive maturity to understand and contribute to their own treatment decisions. More important, Gallagher argued that patients would be more willing to comply with medical advice if they received a full and honest explanation of their prognosis. He therefore insisted that physicians talk to patients directly, rather than relaying diagnosis and treatment information to parents. *Courtesy of Children's Hospital Archives, Boston, Massachusetts.*

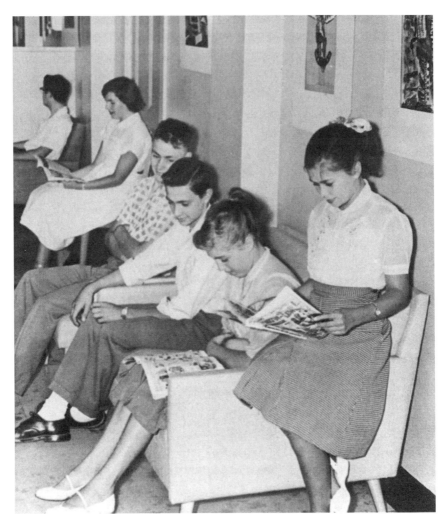

Adolescent Unit waiting room. Gallagher believed that the physical environment of the Adolescent Unit should offer "tangible evidence" that the unit
took a special interest in teenagers. Nowhere was this more evident than in the
waiting area, which had a separate entrance from the rest of Children's Hospital, was decorated with artwork by local teens, and was stocked with a plentiful
supply of teen magazines and comic books. *Courtesy of Children's Hospital
Archives, Boston, Massachusetts.*

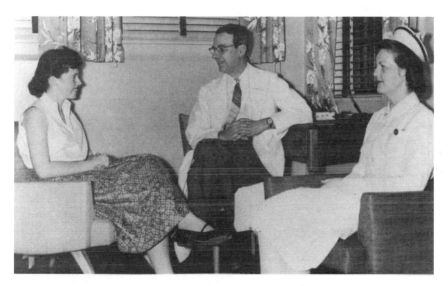

Patient, Dr. Sturgis, and Nurse Margot Lane. Although the Adolescent Unit offered treatment for gynecological problems, female patients generally did not receive pelvic examinations because Gallagher and gynecological consultant Somers Sturgis believed the procedure would cause psychological trauma. Instead, Gallagher and Sturgis recommended performing a rectal examination. If a pelvic examination was necessary, Gallagher and Sturgis advised performing the procedure under anesthesia. They also insisted that a female nurse chaperone be present during all gynecological consultations. *Courtesy of Children's Hospital Archives, Boston, Massachusetts.*

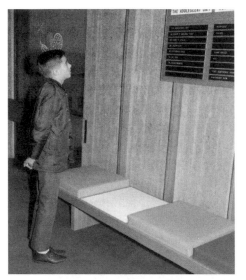

Boy outside Adolescent Unit. Although parents were the ones who paid for medical care, patients were allowed and encouraged to visit the Adolescent Unit without their parents. Gallagher believed that this would help the young person accept responsibility for his or her own health care. *Courtesy of Children's Hospital Archives, Boston, Massachusetts.*

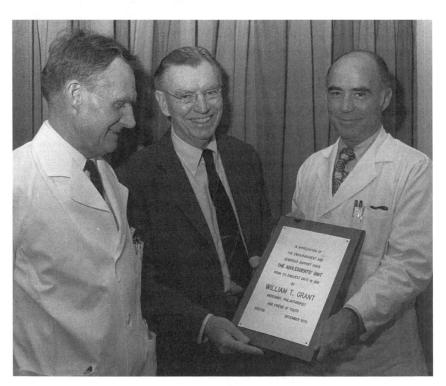

Dr. Janeway, Dr. Gallagher, and Dr. Masland receiving an award from the William T. Grant Foundation in 1970. *Courtesy of Children's Hospital Archives, Boston, Massachusetts.*

appearance just as seriously as they would more critical medical problems. Gallagher even suggested that a relatively minor physical disorder, such as acne or obesity, could in the long run pose just as much threat to an adolescents' self-esteem and progress toward adulthood as could serious physical diseases such as diabetes or cystic fibrosis. If minor problems were "merely brushed off as unimportant," warned Gallagher, then "that division between the adolescent child and the adult world which is always in danger of becoming an impassable gulf, is once more widened."[38]

Gallagher's approach to adolescent problems could be viewed as a subtle criticism of the conformist tendencies of the postwar period. Although historians have acknowledged that the popular image of the 1950s as a "placid decade" of unrelenting conformity has been overdrawn, they do agree that individuals who deviated from the "norm" were frequently stigmatized by mainstream society. American social scientists were ambivalent, however, about the idea of conformity: on the one hand, sociologists such as David Riesman, William Whyte, and Talcott Parsons praised the social stability created by "other-directedness" and solidarity with the group. On the other hand, they warned of the dangers to American democracy posed by conformist movements such as communism, fascism, and McCarthyism, and condemned what they viewed as the shallow and manipulative aspects of mass culture.[39]

Throughout his writings, Gallagher expressed similar concerns about the dangers of conformity and the necessity of encouraging "the idea of uniqueness and the importance of the individual." Gallagher realized that such a task was not easy, since "to promote the idea of the individual" among adolescents "whose world, while protesting the belief in freedom, bombards them with talk about, and the rewards of, average sizes, behavior, and attitudes, and unwittingly sets conformity on a pedestal," was "as difficult as it is desirable." Nevertheless, Gallagher believed that convincing adolescents that even "wide variations" from the average were normal was essential to their emotional well-being. Gallagher's critique of conformity had wider social implications, as well. Quoting the noted circuit court judge Learned Hand, Gallagher argued that the most serious threat to American democracy came "'not from the outrageous, but from the conforming; not from those who rarely and under the lurid glare of obloquy upset our moral complaisance or shock us from unaccustomed conduct, but from those, the mass of us, who take their virtues and their tastes, like their shirts and their furniture, from the limited patterns which the market offers.'"[40]

Gallagher's concerns about the "sin" of difference were echoed by the young patients who came to the Adolescent Unit for disorders that affected their interaction with other teenagers. Those with serious illnesses had the most difficult time fitting in with other teens: not only did they have to take medical treatments that stigmatized them as "different," but frequent absences from school and social events severely inhibited their acceptance by other teenagers. Cindy Wilson, a thirteen-year-old girl with ulcerative colitis, not only experienced extreme physical discomfort from her illness, but found "the social challenges of adolescence a more than usual threat" because of the limitations imposed by the disease. Cindy described herself as "nervous" and "fearful" around other teenagers, adding that she "wanted to belong" but was not accepted by her classmates.[41] Likewise, twelve-year-old Pamela Cartwright was brought to the clinic in a complete panic about her epilepsy because doctors at another hospital had informed her that the disease would "change her facial expression and perhaps retard her." Worried that this would affect her popularity with boys, Pamela had become depressed and anxious, prompting her parents to bring her to the Adolescent Unit.[42] Ron Houston, a thirteen-year-old diabetic patient, expressed similar despair about his illness, telling his physician that "sometimes I'd like to get away from my diabetes completely" and be like "normal" kids.[43]

Even adolescents with comparatively minor, non-life-threatening complaints often experienced great emotional distress. Annette Miller, a seventeen-year-old girl with a mild acne and weight problem, described herself as "repulsive" and lamented that she had "no friends" in high school.[44] Eighteen-year-old Brian Defoe was equally upset by his poor complexion, complaining that he was tired of doing "nothing but watch my skin." Like Annette, Brian was extremely unhappy about his fate, adding that "for years now I have had no friends, no girl, no fun, no anything . . . I feel empty from head to foot just like a hollow shell."[45]

Patients with accelerated or delayed physical development were particularly distressed by their appearance and its effect on their social adjustment. The cases of Betty Markel and Arnie Goldman demonstrate the anxieties of adolescents who worried about being "abnormal." Betty was only fifteen, but had already reached a height of 6 foot 2 inches and weighed over 200 pounds. Betty was so upset by her excessive height and weight that she refused to go to school out of fear of her classmates' ridicule.[46] Arnie represented the opposite end of the growth spectrum: although he was almost fourteen years old, he was only 4 feet 8 inches tall, weighed less than sixty pounds, and showed no evidence of sexual maturation. During therapy, Arnie drew a picture of himself as a "mouse in a zoot suit" to symbolize his distress with his extremely short height as well as his desire to fit in with other teenagers.[47]

In cases like those described above, physicians tried to convince patients that failure to be like "average" teenagers did not mean they were "abnormal." Physicians insisted that no problem, no matter how serious, should prevent a young person from participating as fully as possible in the peer culture. Although they were realistic about the degree to which a seriously ill teenager could engage in strenuous activities, Gallagher and his staff recommended that every attempt be made to find some way for a teenager to fit in with his or her peers. When a physical illness made rest and restriction unavoidable, "there should be serious attempts to offer alternative sources of success or at least an open acknowledgment and discussion of the unfortunate aspects of restriction." To do otherwise, Gallagher warned, would thwart an adolescent's achievement of independence, self-confidence, and healthy personality development.[48]

Patients usually responded positively to the news that their problems would not prevent them from leading a normal teenage life. Pamela Cartwright, for example, was elated when doctors told her epilepsy could be controlled with medication, thereby allowing her to date and engage in other teenage activities.[49] Similarly, Ron Houston's behavior at home and school improved drastically after his doctor told him that the disease would not prevent him from participating in sports and going out with his friends.[50]

Of course, not all adolescent patients responded so well to the chipper suggestion that if they would "just be themselves," they would eventually be accepted by other teenagers. Susie Barnard, a thirteen-year-old scoliosis patient, objected to any kind of physical therapy or psychological counseling for her back problems. Susie refused to wear a brace or attend physical therapy sessions because they made her feel "crippled and different from everyone else," nor would she talk with physicians about her feelings because she did not think she was a "mental case." Although Susie's mother continued to consult physicians at the unit for advice on how to help her emotionally distraught daughter, Susie herself never returned for another visit.[51]

Physicians thus did not always diminish the psychic pain caused by the "sin" of being different, but they were much more tolerant of individual differences than were teenagers themselves. Gallagher and his staff insisted that no physical flaw or illness should prevent an adolescent from enjoying all the pleasures of teenage life. By helping adolescents accept themselves they way they were, rather than trying to make them be more like "average" teenagers, unit physicians expressed a sympathy for individual difference that was a refreshing exception to the conformist tendencies of the early cold war period.

"The Difficult Line between the Psychological and the Physical"

The focus on the adolescent patient created a dilemma for Gallagher and other physicians who worked at the Adolescent Unit, since parents were the ones who paid for medical care and were usually the ones who initiated treatment. Typically the physician would interview the parents a day or two ahead of time to get their perspective on the patient's problem. Parents also had their own reasons for consulting the Adolescent Unit. Although the unit was ostensibly a medical clinic and advertised itself as such, only a small portion of the cases sampled involved strictly medical problems.[52] Instead, parents most commonly sought the services of the Adolescent Unit for school-related problems, which made up over half of the cases examined for this study.[53]

This statistic grew partly out of Gallagher's earlier work on specific language disability at Phillips Academy. Gallagher continued his work on SLD at Children's Hospital, serving as a consultant to a number of private schools in the Boston area, most notably his former employer. Soon after his arrival at Children's Hospital, Gallagher set up a small language disability division within the Blood Grouping Laboratory of the Adolescent Unit. The language disability division was located in the Blood Grouping Laboratory because Gallagher believed that SLD was hereditary. The language disability division was devoted to diagnosing patients with language disabilities and training teachers to recognize and treat students with these learning problems. Gallagher hoped that by studying blood samples from patients and their families, he would be able to determine the genetic marker for SLD and predict which individuals would inherit this trait so that remedial measures could be taken in elementary school.[54]

The language disabilities division of the Adolescent Unit was staffed by a psychologist who administered an intelligence test, perceptual tests, and examinations of the child's reading and spelling abilities. Also on the staff was Helene Dubrow, a language therapist who had trained under Samuel T. Orton, one of the first psychologists to describe a condition he called "reading disabilities." Dubrow was mainly responsible for training the volunteer staff of tutors, many of whom were women who had children with SLD. After an adolescent was diagnosed, doctors at the unit would assign one of their specially trained tutors to the patient, and would inform the patient's guidance counselor and principal that the youngster's school difficulties were due to SLD rather than to laziness or lack of intelligence.[55]

Gallagher and his staff promoted their research on SLD through dozens of public lectures at public and private schools in the greater Boston area. Gallagher's skills in public relations quickly gained him the respect and cooperation of many local teachers and school administrators, who recognized his expertise in this area and began referring students to the language disabilities division of the Adolescent Unit soon after it opened in 1953.[56]

Gallagher's public relations skills only tell part of the story, however. Evidence from patient case records indicates that use of the Adolescent Unit for treatment of school problems also grew out of the social ambitions parents had for their children. Parents who turned to the Adolescent Unit for help with their children's school problems knew that education was the main vehicle of social mobility in American society. In the postwar world, obtaining a high school and college education was essential to gaining access to the most lucrative and prestigious occupations and professions.[57] Social science research conducted after the Second World War confirmed the association between education and income, further bolstering parents' desire to obtain a good education for their children.[58] Yet more was at stake than the quality of instruction. For the upper- and middle-class parents who frequented the Adolescent Unit, simply obtaining a good education for their children was not enough. As public secondary and higher education became available to increasing numbers of American citizens during the first half of the twentieth century, attendance at elite private boarding schools became one of the most important signs that set the upper classes apart from lower socioeconomic groups. Agreeing with the sociologist C. Wright Mills's assessment of the elite boarding school as "the most important agency for transmitting the traditions of the upper social classes and regulating the admission of new wealth and talent," these parents sent their sons and daughters to prestigious private schools not only to receive a high-quality education but also to facilitate admission to an Ivy League university, ensure future business success, and/or help them marry into families with a socioeconomic background similar to or better than that of their parents. Given the status and social contacts that attendance at an elite private school provided, parents made every effort possible to keep their children in private school.[59]

The second most common problem seen at the unit was unacceptable teenage behavior such as smoking, drinking, strange hair and clothing styles, conflicts with parents, and similar signs of teenage rebellion, which made up about one-third of the cases sampled. A small number of these patients were referred to the clinic by juvenile courts and other social service agencies for more serious forms of rebellion, such as car theft, robbery, running away, sexual delinquency, or alcohol abuse.[60]

The behavior of postwar teenagers was especially troubling given the family-centered nature of American culture during the 1950s. As the historian Elaine Tyler May demonstrates, the domestic ideology of the postwar decades served as a "buffer" or "psychological fortress" against such disturbing tendencies of the age as communism and the threat of nuclear war. Emerging from the unsettling events of the Depression and World War, Americans were anxious to return to the security of hearth and home and the comfort of a "normal" family life.[61] Within this context, the rebellious teenager who rejected parental values was seen as a threat to the image of domestic tranquillity and harmony represented in American popular culture. Some social scientists suggested that juvenile delinquents came from unstable home environments where parents failed to provide the emotional nourishment necessary for the development of well-adjusted children. Since a broken home was usually seen as characteristic of lower-class families, having a delinquent child was a sign that the parents had failed to cultivate middle-class standards of child nurture and parental conduct.[62]

To many middle- and upper-class parents, therefore, rebellious teenage behavior posed a threat to the family's respectability and the social ambitions these parents had for their children. The case of Harry Richardson illustrates the kinds of unacceptable behavior that led parents to turn to the Adolescent Unit for help. Harry's mother described her son as a "typical Presley type" who combed his hair into a D.A. style, wore pointed suede shoes, and was interested in little more than driving fast cars and chasing girls. Harry also smoked, carried a gun and a switchblade, shoplifted, and did other things to win the approval of the "tough" kids who hung around his high school. After several encounters with the juvenile court over Harry's behavior, Mrs. Richardson became worried that her son was turning into a "protodelinquent." Rather than allow her son to continue on his downward spiral toward reform school, Mrs. Richardson brought him to the Adolescent Unit.[63]

Even patients who were referred to the unit primarily because of a medical problem frequently manifested behavioral problems that were the cause of much parental anguish. The case of Tom Beimers is a good example of how adolescent patients rebelled against the restrictions posed by their illnesses. Tom was a fifteen-year-old boy with celiac disease, a chronic inability to digest starches and fats that resulted in a foul-smelling diarrhea, poor nutrition, and irritability. Tom complained that throughout his childhood his mother had been extremely restrictive about his eating habits, but never explained to him what celiac disease was or why it was necessary to adhere to certain dietary restrictions, other than to say that certain foods would "poison" him. Tom responded to these restrictions by misbehaving at home and school: not only did he refuse to adhere to the dietary limitations imposed by his illness, he frequently stole money from his parents and family friends in order to buy forbidden snacks. In early adolescence, Tom's behavior became increasingly disturbing and dangerous. He was expelled from boarding school for lying and stealing books from the library. When Tom was caught trying to strangle his younger brother and then attempted to run away from home, Mr. and Mrs. Beimers realized that Tom's behavior was beyond their control and brought him to the Adolescent Unit for treatment.[64]

The kinds of problems for which parents sought help were also shaped by the gender roles of the period. Like most parents in the 1950s and early 1960s, those who frequented the Adolescent Unit believed that marriage and motherhood was the proper goal for most women, while boys were supposed to pursue careers that required high levels of education. Consequently, the majority (over 80 percent) of patients referred for school problems were boys. In fact, the school problems of adolescent boys made up such a large proportion of the case load at the Adolescent Unit during the 1950s that the total number of male patients seen at the clinic was more than twice the number of female patients.[65]

Parents were also concerned about their daughters' performance in school, but only as it affected the girls' marriage into the proper socioeconomic class. Most parents who visited the Adolescent Unit were primarily concerned with how school attendance affected a young woman's marriage prospects. Parents were particularly alarmed when a daughter's school failure was combined with having the "wrong" sort of friends, that is, those from lower-class backgrounds and/or those who were not in a college-preparatory track.

The case of Diane Reynolds demonstrates typical parental concerns. Both of the parents were described in the case record as "status-seeking" individuals who had attended elite colleges and who were distressed by their daughter's poor performance in school and what they considered to be an excessive interest in boys and dating. They were even more disturbed by the fact that Diane tended to prefer "less well motivated" and "non–college bound" boys. Although both parents eventually resigned themselves to the fact that their daughter would always be "more interested in boys than books," they sought help from the Adolescent Unit in the hopes that their daughter could enter a good college and meet a spouse more suitable to the parents' social ambitions.[66]

A daughter's marriage opportunities were especially critical to parents who aspired to middle-class status. The Archer family illustrates the kinds of expectations parents placed on their daughter's social mobility. Like Diane Reynolds, the Archer's daughter Hope was doing poorly in school and in addition was dating an Irish boy from the "projects." Unlike the Reynolds, the Archers were on the fringes of the middle class: the father made a comfortable living in a blue-collar job, but both parents came from working-class backgrounds and were therefore upset when their daughter's behavior threatened to upset their social ambitions. Hope's mother was particularly anxious about her daughter's academic and social success: Mrs. Archer's parents had divorced when she was young, and she described herself as being something of a "juvenile delinquent" as a child. In her interview with Masland, Mrs. Archer expressed her wish that her daughter would attend private school in Wellesley and eventually go to a college where she could find an upwardly mobile spouse, adding that she would "die" if her daughter married what both parents considered to be a socially unsuitable boyfriend.[67]

Parents' concerns about their daughters' marriageability also meant that girls were just as likely to be referred to the Adolescent Unit for problems affecting their physical appearance as they were for school problems.[68] This fact confirms work by Joan Jacobs Brumberg and Wini Breines on the affect of postwar beauty standards on the lives of adolescent girls. Both argue that during the postwar period, the pressure to marry within or above one's social class increased parents' scrutiny of their daughters' physical appearance and stigmatized those whose bodies and faces did not conform to white (and Anglo-Saxon) middle-class standards of physical attractiveness. Having a daughter who failed to embody these beauty standards was especially threatening to middle- and upper-class mothers: not only did a faulty physical appearance threaten a daughter's social mobility, but also gave the impression that a mother was failing to care for her child adequately.[69]

The case of Jean Berkman is typical example of the intense emotional investment that parents—especially mothers—made in a daughter's physical appearance and marriageability. Jean was described as a mildly overweight, fourteen-year-old girl with acne and tooth decay that resulted from her fondness for candy and other sugary snacks. Jean's mother was especially disturbed by her daughter's weight problems because she had also been overweight as a child. After numerous strategies "both strict and lenient" to get Jean to lose weight and take care of her skin and teeth, Mrs. Berkman turned to the Adolescent Unit in desperation, convinced that her daughter would be more attractive to boys "if her skin and fat could be better controlled." Mrs. Berkman also worried that her daughters' physical flaws were a sign that she was failing in her duties as a mother.[70]

Why did parents consult the Adolescent Unit for adolescent emotional and behavioral problems? It is not surprising that parents went to the Adolescent Unit for help with diseases and other physical problems in adolescence: there were no other facilities in the Boston area that were prepared to offer this kind of medical service, at least not on the scale offered at Children's Hospital.[71] Likewise, Gallagher's reputation as an expert on adolescent school problems explains why parents used the Adolescent Unit for this purpose. What is less clear is why parents relied on the Adolescent Unit for adolescent emotional and behavioral problems when there was already a facility just down the street from the Children's Hospital—the Judge Baker Child Guidance Center—that handled issues of adolescent mental hygiene. Founded in 1917 as a memorial to Harvey H. Baker, the first judge of the Boston Juvenile Court, the Judge Baker was originally designed to provide psychological counseling to juvenile offenders and their families, most of whom were from Boston's poorest neighborhoods. During the 1920s and 1930s the socioeconomic background of the clientele at the Judge Baker began to diversify as a result of middle-class parents' anxieties about the changing behavior of youth during this period. Learning of the Judge Baker's reputation as an institution for treating the underlying psychological causes of rebellious behavior, middle-class parents began to consult the clinic about their problem children. By 1935 nearly 50 percent of the clientele at the Judge Baker were middle class, and by the end of the 1940s, the number of middle-class patients had exceeded 60 percent of the total patient load.[72]

Gallagher used two strategies to convince parents to use the Adolescent Unit rather than the Judge Baker or other child guidance facilities. First, he drew on lingering fears about psychiatry and the social stigma attached to mental illness that persisted during the post–World War II period. Although the popular image of psychiatry became more positive after the Second World War, studies of how Americans actually used psychiatric services indicate that most individuals remained ambivalent about relying on the expertise of mental health professionals.[73] In his popular and professional writings, Gallagher used these misgivings about psychiatry to build up a clientele for his new service. In his textbook, *Medical Care of the Adolescent* (1960), for example, Gallagher wrote that even though some adolescent emotional problems "require a psychiatrist's care and though many of them would be more effectively managed by one, the fact is that . . . many of these patients (and/or their parents) will, because of prejudice, refuse to seek a psychiatrist's care." It was therefore up to doctors like himself to treat adolescent emotional problems in cases where patients and their parents were afraid of consulting a mental health professional. Gallagher's treatment of adolescent emotional problems, however, did not differ significantly from that of the Judge Baker and similar child psychiatric facilities: like these institutions, Gallagher relied heavily on psychoanalytic concepts and frequently framed adolescent emotional problems in Freudian terms.[74]

Gallagher also employed a second tactic to distinguish his service from adolescent psychiatry, which involved an approach to health care delivery rather than therapeutic methods. According to Gallagher, child psychiatry was a one-sided approach to adolescent health problems because it overlooked the totality of an adolescent's health needs. In particular, Gallagher believed that child psychiatrists were unable to detect underlying physical causes that contributed to adolescent emotional states and behavioral problems. As Gallagher remarked, child psychiatrists "didn't have as good a feeling [as the physicians at the Adolescent Unit] for the difficult line between the psychological and the physical."[75] Consequently, said Gallagher, child psychiatrists tended to overlook physiological problems that might contribute to adolescent misbehavior. In contrast, Gallagher claimed, the staff at the Adolescent Unit looked at the way in which physical and psychological complaints were interrelated, and therefore addressed not only their patients' psychological needs, but their medical ones as well.[76]

To underscore the difference between child psychiatry and the Adolescent Unit, Gallagher filled his popular writings with "success stories" describing how he and his staff were able to cure a particular teenage patient whom psychiatrists had failed to help. In an advice manual for parents entitled *Emotional Problems of Adolescents* (1958) Gallagher described the case of "Judy," whose parents had taken her to a psychiatrist because "she was destructive, she refused to do her schoolwork, [and] she was insolent." Judy also refused to eat, and had grown alarmingly thin. These symptoms led her psychiatrist to suggest that the girl's hostile feelings toward her parents "were the reasons for her destroying things they had given her and for her refusing to accept their advice or food." Intensive psychotherapy did not appear to help the girl, and so the parents decided to have a complete medical examination. "In this instance they were wise," remarked Gallagher, for the girl's "very dry skin, emaciation, coarse hair, thin eyebrows, all suggested hypothyroidism and subsequent laboratory tests bore out this diagnosis." Judy's condition "rapidly improved after she was given glandular therapy." Gallagher used this case to illustrate that "medical factors or causes are not to be slighted just because emotional ones are present." Gallagher added that "only a well-trained physician" could "distinguish between the organic and emotional elements" of psychosomatic disorders like peptic ulcer, migraines, ulcerative colitis, and enuresis or bed-wetting.[77]

Conversely, Gallagher argued that only he and his staff could tell when an adolescent's problems were due to psychological rather than physical causes. In an article for *Children,* Gallagher described the case of "Sam," who had been brought to the clinic for symptoms of apparent heart disease. When Sam was allowed to talk to a physician without the presence of his mother, Gallagher discovered that the boy's heart symptoms grew out of guilty feelings about masturbation. Gallagher concluded from this case that while "variation from the normal character of heart sounds or of the heart rate or rhythm must not be overlooked . . . it is important for physicians to remember that factors other than heart disease may be involved and that the worries which cause adolescents confusion and anxiety can also produce pain over the heart or a rapid beat."[78]

Gallagher's complaints about the alleged pitfalls of child psychiatry were not entirely unfounded. There is evidence in the case records that Gallagher and his staff were in some instances better able to distinguish between psychological and medical causes of adolescent problems than were child psychiatrists. Occasionally Gallagher and his staff would get referrals from the Judge Baker and other local psychiatric facilities that involved patients with serious, supposedly psychosomatic complaints that had not responded well to psychotherapy. Cindy Wilson, who as mentioned earlier suffered from ulcerative colitis, was referred by psychiatrists at the Judge Baker to the Adolescent Unit in 1958. Cindy's condition did not respond to psychological treatment alone, but she did improve considerably when psychotherapy was combined with drug therapy at the Adolescent Unit.[79]

It is impossible to tell from the case records whether the Adolescent Unit actually had a higher success rate in treating adolescent misbehavior and emotional difficulties than did child psychiatric services. The more important question here is whether parents *believed* that the Adolescent Unit was more qualified to deal with these problems than were child psychiatric facilities. Evidence from the case records indicates that in this regard Gallagher's persuasive efforts were successful. One of the most attractive features of the unit for many parents was the hope that adolescent misbehavior could be attributed to biomedical rather than psychological causes. Although there were some cases who, like "Mary," had genuine physical disorders that caused or contributed to their antisocial behavior, often the desire for a biomedical diagnosis represented wishful thinking on the part of parents. There are numerous cases in which parents insisted that doctors at the Adolescent Unit find a biomedical cause for adolescent rebellion, even when it was obvious that psychological disturbances or family conflicts were the main causes of their children's problems.

The case of Richard Reinhardt typifies this kind of strategy. Richard was a sixteen-year-old, adopted boy who had been exhibiting hyperactive, obnoxious behavior in school that was too difficult for his teachers at his local high school to handle. At first, his mother sent him to a private academy that Richard described as an "expensive reform school" with round-the-clock psychiatric care and constant supervision of students. Dismayed with the inability of the staff at the school to help her son, Mrs. Reinhardt brought the boy to the Adolescent Unit to see if his "metabolism" was to blame for his rebellious behavior. When Masland informed her that the problem was psychological and not somatic, Mrs. Reinhardt refused to have her son see a psychiatrist, complaining that "although I'm not opposed to psychiatry at all . . . too often the well-meaning psychiatrists [*sic*] can frighten people out of proportion to common sense. Well, I prefer to use the middle road, sir. I'll cooperate with any sound plan, but I will not consent to nonsense."[80]

Parents' desire for a purely biomedical diagnosis extended to other adolescent problems as well. Gallagher's publications on special language disability attracted numerous parents who were eager to have their children's school problems attributed to a biomedical condition, rather than to other causes such as mental retardation or emotional conflicts within the home. Although Gallagher argued that SLD was rooted in an organic brain disorder, it offered a far more optimistic prognosis than did mental retardation. Gallagher claimed that, unlike mental retardation, a diagnosis of learning disability "does not suggest any abnormality or deficiency of the brain or its language mechanism, but only an hereditary tendency to fail to develop complete dominance of one cerebral hemisphere." SLD could therefore be cured by designing teaching techniques "to impress and reimpress visual, auditory and kinesthetic memories of letters, syllables and words upon one hemisphere in such a way as these records will become vivid and dominant."[81]

The SLD category also allowed parents to escape responsibility for causing their children's school problems. Most psychologists and psychiatrists during the postwar period argued that school failure or underachievement in children of normal intelligence was due to poor parenting skills, a turbulent family setting, or other upsetting features of the child's environment. By blaming school failure on an organic deficiency within the individual child rather than on parental shortcomings, the SLD category absolved parents from responsibility for their child's failure in school.[82]

Many of the parents who came to the Adolescent Unit for treatment of school problems were eager to obtain a diagnosis of SLD because it provided a more favorable alternative to other explanations for school failure. Few of the school problem cases actually involved patients with genuine cases of SLD, however. In fact, less than 14 percent of the school problem records surveyed involved cases where a learning disability was actually diagnosed.[83] Instead, many school problem cases involved instances where the parents tried to get doctors to attribute their children's academic difficulties to learning disability, when in fact their children's school failure was due to some other cause. The parents who were the most desperate to obtain an SLD diagnosis were those whose children were mentally retarded or had below-average intelligence. Often these parents would bring their children to the Adolescent Unit with the hope that doctors would change the diagnosis from mental retardation or low intelligence to SLD. The cases of Howie Baker and Janice Boyd demonstrate the lengths to which parents would go to preserve their children's chances for a successful academic career. Mrs. Baker refused to believe that her son's school problems were due to low intelligence. When doctors failed to diagnose SLD, Mrs. Baker demanded that her son be tested for muscular dystrophy, cerebral palsy, or some other diagnosis that might preserve the hope that her boy could eventually be made into "college material."[84] Likewise, Mr. and Mrs. Boyd desperately sought an SLD diagnosis for their daughter Janice, even though the girl had an IQ below fifty. Masland described Mrs. Boyd as particularly reluctant to accept her daughter's handicap, saying that she "would not rest" until a psychological evaluation was done to see if her daughter was suffering from an "emotional block" or a "learning disability." Even after they accepted Janice's limitations, the Boyds insisted that their daughter "did not appear retarded" and therefore should not be forced to attend school with "morons and idiots" whose mental handicaps were more visibly apparent.[85]

Other parents sought an SLD diagnosis for teens who were acting up at home or at school. Some of these cases, in fact, turned out to be genuine instances of SLD. Jenny Parker, for example, was originally referred to the unit for rebelling in school, which she claimed had "too many rules." After administering the diagnostic tests, doctors soon found that SLD was indeed the main cause of her frustrations in the classroom. Once Jenny received tutoring to bring her reading skills up to the same level as her classmates, her problems in school disappeared and her behavior at home improved dramatically.[86]

Far more often, parents' requests for a learning disability diagnosis grew out of their attempts to disguise familial disputes that were the actual cause of their children's school troubles. The case of Tom Boucher was a typical example of parents' attempts to use the learning disability category as a dodge for family problems. Tom's parents specifically requested that the boy be tested for SLD, but it only took a brief conversation with the boy for Masland to discover that the real root of Tom's school difficulties was an abusive, alcoholic father and the imminent divorce of his parents.[87]

Even in cases that involved physical illnesses, growth and development disorders, or problems involving physical appearance, parents sought an uncomplicated biomedical solution for their children's problems. For example, the mother of Lois Kent, a young obesity patient, was described as "having little insight" into the psychological nature of her daughter's weight problems. Instead, Mrs. Kent wanted her daughter's problem to be considered strictly a "physical handicap that can be treated with medication." When Masland refused to give her the kind of advice she wanted, Mrs. Kent went elsewhere to search for a more acceptable diagnosis.[88]

Gallagher's sales strategy therefore attracted a variety of parents to the Adolescent Unit for problems that might otherwise have been treated by adolescent psychiatric clinics. By claiming that the unit was the only place where doctors were able to discern the "difficult line between the psychological and the physical," Gallagher and his staff offered the hope that complex teenage problems could be "cured" in a manner that did not involve a challenge to their performance as parents.

"Your Primary Emphasis Should Be on the Young Person"

Parents who came to the Adolescent Unit in search of a biomedical quick fix for their children's problems were frequently disappointed, because this kind of solution violated Gallagher's therapeutic outlook. In his textbook on adolescent medical care, Gallagher insisted that "the physician's task and privilege is to help a *person;* he loses much of his opportunity when he confines his attention to his patient's disease." Gallagher therefore argued that physicians should look at the "total life picture" of the young patient, including emotional factors and family environment, not just at a particular disease or problem.[89]

Treating the adolescent patient as a person also meant that physicians did not let parental demands supersede the best interests of the patient. "This does not mean that parents no longer play a part," Gallagher said: "their story, their anxiety, their questions will have to have attention." However, Gallagher advised physicians that their primary emphasis should be "on helping this young person in your role as his or her physician."[90]

In practice, this meant that the welfare of the teenage patient often came before the wishes of parents. Unit physicians, for instance, refused to allow parents to coerce adolescents into coming to the clinic. Doctors justified this policy by pointing out that an adolescent who did not come to the clinic willingly was extremely unlikely to comply with medical advice or develop a beneficial relationship with a physician. Physicians also believed that parental coercion interfered with the more central task of encouraging the development of adolescent independence. In addition to providing medical care, Gallagher argued that physicians should encourage autonomy in their young patients. Referring to the work of Erikson, Gallagher wrote that "[t]o foster independence, to help build confidence . . . and to persuade parents that their function is to produce an adult not just a child, are important parts of the doctor's job."[91]

Parents did not necessarily share Gallagher's views: although most parents agreed that their teenage children were old enough to see the doctor by themselves, some parents were uneasy about allowing their teenage children to build a confidential relationship with their physicians. To parents, the adolescent peer group culture had already eroded much of their authority over their children's lives. The confidential relationship between their teenage children and the doctors at the Adolescent Unit added yet another layer of interference between parent and child. Many parents who consulted the Adolescent Unit for help were thus naturally resentful when doctors appeared to value the opinions of teenage patients more than those of parents. Whenever possible, physicians tried to work out compromises that pleased both parents and adolescent patients. Physicians' concern with fostering adolescent independence, however, limited the degree to which they accommodated parental wishes.

In the school problems cases, unit physicians were willing to attribute school failure to SLD whenever appropriate. Masland, for example, wrote the headmaster of a local private school that it was unfair for doctors and school officials to place the blame for children's school problems entirely on parents, adding that "the longer I work with these young people [with SLD], the more convinced I am, that the genetic background is far more important, at least so far as scholastic achievement is concerned, than is the environment." [92]

Physicians also acknowledged that an SLD diagnosis should not overshadow other factors that might contribute to a youngster's academic difficulties. Mike Barton's case is a particularly striking example of how harsh child-rearing standards could do far more damage than SLD. Although doctors found that Mike did have a mild case of SLD, they also found that the father's rigid and perfectionist parental style was the main cause of the boy's problems. [93] In cases like Mike's, doctors would try to get parents to accept some degree of responsibility for the emotional upset that might be contributing to their child's problems in school.

Physicians also refused to provide parents with an SLD diagnosis when it was not warranted. In cases of mental retardation or low intelligence, physicians tried to persuade parents to accept their children's limitations and helped refer parents to schools that were more suitable for their children's intellectual abilities. When an adolescent's school problems were due to underlying emotional problems, physicians tried to convince parents that psychological treatment was needed. At the very least, physicians insisted that parents set realistic educational goals for their children.

The case of Donald Edwards is a good example of how doctors mediated between parental expectations and patients' abilities and interests. Donald was performing poorly at his private school in spite of an above average IQ. When Donald's parents brought him to the Adolescent Unit for help with his academic problems, the boy told Masland that he did not really want to go to college, but would rather go into farming. Donald was afraid to tell his highly educated parents of his career intentions, asking, "How would it look for me to be a farmer when my Dad's a professor?" Masland agreed that the boy would be much happier if he attended high school near a farm he had worked at the previous summer.[94]

Parents were not always willing to surrender their academic aspirations for their children. The parents of Derrick and Sam Benson were particularly adamant about finding a solution to their sons' school difficulties that did not challenge their parenting abilities. In a letter to the boys' psychologist, Masland wrote that both boys were under "terrific pressure both at home and school" and that unless "something is done about this pressure" both boys would continue to fail in school. Rather than accept Masland's advice to go easier on their sons, the Bensons continued to "shop around" for a strictly biomedical diagnosis, and had thereby "nearly exhausted the patience" of most of the unit's staff and other experts in the Boston area.[95]

Other parents took the advice of unit physicians, although this frequently came after much soul-searching and anguish. Mr. Bramble, for example, had "tears in his eyes" when he finally admitted to himself that his son Joe would never be a "college man." Despite his sadness, Mr. Bramble found a marked improvement in Joe's attitude once he reduced his demands on him and allowed him to transfer from an elite boarding school to a less demanding vocational-technical high school.[96]

When doctors did convince parents to lower their expectations and allow their child to choose his or her own career path, doctors usually had a good success rate in getting the adolescent to at least finish high school. Masland told an interviewer for *Seventeen* that since its inception, the unit's "success rate in salvaging youngsters to finish high school" had been about 80 to 90 percent, provided that doctors "try to find a school which will adapt to him . . . instead of getting him to adapt to the school."[97]

Physicians showed a similar respect for the patient's perspective in cases involving conflicts over adolescent behavior. Like Erikson, Gallagher tried to convince parents that a certain degree of rebellion was a critical part of normal adolescent development. In his numerous articles and books of advice for parents, Gallagher wrote that it was "natural and proper" for adolescents to rebel. Instead of focusing so much attention on adolescents who defied parental authority, Gallagher claimed that parents and other adults should be more worried about the youngsters who remain overly compliant and dependent on parents, since they rather than "teen rebels" were the real threat to American democratic institutions. According to Gallagher, "fear of responsibility" and a "preference for dependence" are "a more disheartening spectacle than is defiance. Few of us can view complacently the prospect of the spiritless boy or girl accepting today oversolicitude and domination who thereby gives promise of tomorrow relinquishing their remaining hope of independence to the blandishments of a dictator."[98]

Rather than submit to parents' demands for an uncomplicated biomedical solution to their children's misbehavior, Gallagher and his staff presented an image of adolescent development that "normalized" adolescent rebellion. Within this model, teenagers who showed initiative and established autonomy from parental control were depicted as well on the road to healthy adulthood, while those who failed to move beyond their parents' values were viewed as abnormal. As Gallagher himself phrased it, "it is better to have bizarre hair-dos and slammed doors, unheeded warnings and monosyllables, than no evidence of a desire to stand alone . . . To continue to protect adolescents, to continually thwart their attempts to develop independence," concluded Gallagher, "is to rob them of abilities, confidence, and resiliency they must have in the demanding and unpredictable adult world they face."[99] Although unit physicians realized that occasionally adolescent rebellion could go too far and cross the boundary into delinquency, they nevertheless made rejection of parental values and identification with those of peer group essential to normal adolescent development.

Instead of condemning teenage rebellion, Gallagher and his associates argued that adolescents who did not achieve autonomy from their parents and identify with their peer group were the ones who needed professional attention. In a letter to Boston Juvenile Court Justice Frederick T. Iddings, Gallagher observed that his contact "day after day with youngsters and their parents" made him realize the importance of "giving young people increasing opportunities over the years to increase their responsibility and independence. Neither parents nor teachers, in general, seem to pay much attention to this, and go about protecting or spoon-feeding them." Then, when these young people went off to college or work and were free from parental control, Gallagher noted, they were "completely unprepared" for it, and lacked the "experience or confidence" to make decisions on their own.[100]

Although physicians did not encourage adolescents to openly defy their parents, much of the unit doctors' interactions with parents consisted of persuading parents that rebellion was usually a sign of their child's progress toward independent decision making. For example, in the case of Ted White, a twelve-year-old boy brought to the clinic for lying to and stealing from his parents, Masland advised the father to "be more of a friendly figure" rather than harshly punishing the boy for misbehavior, and added that the "boy should and could respond to kindness" by acting in a more mature fashion.[101]

Doctors found that both parents and teenagers could benefit from the kind of intergenerational mediation offered at the unit. In the case of Amy Darling, a seventeen-year-old who was brought to the clinic because she had been caught going on wild drinking sprees with her friends, the girl's mother reported after just a few chats with Dr. Masland that "my husband and I have a much more realistic attitude toward Amy, and, oddly enough, a much greater respect for her." Amy, in turn, responded to growing parental trust with a "new understanding of herself" and a "blossoming sense of her self-worth." As a result of her parents' new-found confidence in her, Amy eventually gave up her outlandish behavior and "erstwhile friends," instead pursuing more wholesome pastimes such as "shopping, [and] going to folk-singing concerts, or museums."[102]

Frequently doctors would recommend boarding school as a means of circumventing parent-child conflict and encouraging more mature behavior in the adolescent patient. In the case of Gary Sands, for instance, Masland told the boy's parents that Gary's "failure in school may be the only way that he feels he can assert his independence during the rebellious adolescent years." Since the boy "has a lot of maturing to do, Masland wrote, "perhaps this maturing process can occur at a more even pace in an atmosphere of lower emotional tension" provided by a private boarding school.[103]

Doctors also recommended boarding school or a similar move away from the parents in cases where parents were particularly unwilling to allow their children any degree of personal autonomy in the home, or where familial turmoil was so great that it interfered with the adolescent's maturational process. For example, in the case of Lloyd Bartley, Masland observed that boarding school was the "only answer" to the boy's emotional problems "unless the father will listen to me and relent his discipline."[104]

Patients often flourished once they were free from a tense home environment, as is apparent in the case of Deborah Henson. Debbie was originally brought to the clinic because she had run away from home in order to be with a boy her parents did not like. After interviewing Debbie, Masland found that many of her problems were due to an overbearing father who insisted on "programming" all her affairs, and to parents who constantly took their hostility toward each other out on their daughter. Finding the family situation intolerable and unhealthy for the girl's development, Masland recommended that the girl be sent to live with her grandparents in another city. Once there, Debbie's grandparents reported that the girl began to respond remarkably well to adults who trusted her and expressed their confidence in her ability to make her own choices. Debbie herself wrote that "it's great to make a decision on your own with no interference from parents or friends and to feel that you have made the right choices . . . I am thinking for myself and am succeeding in a world of new-found maturity." Debbie reported that her parents were equally pleased with her change in attitude, writing that "when I told Mom and Dad they were very happy and I think they are getting along better too."[105]

Doctors showed the greatest sympathy for the patient's point of view in cases involving problems affecting a young person's physical appearance. Gallagher's critique of conformity extended to parents who demanded that he make their children appear more "normal" by accelerating or delaying their growth, clearing up their skin, or helping them to lose weight. Gallagher's classic statement "there is no average boy" was a thinly veiled criticism of status-conscious parents whose desire to "keep up with the Joneses" extended to having an attractive, socially successful child. In contrast, Gallagher and his associates showed a respect for the rights of the individual adolescent patient that superseded the ambitions of parents. Gallagher continually reminded physicians to keep in mind that it was the *adolescent's* body, not the parent's, that was being manipulated through medical intervention. Physicians should be "reluctant to attempt a change" based primarily on parents' wishes, said Gallagher, since doing so would be to extend a parent's authority over an adolescent's "shape and design to a point which usurps another's rights." Instead, Gallagher argued, treatment should be based on the *adolescent's* feelings about his or her body.[106]

Physicians frequently found that parents were more upset about an adolescent's appearance than were patients themselves. In Cindy Welter's case, for example, Masland observed that the girl had a rather severe case of acne, and was already 5 foot 4 inches at the age of eleven. Nevertheless, Masland found that Cindy was relatively "undisturbed" by problems that obviously distressed her mother. In fact Cindy's height and skin problems "did not affect her socially" or prevent her from having plenty of friends in her local high school.[107] Likewise, thirteen-year-old Ron Horowitz was described as a "happy, well-adjusted lad" despite the fact that he was much shorter and chubbier than most boys his age.[108] In such cases, "when the boy or girl shows little anxiety or embarrassment . . . or when reassurance gives promise of success," Gallagher advised that treatment should be deferred unless evidence of severe hormonal imbalances or other physical disease was present.[109]

Gallagher advocated therapeutic conservatism even when an adolescent's appearance was inappropriate for his or her gender. In the case of "unfeminine" girls, for example, Gallagher argued that efforts to limit a young girl's height, increase the size of her breasts, or stimulate menstruation "should never be made" without first attempting to "get the girl to accept herself the way she is" and to relieve parental anxiety about the daughter's appearance. Gallagher was even tolerant of "excessive tallness" (over 6 feet 2 inches) in girls, pointing out that "there are today so many tall girls who are successful in business, on the stage, in television, and in athletics—and who along with this have obviously also achieved social success and acceptance—that it has become increasingly easy to reassure those girls who seem destined to be quite tall."

Similarly, Gallagher was reluctant to use therapies to correct the appearance of "feminine-looking" boys or to stimulate the growth of boys who were below the height and weight standards for their age. As with girls, boys who failed to live up to the average should be told that wide variations in growth were normal and that eventually they would catch up to their peers. Even if all these attempts at reassurance failed, Gallagher continued, attempts to limit or stimulate growth through hormone therapy should be used with caution, since doing so could affect "other physiologic processes in ways which may not be harmless and which may result in substituting one physiologic difficulty for another."[110]

These cases show that the staff did not always submit to parents' requests to make their children appear more "normal." To be sure, Gallagher did not overlook the anguish that adolescents felt about being different from their peers, nor did he refuse treatment in cases where an adolescent's difficulty was due to some underlying medical disorder. However, Gallagher was also aware that parental demands to be "normal" were as much a problem as peer pressure, and was strongly opposed to any medical intervention that grew solely out of a parent's request to make their child "be like other kids."

Tomboys and Short Boys

Gallagher's tolerance of individual difference only went so far, however, and was constrained by prevailing notions about gender and sexuality during the 1950s and 1960s. After the social upheaval caused by Depression and war, enforcement of traditional gender roles was an integral part of establishing a sense of stability. Within this context, gays, lesbians, and heterosexual women who rejected marriage and motherhood were depicted as dangerous to national security. Politicians and behavioral scientists alike made deliberate links between the threat posed by deviant individuals and the menace of international communism. Senator Joseph McCarthy, for example, delighted in pointing out the "masculine" characteristics of Soviet women and blamed the "fall" of China and other communist victories on "pansies" who had infiltrated the U.S. State Department and armed forces. Defense of American democratic institutions therefore entailed enforcing traditional notions of masculine and feminine heterosexuality.[111]

The sexuality of American young people was an especially volatile issue during this period. Public health statistics indicated alarming rates of venereal disease among young soldiers and the "Victory girls" who sought their company. Studies of male and female sexuality made by Alfred Kinsey in the late 1940s and 1950s confirmed that premarital sexual activity among adolescents and young adults was on the rise. Finally, medical statistics from the war indicated what many considered to be alarmingly high rates of homosexuality and "effeminate" reactions to combat among young military recruits.[112]

Concerns about adolescent sexuality were not new, of course, but dated back to at least the late nineteenth century. The cold war simply intensified preexisting fears, making a direct link between uncontained teenage sexual behavior and national security. As always, young women took the brunt of criticism. Female adolescent sexuality was particularly threatening not only because of the prevailing sexual double standard but also because it challenged the primacy of home and family, which were the centerpieces of America's defense against the subversive forces of the era.[113]

Child-rearing experts blamed this unacceptable behavior on bad parenting and, more specifically, on the inadequacies of American mothers. Women were simultaneously accused of being both inattentive and overindulgent: maternal neglect and work outside the home was thought to lead to rampant premarital sexual activity among teenagers. However, too much maternal attention supposedly created weak and "effeminate" sons who would be unable to protect the nation from communist subversion. This negative image of American mothers was first introduced by the psychoanalyst David Levy in 1939 and popularized by Philip Wylie's best-selling book *Generation of Vipers* (1942). Wylie warned of the noxious affect of "Momism" on America's children, particularly its sons, arguing that mothers who "smothered" their sons with maternal love and control would make them weak and feminine. Wylie's claims appeared to be legitimated by the psychiatrist Edward Strecker's study of young men who were rejected for military service on psychiatric grounds. Like Wylie, Strecker claimed that overprotective mothers were to blame for their sons' emotional difficulties. Strecker's ideas were further promoted by the writings of Erik Erikson, Margaret Mead, and other writers on adolescent male psychological development.[114]

Gallagher shared similar views about the relationship between gender roles and the integrity of the American social order: for example, his ideas on adolescent female sexuality drew upon the work of the Viennese psychoanalyst Helene Deutsch, who served as one of the psychiatric consultants to the Adolescent Unit. Like her mentor Sigmund Freud, Deutsch believed that the central task of female psychological development was the resolution of penis envy. According to Deutsch, girls who identified too closely with their fathers and refused to accept the feminine role of wife and mother were considered psychologically disturbed or immature in their psychological development. "True motherliness," wrote Deutsch, "is achieved only when all masculine wishes have been given up or sublimated into other goals. If 'the old factor of lack of a penis has not yet forfeited its power,'" warned Deutsch, "complete motherliness remains still to be achieved." [115]

According to this theory, a mother could inhibit her daughter's progress toward adulthood by being too "masculine" in appearance, attitude, or behavior. Therefore mothers who worked outside the home, who tended to dominate their husbands, or who were otherwise "unfeminine" could "turn off" an adolescent girl from femininity and make her unwilling to accept an adult feminine role. Mothers could also thwart their daughter's development by failing to instruct their daughters in the hygiene of menarche out of fears that this would encourage premature sexual awakenings in their daughters. Girls who menstruated without adequate maternal preparation, Gallagher noted, could become so frightened by their menses that they would reject their femininity altogether. [116]

Gallagher applied these ideas about adolescent gender role identity not only to menstruation but to physical growth. In the case of girls, Gallagher claimed that one of the most certain signs that a young woman feared adult femininity was if she experienced excessive pain (dysmenorrhea) or bleeding (metrorrhagia) during menstruation, or if she failed to menstruate at all (amenorrhea). One of the major research projects at the Adolescent Unit involved a study of menstrual difficulties in adolescent girls conducted by Gallagher, staff physicians Heald and Masland, and gynecological consultant Somers Sturgis from the Department of Gynecology at the Brigham and Women's Hospital. Financed by the Commonwealth Fund, this project was guided by the belief that conflicts over femininity were the main cause of menstrual disorders in both adolescent and adult women. [117]

When physicians treated adolescent girls with menstrual difficulties or unfeminine physical characteristics, they looked not only for hormonal anomalies but for problems in the home that might be interfering with a young woman's feminine role identification. The cases of Lois Kent and Martha Humphrey demonstrate these ideas in practice. Masland described Lois as an unhappy, obese young girl with dysmenorrhea. Although laboratory tests indicated a mild thyroid problem, Masland attributed most of Lois's troubles to a domineering mother with a "masculine-type personality," whose social ambitions and "shrewish" behavior had allegedly driven her husband to an early grave. Lois's physician recommended that rather than give the girl thyroid treatment, she should be removed from her mother's "bad influence" and placed in the home of a paternal aunt who would provide a more appropriate feminine role model.[118]

Martha Humphrey's case record demonstrates how physicians treated girls with menstrual difficulties that grew out lack of preparation for menstruation. Martha was described as a "thin, tense, anxious girl with more masculine than feminine look," who was experiencing extreme pain, emotional distress, and cardiac irregularities during her menstrual period. Sturgis attributed Martha's complaints to the girl's mother, who had told her "little or nothing" about menstruation. As a result, Martha was "bewildered by her menses" and exhibited this distress by rejecting anything having to do with femininity. Once Sturgis gave Martha a better understanding of menstruation, her anxiety was alleviated, and she began to adopt a more appropriately "feminine" appearance.[119]

Informing a young woman about menstruation, however, did not entail approval of sexual activity. Although Gallagher felt it was necessary to give a young woman a "healthy" knowledge of and attitude toward menstruation and reproduction, he shared the prevailing belief that adolescent girls were too young to engage in sexual intercourse. In fact, he suggested that girls who were obsessively interested in the genital area could have problems with their feminine orientation. These concerns about the dangers of sexual awareness in adolescent girls are particularly apparent in his publications on adolescent masturbation: although Gallagher considered masturbation an "infantile" and "regressive" practice for both sexes, he argued that it was particularly disturbing in adolescent girls, since it showed a lack of proper feminine development. In *Emotional Problems of Adolescents,* Gallagher and Harris wrote:

> In girls' development masturbatory activity is less frequent than it is in that of boys. When similarity to the mother has been accepted and the drive to be like her grows, the girl appears to direct her attention and feelings toward her whole body rather than to the genital area. Hence, at this period, her interest in dress, hair ribbons, and dolls and their clothing increases. Girls who masturbate may have difficulty in developing the wish to be like their mothers, and among them will be found the tomboys who compete with boys and who seem to be

saying by their aggressive behavior, 'I am just as powerful if not more so than you.'[120]

When female patients were brought to the unit for problems related to sexual activity, physicians also tried to attribute this behavior to lack of maternal preparation or poor maternal example, as is illustrated by the case of Josie McDonald. Josie's mother was described as a masculine, "sporty"-looking woman, who worked as a coach for a local women's college swim team and had separated from her husband ten years earlier. The mother had prepared Josie for menstruation, but she had also given her a frightening version of intercourse and reproduction. As a result, Josie both feared and craved sexual activity. Although she experienced extreme pain and emotional upset during menstruation because of her mother's warnings, Josie nevertheless engaged in several affairs with older men. Although Masland tried to give her a "healthier" view about menstruation and told her to wait until marriage to have intercourse, Josie's problems continued through late adolescence. Several years later, when Masland learned about Josie's divorce after only several months of marriage, he attributed the breakup to her mother's hostile attitudes toward men and sexuality.[121]

Gallagher's interest in preventing premature sexual activity in girls made him particularly concerned about the fate of girls who matured earlier than other adolescents their age. "Girls who are taller (and more mature sexually) than boys of their same chronological age," wrote Gallagher, "will not go out with them and tend to seek the companionship of boys considerably older." The older boy, warned Gallagher, "is not only tall and sexually mature from a physical standpoint but also has a sexual drive far in excess of the girl's and of a degree most girls will not experience until they are considerably older." Gallagher believed that it was therefore the duty of physicians and parents alike to make sure that early maturity in girls did not lead to sexual activity.[122]

Gallagher's desire to protect the sexual virtue of female adolescents also led him to oppose vaginal exams for this age group. "These young girls are going through a period in their emotional development which involves their attempting to discard their tomboyishness and to accept a feminine way of life," Gallagher argued. Therefore, "at this particular time a maneuver such as a vaginal examination may represent a sexual attack and have a regrettable emotional effect." Instead of performing pelvic examinations on adolescent girls, Gallagher believed that physicians could obtain all the information they needed from a rectal examination. If a vaginal examination was absolutely necessary for diagnosis, then it should be performed under anesthesia so as not to unduly traumatize the patient.[123]

Gallagher suggested that psychological conflicts about femininity not only could affect menstruation, but could also interfere with a girl's physical growth. In his textbook on adolescent medical care, Gallagher wrote that "those whose contours are less feminine," or those who experience menstrual difficulties "may present attitudes and behavior which suggest that they are avoiding their adult feminine role." Although Gallagher admitted that often these ambivalent attitudes toward femininity represented young women's "defense against a physical state they dislike," he also observed that "fears about becoming feminine" could affect physical maturation by interfering with the secretion of hormones required for development of breasts, pubic hair, and other secondary sexual characteristics. "Regardless of which is cart and which is horse," Gallagher concluded, "these girls may need an opportunity to work out their feelings and to adjust their attitudes so that they will no longer persist in their defensive tomboyishness and in efforts to become more like their fathers, and will become able to relinquish those fears of femininity which may be inhibiting their development."[124]

Even in cases where a young woman's "unfeminine" body type was obviously caused by hormonal or genetic disorders, physicians believed that emotions played a major role in determining an adolescent girl's feminine orientation. This view was particularly apparent in the unit's research on Turner syndrome, a genetic disorder of the X chromosome which causes ovarian dysfunction, little or no estrogen production, amenorrhea, and extremely short stature. Although Sturgis acknowledged the need to give these patients estrogen supplements to prevent osteoporosis he also stated that simply giving estrogen would not change these "neuters" into "little girls interested in boys and dating and all." Instead, their gender identity was determined by the "mature adult figure that they have identified with, whether it is a father in one case and they're little tomboys, or whether it's a warm, feminine mother or mother figure in the other case where they are 'little girls.'" To illustrate this point, Sturgis gave an example of two Turner patients: one was an XX-XO mosaic, which meant her ovaries produced some estrogen. Despite the presence of female hormones, this patient was a "tomboy" because her mother "was out working all day, paying no attention to this youngster, but she was very close to her father." The girl seldom wore dresses, and "had a couple of brothers and she loved to play sports with them." The other patient was a "doll-like" girl who liked to wear frilly dresses and hair ribbons, despite a complete absence of estrogen in her system. The feminine behavior in the second patient, Sturgis argued, was modeled after a mother who gave the girl an appropriate role to follow by choosing to be a housewife rather than pursuing a career outside the home.[125]

Although mothers came under the most criticism, Gallagher and his staff also believed that fathers could also have a negative effect on a young girl's physical and psychological development. The case of Carolyn Douglas represents what physicians considered to be the dangers of excessive paternal authority. Like Martha Humphrey, Carolyn had not been prepared for menstruation and found the experience to be frightening. Carolyn's mother had at least attempted to tell Carolyn the "facts of life" ahead of time, but the girl herself had been too embarrassed to talk about the subject. Masland attributed some of Carolyn's problems to lack of maternal preparation, but added that Carolyn's fears of her strict father "and his discipline" contributed to her menstrual difficulties.[126]

Physicians believed that a father's influence was particularly harmful if it involved inappropriate gender expectations: for example, in the case of June Goldwin, a twelve-year-old girl treated for menstrual and school difficulties, Masland observed that much of the girl's troubles were due to a father who "treats her like a boy" and expected her to fulfill his ambition of going to MIT. Masland noted with relief that the mother was more willing to "see what the girl wants to do." June was considered "cured" when she began to wear "feminine" hairstyles and clothing and began dating a boy from her junior high school.[127]

The Adolescent Unit had a similar psychosomatic theory for boys, which grew out of Gallagher's earlier work with the Grant Study. Gallagher continued his interest in the relationship between personality and body type during his years at Children's Hospital, and became involved in a comparative study of delinquents and nondelinquents that was led by Carl Seltzer and William Sheldon of Harvard University and Emil Hartl at the Hayden Goodwill Inn for delinquent boys. One of the major findings of this study was that delinquent boys tended to lag behind nondelinquents in height and weight during the early years of adolescence. After the age of fourteen, delinquents usually caught up with nondelinquents developmentally, but showed a greater degree of mesomorphy (muscular body build) than did nondelinquents. In other words, delinquents in late adolescence and adulthood were "hypermasculine" when compared with nondelinquents.[128]

As in the case of masculine girls, Gallagher was unclear about which came first, the body type or the personality traits. The most important issue for Gallagher and other physicians at the unit was how the boy felt about his body, and how his distress about his appearance could manifest itself in unacceptable and even delinquent behavior. Among the more common reasons for visits to the clinic was what Gallagher referred to as the "short boy syndrome"—boys who dressed and acted "tough" as a way to make up for their short stature or sexual immaturity. Such boys, noted Gallagher, "doubting their masculinity, seek to prove it to themselves by behavior they would not otherwise choose."[129]

Gallagher warned that mothers could exacerbate the emotional consequences of the "short boy syndrome" by "coddling" their sons and preventing them from engaging in appropriately masculine activities with other boys their age. Boys who identified too closely with overprotective mothers, Gallagher and Harris argued, could fail to develop a healthy interest in girls. This "attachment to their mothers causes many to approach all girls as symbols of their mothers and consequently taboo." If this situation were allowed to continue, argued Gallagher and Harris, such boys might become homosexuals.[130]

Gallagher and Harris insisted that if caught in time, even "feminine-looking" boys could be steered along the correct path to masculinity. Indeed, they noted that a "rather pretty, not very athletic, unaggressive boy should no more—on the basis of such traits—be labeled a homosexual than the football player." Unfortunately, noted Gallagher and Harris, an effeminate boy was often rejected by his peers "and forced to fill his needs for companionship by associating with those who have no other friends— perhaps the true homosexuals."[131]

The case of Steve Sussman demonstrates these fears about the relationship between maternal overprotection and effeminate behavior in boys. Steve was described as having a "small, slight figure" and a "waltzing, mincing" manner. Although Masland blamed some of the boy's problems on a "high titre of estrogens," he also attributed Steve's effeminacy to an "oversolicitous" mother with a "borderline personality." After two years of androgen supplements combined with psychotherapy with Masland to help him break his attachment to his mother, Steve showed "definite progress in his sexual growth and development" and a significant lessening in his effeminate characteristics.[132]

Warnings about the negative affect of "Momism" on adolescent boys extended to female physicians as well. Gallagher and Harris argued that examination by a female physician could cause or exacerbate "castration anxiety" in boys. Although this was particularly true of boys with disorders of growth and development, Gallagher argued that even normal boys could be traumatized by having their bodies scrutinized by a woman. Therefore, Gallagher did not permit any of the female physicians who trained at his unit to perform physical examinations on boys. Male physicians were allowed to examine adolescent girls, but were required to have a female nurse as a chaperone. Girls also had the option of requesting a female physician if they were uncomfortable about being examined by a man.[133]

Although Gallagher focused much of his attention on Momism, he also recognized that fathers could have a detrimental affect on a boy's gender identity. According to Gallagher and Harris, "fathers who plan too much, who are too ambitious for their sons, who want them to succeed where they have failed, can unwittingly do just as much harm" as overly restrictive mothers. Boys who were continually badgered by an authoritarian father would either become "fearful of being a man" and retreat into passive pursuits to avoid their father's wrath or become "hypermasculine" by engaging in delinquent activities to "prove their manhood." Fathers could also foster effeminacy in boys by providing a poor male role model, and were especially harmful if they harbored homosexual tendencies themselves.[134] The case of Bob Russell illustrates what Gallagher believed to be the dangers of inappropriate paternal influence. Like Steve Sussman, Bob was described as a small, effeminate boy who was "too much under Mama's jurisdiction and [has] too little association with Dad." However, Masland also laid much of the blame on Bob's father, who placed extraordinary demands on the boy to be an "A student" and a "great athlete." After a visit with Bob's father, Masland speculated that Mr. Russell might be "a latent homosexual who can't stand the effeminate streak" in his son.[135]

Physicians insisted that discouraging homosexual or effeminate traits in boys should not entail approval of sexual behavior. Rather than being a sign of healthy masculinity, promiscuity was just as much a sign of disordered sexual identity in boys as it was in girls. Gallagher and Harris argued that a sexually promiscuous boy, like an effeminate one, "is often one who has never given up his childish attachment to his mother. Such an attachment is accompanied by strong desires to be feminine like her, urges whose fulfillment is intolerable in a male society whose mores all conspire to frown on the slightest suggestion of femininity. Driven by these forces, and unaware of their nature, he strives desperately to prove his masculinity by what he considers a virile form of behavior—promiscuity."[136] One of the main reasons Gallagher advocated athletics for boys was because it provided them with "a socially acceptable outlet for their sexual drive."[137]

The case of Ronnie Feinstein illustrates how physicians approached the issue of sexual activity in adolescent boys. Ronnie's mother brought him to the unit because he was hanging around with "tough" older boys, frequenting strip clubs in Boston's Combat Zone, and picking up "loose" girls from working-class neighborhoods, all of which upset the sensibilities of his socially ambitious parents. Although Masland thought that this behavior and interest in sex was "not unusual for a sixteen-year-old boy" he did recommend sending Ronnie to private school in order to contain the boy's sexual impulses.[138]

The treatment style at the Adolescent Unit thus offered a mixture of progressive ideas about adolescent independence and conventional ideas about gender roles and sexuality. On the one hand, Gallagher realized that both boys and girls needed to achieve autonomy from their parents and become "self-reliant men and women." "Demure, dependent little girls are not truly feminine," wrote Gallagher and Harris. "They are just as much to be pitied as their seemingly courageous sisters who escape into masculine pursuits to avoid those accompaniments of womanhood which they secretly fear." Likewise, a boy who was dependent on his parents and a "low nuisance value" in the classroom and home might be a blessing to grownups, but would ultimately prove be a weak, ineffectual adult. "It may be painful to watch" a boy mature and make decisions on his own, "but it isn't half as disheartening as to find he doesn't want to do so."[139]

Autonomy from parental control did not mean the same thing for girls, however, as it did for boys. As in his earlier work with the Grant Study, notions about appropriate gender roles permeated Gallagher's theories of adolescent medical care. Like most Americans, Gallagher saw traditional gender roles as a island of security in the political and social turmoil of the cold war era. Consequently, the medical care that adolescents received at the unit during the 1950s and early 1960s tended to reflect the gender-role expectations of the postwar years.

Nevertheless, the Adolescent Unit at Boston Children's Hospital was the first facility to recognize that adolescents needed a "doctor of their own" who considered the young person's needs and opinions more important than those of the parents. As doctors weakened parental authority, they simultaneously empowered adolescents by giving them more of a voice in the clinical setting. This unique doctor-patient relationship provided the foundation for further developments in the rights of adolescents in the ensuing decades.

Adolescent Medicine since the 1960s

The year 1968 is usually depicted as a watershed in American history, a turning point in a decade of protests and activism.[1] 1968 was also a critical year for the field of adolescent medicine: in March of that year, physicians from adolescent clinics throughout North America voted to create a Society for Adolescent Medicine (SAM) that would serve as the professional organization for physicians involved in adolescent health care. The founding of SAM was the culmination of over a decade of growth in the number of facilities treating adolescents. According to a survey of 225 hospitals in the United States and Canada conducted by Dale Garell of the Children's Hospital of Los Angeles in 1964, 55 hospitals of those polled already had adolescent medical services, and another 4 were planned to begin within the next two years. Of those hospitals without adolescent services, 70 percent of those surveyed reported an interest among the staff in starting an adolescent service.[2] This rapid expansion of clinics and training programs led Garell to quip that his field had entered its own "adolescence."[3]

Growth continued throughout the next two decades: by the mid-1970s nearly half of all pediatric departments in the United States had adolescent inpatient wards and/or outpatient clinics, and by the 1980s more than half had adolescent services of some kind. The demand for services was accompanied by an increase in training opportunities in adolescent medicine: the number of fellowship programs grew from sixteen in 1969 to twenty-eight in 1974, forty in 1978, and fifty-one by the mid-1980s. Adolescent medical care became an integral part of the medical school curriculum and residency training programs of medical schools and hospitals around the country.[4]

This increase in the number of adolescent medical services was the result of a combination of forces, not the least of which was Gallagher's own "missionary" work. Gallagher gave lectures on adolescent medical care to groups of parents, physicians, and teenagers around the country, which prompted interest in developing new clinics devoted to the health care of adolescents. Physicians from all over North America soon came to study under Gallagher and learn how they could set up their own adolescent service. Demand for advice became so great by the late 1950s that Gallagher decided to create a more systematic method of training physicians in the health care of adolescents. In 1958 the Adolescent Unit began offering a postgraduate course in adolescent medicine for physicians interested in adding adolescents to their private practices, practicing college or school health, or starting similar adolescent units at other hospitals and medical facilities. Two years later, Gallagher published the first edition of his textbook *Medical Care of the Adolescent*, which was aimed at pediatricians who wanted to include teenagers in their practices.[5] The Boston Adolescent Unit thus served as a fountainhead for other adolescent programs throughout the country throughout much of the 1950s and 1960s: many of the founders of the newer clinics had either studied under Gallagher or had modeled their ventures after his unit in Boston.[6]

Although physicians were inspired by Gallagher to create new clinics for adolescents, many soon departed from both Gallagher's professional ideology and his model of patient care. Physicians who entered adolescent medicine during the late 1950s and 1960s were educated in a professional climate that valued specialization and technical skill over general practice. Although they often shared Gallagher's holistic perspective on adolescent health care, they also realized that in order to enhance the image of adolescent medicine, they had to bring the field more in line with the professional model provided by the organ- and technology-based medical specialties. This meant establishing a standardized curriculum in adolescent medicine, a professional association, and procedures such as board certification that would regulate entry into the field.

The movement toward specialization was shaped by trends outside of medicine in the late 1960s and 1970s. It was no coincidence that SAM was founded in the same year as widespread demonstrations against racism, poverty, and the war in Vietnam: the creation of SAM was intertwined with the social unrest of the decade. Although demands for reform came from all age groups, young people were at the center of many of the social movements of the 1960s and consequently became a target of special national concern. Physicians in adolescent medicine repeatedly observed that they wanted to remain "socially relevant" and responsive to the changing needs of American youth. This meant developing new kinds of services and training nonphysicians to deal with the vast array of adolescent health problems that emerged in the late 1960s and early 1970s. Early meetings of SAM also reflected this desire to be in touch with the times: in addition to examining the scientific aspects of adolescent growth and development, meetings included sections on substance abuse, abortion, contraception, and legal issues in the treatment of minors.[7] There was some self-interest in this desire to be socially relevant, since adolescent clinics benefited greatly from the federal programs that emerged in response to the new morbidities affecting adolescents in the late 1960s and early 1970s. Yet these professional concerns were matched by a sincere desire to improve the quality and availability of adolescent health services. Indeed, physicians in SAM believed that professional interests and the quality of adolescent health care were interdependent: improving the professional standing of adolescent medicine in relationship to other medical disciplines, physicians believed, would attract federal dollars and institutional support for adolescent health care, thereby improving the quality of medical care available to all adolescents. The creation of SAM not only symbolized that the field of adolescent medicine had "come of age" professionally: it also represented a recognition that meeting the health needs of adolescents required a formal professional organization dedicated to advocating health reforms for this age group.

Critics outside of medicine saw subspecialization as elitist and counterproductive, however, and blamed many of the inequities in health care on the tendency toward overspecialization in the postwar era. To address these concerns, physicians in adolescent medicine were faced with a dilemma: how to increase the number of health care professionals—not just physicians—who were trained to take care of teenagers, while at the same time maintaining a unique professional identity for the field of adolescent *medicine?* Balancing these two competing goals would not be an easy task.

At the same time, young people themselves produced a scathing critique of American society that many practitioners who worked with adolescents took to heart. Drawing upon the language of the civil rights movement, teenagers and young adults argued that the time had come to eliminate the "institutionalized paternalism" that restricted the freedom of American youth, much in the same way that other activists had attacked institutionalized racism and sexism. In response to the demands of young people themselves, adolescent medicine developed new methods of health care delivery that challenged traditional medical models and gave teenagers even more of a voice in how their health needs were met.

"The Garbage Pail of Medicine": Status Anxiety and the Emergence of the Society for Adolescent Medicine

According to Halpern's analysis of the history of pediatrics, pediatric subspecialties began as separate departmental divisions within teaching hospitals and medical schools. In this sense, adolescent medicine was similar to other pediatric subspecialties, which also created new facilities and departments as precursors to subspecialization.[8] The emergence of new adolescent clinics was also a reflection of broader demographic changes: during the late 1950s and early 1960s, the first wave of baby boomers reached puberty, thereby justifying additional medical facilities for this age group.[9] In the same period, changes in the nature of pediatric medicine prompted a search for new medical consumers: like Boston Children's Hospital, many pediatric departments turned to adolescents as a way of increasing the market for their services. At Columbus Children's Hospital, for example, the idea for an adolescent clinic grew partly out of the hospital's need to find a use for an expensive polio rehabilitation facility that had been rendered largely obsolete by the development of a vaccine for the disease.[10] Similarly, the Adolescent Unit at Cincinnati Children's Hospital grew out of a special cardiac service for children, which was developed to attract paying patients from the entire state of Ohio as well as the surrounding states of Kentucky and Indiana.[11]

The need to find new medical markets was particularly apparent at university hospitals located in impoverished inner-city areas that were trying to attract more middle-class, paying patients. At the National Children's Hospital in Washington, D.C., the hospital's tradition of treating patients regardless of ability to pay had led to major economic problems by the late 1950s, difficulties that were exacerbated by growing competition with suburban hospitals for pediatric patients. Although administrators at National Children's Hospital wanted to continue their tradition of providing medical care to impoverished children, they also realized that they needed to attract more paying patients if they were to remain in business. As physician-in-chief Robert Parrott recalled, "the hospital was losing money" at the time, and "we needed to fill beds" with paying patients to make up the deficit. Parrott and other administrators therefore saw the development of an adolescent service as a way of distinguishing the National Children's Hospital from suburban hospitals, thereby attracting more paying patients from these areas.[12]

The commitment to adolescent medical services at many of the parent facilities was rather half-hearted, however, particularly when compared with other pediatric subspecialties. Most of the hospitals surveyed in the 1960s did not have full-time personnel and services devoted to adolescents: of the 131 staff physicians in the twenty-four clinics Garell surveyed, only 10 percent were assigned full-time to adolescent medical care. Many of the clinics were only open for adolescent care a few mornings or afternoons a week, spending the rest of the time as general outpatient clinics for either pediatrics or internal medicine. Although a substantial number of hospitals (84 percent) were "interested" in adolescent medical services, half of them also reported that they "could not justify such a program" because of "more 'acute' needs, and an impression that the adolescent's medical problem did not constitute a significantly large fraction of the medical problems of the community."[13]

Of those hospitals that did have adolescent medical services, the relationship between the adolescent clinic and other services in the hospital was frequently tense. Gallagher's tug of war with other pediatric subspecialists was not unique: Garell's survey in 1965 indicated that many hospitals were reluctant to start adolescent programs because they "believed that these programs would remove patients from the general clinic population or from specialty teaching clinics," thereby upsetting the physicians who headed these services.[14]

Competition with other pediatric departments could quickly lead to the demise of an adolescent unit, especially since most adolescent facilities were expected to generate their own funding through patient fees. The fitful history of adolescent services at Columbus Children's Hospital illustrates some of the hardships faced by adolescent clinics as they competed with other pediatric services for patients. Thomas Shaffer first started a part-time adolescent outpatient clinic in the mid-1950s, but had trouble attracting patients because the other pediatric services were reluctant to refer adolescents to him unless they were especially troublesome or non-compliant. This situation made economic survival difficult for the adolescent clinic, since it was supported entirely by patient fees and received no funding from the hospital. Shaffer eventually became so frustrated that he left Children's Hospital to direct the health services at the Ohio Juvenile Diagnostic Center, a local residential facility for delinquent youth. During the early 1960s, an attempt was made to start an adolescent inpatient ward called "Suite 13–19." However, this ward also soon encountered difficulties, as specialists from surgery and other pediatric subspecialties complained that it was too inconvenient for them to have their adolescent patients on a separate ward.[15]

Even when other specialists were willing to hand over patients to adolescent wards and clinics, they seldom gave physicians in adolescent services the same respect accorded other medical specialists. The attitude toward adolescent services is summed up by observations made by Dale Garell of Los Angeles and Robert Blum of Minnesota in an oral history interview conducted in 1993, in which they described the hardships they encountered when they first began their adolescent medicine services. Garell recalled that his colleagues at Children's Hospital of Los Angeles were incredulous at his willingness to work with teenagers, a class of patients they found too troublesome and unwieldy to handle. Blum recounted a similar experience, and recalled that when he proposed beginning an adolescent program at the University of Minnesota in the early 1970s, the chief of otolaryngology sarcastically agreed that an adolescent clinic was a "great idea" but first they should create a unit for "elderly chiefs of departments," and another colleague chimed in that a unit for "individuals who were left-handed" should take precedence over a service for teenagers. In short, observed Garell and Blum, most of their colleagues thought what they were doing was "absurd," the "garbage pail" of medicine.[16]

The experiences of Blum and Garell were not uncommon among adolescent clinic directors: their counterparts at other hospitals reported feeling underappreciated by their colleagues in other areas of medicine, particularly those in high-powered, prestigious bench subspecialties such as cardiology, neonatology, and endocrinology. Although their colleagues in other departments realized that the adolescent services attracted new patients and increased revenue for the hospital, they also tended to regard adolescent medicine as a relatively unprestigious branch of pediatrics. For example, the director of the adolescent clinic at Jewish Hospital of Brooklyn, Joseph P. Michelson, observed on the fifth anniversary of the clinic that while "conception" of the clinic was "easy" because of Gallagher's assistance, "delivery was much more difficult since the Medical Department of the hospital was not ready for the accouchement."[17]

The subject matter of adolescent medicine—teenagers—dealt a further blow to the image of the field among other pediatricians. Although some subspecialists liked to hold onto adolescent cases that were interesting from a research perspective, they were reluctant to treat teenagers as a class because of their reputation as uncooperative patients. As Garell put it, pediatricians were "afraid of pubic hair" and the attendant problems of adolescence, so they were more than happy to send their most unmanageable teenage patients to the adolescent service. Consequently, adolescent clinics typically became "dumping grounds" for patients that no other service in the hospital wanted or found interesting.[18]

Gallagher's position on specialization tended to reinforce rather than alleviate the low prestige of adolescent medicine in relation to other medical disciplines. One of the central tenets of Gallagher's treatment philosophy was that unlike medical specialties, which tended to focus on specific symptoms and pathology, physicians in adolescent medicine should focus on the patient as a whole. Unfortunately, Gallagher's opposition to specialization put him distinctly out of step with mainstream medicine of the post–World War II era. Although some physicians, most notably those in general practice and family medicine, shared Gallagher's alarm at the negative consequences of medical specialization, highly technical bench specialties were the medical fields that attracted the most research dollars, the highest salaries, and the greatest degree of professional prestige. Adolescent medicine, with its emphasis on psychological and social problems and its focus on the patient rather than a disease or organ, appeared to many high-tech subspecialists to be old-fashioned. As a result, Gallagher's efforts were frequently ignored or even ridiculed by other members of the staff at Children's Hospital.[19]

Among those most sensitive about the status of the Adolescent Unit was Felix Heald. Although Heald shared much of Gallagher's philosophy about adolescent patient care, he gradually became dissatisfied with the relationship between the Adolescent Unit and the rest of the Children's Hospital.

Heald was particularly disturbed by the misconception that the unit was a psychiatric clinic for adolescents. His colleagues in other hospital departments continually kidded him about being an "amateur psychiatrist." Heald was also dismayed by the unit's low publication rate compared with other pediatric departments, and felt that Gallagher placed too little emphasis on research. Thus, when Heald was offered a position as head of the clinic at National Children's Hospital in Washington, D.C., in 1959, he saw it as an opportunity to start a program that would avoid what he considered to be the pitfalls of the Adolescent Unit in Boston.

One of Heald's main concerns was to prevent his clinic from being mistaken for an adolescent psychiatric facility. Heald refused to accept referrals for patients whose complaints were primarily psychological in nature. Although he would attend to secondary psychological problems and disorders that had psychosocial elements as contributing factors, he insisted that each patient's primary complaint be manifested as a physical symptom such as a headache or stomach upset.

Heald's contacts with other physicians at adolescent units throughout the country indicated that they were having problems similar to those that Heald had encountered in Boston. Like Heald, their efforts were frequently met with incomprehension, indifference, or even ridicule. Frequently, the head of an adolescent clinic would be the only physician or one of a very few interested in adolescent health care at his or her particular institution, and often had to face the scorn of colleagues and competition for hospital resources single-handedly. In addition to feeling estranged within their home institutions, clinic directors felt that they were isolated from their colleagues at similar facilities. The most significant problem faced by many directors of adolescent clinics was their lack of training. Few pediatric residency programs covered adolescent health, growth, and development in any detail. Any additional training these directors received usually consisted of several months at the Boston Adolescent Unit, although some visited for as little as a week.[20] This situation often led to a sense of frustration and isolation that Adele Hofmann, director of adolescent services at Beth Israel Hospital in New York City, likened to being an "orphan in the storm," with no one who shared the same experiences to turn to for guidance.[21]

In order to combat the professional isolation of physicians in adolescent medicine, Heald and a small group of other adolescent unit directors began a series of initiatives aimed at promoting cohesiveness among members of the field. In 1960 they organized a Joint Adolescent Clinic Conference at the University of Colorado Medical Center. Funded by a grant from the United States Children's Bureau, which also provided financial assistance to several adolescent clinics during the 1950s and 1960s, the conference was used as a forum to discuss common problems and needs of practitioners in the field.[22] In 1965 several clinic directors who attended this conference put together a newsletter entitled *Adolescent Medicine*, which was intended to foster connections between adolescent medical programs and to keep practitioners abreast of current developments in the field.[23] That same year Heald convinced the Children's Bureau to fund a series of yearly seminars devoted to specific topics in adolescent medicine. Each seminar was devoted to a single topic (legal aspects, nutrition, growth, and so on) and "was designed to improve the knowledge of physicians who were giving a major portion of their attention to teaching others the basics of Adolescent Medicine."[24] The first such seminar, held in March of 1965, attracted a small group of about thirty young physicians who were directors or staff members of various adolescent clinics around the country.[25]

The yearly seminars in Washington, D.C., proved to be extremely popular among directors of adolescent clinics. An informal survey published in the newsletter *Adolescent Medicine* in 1965 indicated that most clinic directors were "uniformly in favor of an annual meeting to exchange ideas between people who are providing adolescent medical care throughout the country." Clinic directors found the Washington seminars an excellent forum in which to upgrade their knowledge about adolescence, discuss problems of mutual interest, and make contact with their counterparts at other facilities around the country.[26]

It soon became apparent to some attendees at the Washington seminars that they needed more than an annual mutual support meeting: they also needed a formal national organization that would represent their interests and advance their standing in the medical profession as a whole. As Garell observed in an editorial written after the first Washington seminar, if adolescent medicine was going to successfully meet "the challenge of establishing itself as an integral and accepted member of the medical community," then the creation of an adolescent medical society was in order. The purpose of such an organization, said Garell, would be similar to that of other medical societies such as the American Medical Association and the American Academy of Pediatrics: to define the boundaries of adolescent medicine, to establish definite standards for education and training, to encourage medical students and residents to consider a career in adolescent medicine, and to investigate adolescent health problems and offer medical consultation for such problems on a national level.[27]

At the second Washington seminar, held in March of 1966, a small group of physicians, including Garell, Joseph Rauh from the University of Cincinnati Children's Hospital, Sherrel Hammar from Seattle, and Andrew Rigg from the Children's Hospital of Washington, D.C., discussed the possibility of forming a society for physicians and other health care providers interested in adolescent medicine. In March of 1967, following one of the Washington seminars, this group of "young turks," as they called themselves, formed an ad hoc committee aimed at developing a plan and a constitution for such an organization. In the fall of that year, they sent copies of a proposed constitution to *Adolescent Medicine* newsletter subscribers soliciting opinions on whether an organization for adolescent medicine was needed and/or feasible.[28]

The subscribers' views about starting a society for adolescent medicine must have been predominantly positive: at the 1968 Washington seminar, "representatives of adolescent clinics throughout the United States and Canada met and unanimously agreed to the formation of a Society for Adolescent Medicine." Attendees at the seminar elected Gallagher president of the society, with Heald as vice president, Rigg as treasurer, Garell as executive secretary, and Rauh, Henry Cooper of the University of Colorado Medical Center, and Joseph Michelson of the Jewish Hospital Medical Center of Brooklyn as members of the executive council.[29] In March of 1969 the first annual meeting of the newly formed Society for Adolescent Medicine was held as part of the fifth annual Washington seminar on adolescent health care.[30]

The formation of a national organization was just the first step in the process of setting professional boundaries for adolescent medicine. The experience of adolescent physicians in hospital and medical school settings made them realize that their existence as a distinct medical field was extremely tenuous. In order to maintain their place in hospital settings, adolescent physicians felt they needed continually to prove the uniqueness of their medical services. Garell noted in a 1967 editorial for *Adolescent Medicine* that the interdisciplinary nature of adolescent clinics often brought "the adolescent clinic directly into competition with any or all of the various sub-specialties and specialty clinics who also may be involved in the care of adolescents." Although in some settings, said Garell, "there has been a healthy, competitive rivalry," in most instances, the competition between adolescent clinics and other hospital services "has been a source of frustration in which the patient usually suffers." If adolescent medicine was to survive, Garell said, it must emphasize its difference from other medical branches. To address these problems, Garell and other clinic directors began actively campaigning to make adolescent medicine a distinct medical specialty with its own knowledge base, educational criteria, and certifying board.[31]

Not everyone was as enthusiastic about making adolescent medicine a distinct medical specialty, least of all the field's founder. To Gallagher, the movement toward specialization violated the original goals of the field: to provide holistic, patient-centered care to adolescents. Since his early days at Children's Hospital, Gallagher had been opposed to making adolescent medicine a specialty. He believed that specialization would eventually lead to the fragmentation of the field, as adolescent medicine splintered into a variety of subspecialties such as adolescent endocrinology and cardiology. Instead of becoming a medical specialty, Gallagher argued, adolescent medicine should be a "set of principles based on an understanding of physical and emotional development to guide physicians in dealing more effectively with teen-age patients." Consequently, Gallagher was ambivalent about forming any kind of professional organization for adolescent medicine and resisted creating even an academic journal for adolescent medicine for a number of years. Although Gallagher agreed to be the first president of SAM, he never accepted the organization's larger professional goal to make adolescent medicine a specialty.[32]

Informal surveys of clinic directors published in the *Adolescent Medicine* newsletter indicated that some clinic directors shared Gallagher's views: although subscribers claimed that they were "uniformly in favor of an annual meeting to exchange ideas between people who are providing adolescent medical care throughout the country," some of them were more ambivalent about allowing adolescent medicine to split off from its institutional base in pediatrics.[33] The director of the Juvenile Diagnostic Center in Columbus, Ohio, stated that he did not "consider this [adolescent medicine] a specialty," and that the main purpose of an adolescent medical organization should be to "point to the opportunities" for adolescent medicine, "not to develop a new field of specialization."[34] Similarly, when asked whether there was a need for a journal of adolescent medicine, fourteen out of fifteen clinic directors surveyed said that there was "no definite need for a Journal of Adolescent Medicine at the present time," and that "it would be a great mistake to segregate the ideas and research of adolescence into a special journal."[35]

Even the "young turks" worried that their attempts to distinguish adolescent medicine from other medical disciplines would in fact destroy the major feature that made adolescent medicine unique, namely, the field's interdisciplinarity and its patient-centered approach to adolescent health care. Moreover, developments outside of medicine made it difficult to justify the creation of yet another medical specialty.

"A Natural Fit": Adolescent Medicine and the Great Society

One of the ironies of the move toward specialty status for adolescent medicine was that it occurred at a time when medical specialization came under increasing attack both from within and outside the medical profession. Critics of medical care during the 1960s and 1970s argued that overspecialization had led to a massive maldistribution of health care services: although the expansion of medical specialties had increased the variety of medical services available to upper- and middle-class Americans, specialization had overlooked the basic health care needs of the poor in rural and inner city areas. Rather than being a metaphor for social progress, observes Paul Starr in his social history of American medicine, the highly differentiated medical profession of the late 1960s was rapidly "becoming a symbol of the continuing inequities and irrationalities of American life."[36]

Many physicians in adolescent medicine were on the front lines of the movement to eliminate the unequal distribution of health services in American society. The founders of new adolescent clinics were frequently prompted by a desire to improve the medical services for the teenagers who lived in the impoverished inner-city areas surrounding many university hospitals. Hospital administrators, however, tended to support adolescent clinics only if they created new sources of funding for their hospitals. The need to generate income from patient fees frequently led administrators to pressure adolescent unit directors into attracting paying clients, even if it meant compromising the care of impoverished patients. This dilemma was especially apparent at the National Children's Hospital, where 97 percent of the clientele were classified as medically indigent. Although the mission of the hospital was to serve all patients in the region, regardless of ability to pay, during the late 1950s the president of the board of trustees, R. B. Slope, requested that all departments find ways to attract and devote more of their bed space and clinic time to paying patients, "the aim being to restore a predominantly private patient service at Children's Hospital." Slope even went as far as suggesting that indigent patients with "no educational value" to residents and fellows be turned away in favor of clients who could generate income for the hospital.[37]

Many physicians who worked with impoverished adolescents saw these kinds of directives as morally objectionable and continued to serve medically indigent clients even if it meant operating under large budget deficits. Some clinics were able to survive economically through contributions from local charitable organizations and wealthy benefactors. The Adolescent Inpatient Unit and Outpatient clinic at National Children's Hospital depended heavily on the generosity of the Washington Junior League, which had provided not only the seed money to start the adolescent inpatient ward in 1957 but a three-year grant to create the outpatient clinic and a training fellowship in adolescent medicine.[38] Similarly, the Adolescent Unit at the University of Cincinnati Medical Center was able to "mature" by receiving funds from the Children's Heart Association of Cincinnati and the Child Health Association, "a local lay-professional organization with a particular interest in adolescence."[39] The Adolescent Unit at Children's Hospital of Los Angeles received most of its funding from a wealthy benefactor named Harriet Bireley, whose husband had made a fortune out of American teenagers' fondness for Pepsi-Cola.[40]

Adolescent clinics also supplemented their incomes through grants from private foundations like the Commonwealth Fund and the Grant Foundation, or from state and federal agencies dedicated to public health and maternal and child health. One of the most significant funding agencies at this time was the United States Children's Bureau. The adolescent clinics were funded largely by special project grants, which were a subset of the child health programs funded under Title V of the Social Security Act of 1935. The special project grants enabled states to "develop new kinds of programs and to include children with diagnostic problems not hitherto included."[41] Although most of the services funded under the special projects grants addressed the needs of children with chronic illnesses and congenital problems such as epilepsy, mental retardation, and heart disease, they also funded projects on school health. Since adolescents fell under the category of school-age children, several adolescent clinics were funded with special project grants, including the ones at Boston Children's Hospital, the University of Washington in Seattle, the Long Island Jewish Hospital, the University of Colorado, and the National Children's Hospital. The special project grants were designed to fund pediatric fellowships to train pediatricians in the health care of adolescents.[42]

Unfortunately, neither the Children's Bureau nor private granting agencies had sufficient funds to assist all of the adolescent facilities that appealed to them for help. The special project funds only received 12 percent of all Title V appropriations and were intended for all age groups, not just adolescents. The Children's Bureau could not begin to fill all requests for financial aid from adolescent clinic directors.[43]

By the mid-1960s, the situation had become critical for many adolescent clinics and their patients: chronic budgetary shortfalls forced numerous clinics to cut back staff and hours of service, thereby forcing patients to wait up to several weeks for an appointment with the adolescent service. Even those clinics with grants from the Children's Bureau and other funding agencies had difficulty fulfilling demands for services, since these grants were designed to fund the training of residents and fellows interested in adolescent health care, not to finance the operating budgets of the clinics. The Adolescent Unit at the University of Washington in Seattle, for example, had to refer patients to other medical services because of large patient backlogs.[44] Felix Heald likewise worried about how his facility could continue to "deliver a high standard of care" to adolescents of all socioeconomic backgrounds given the hospital's chronic financial problems and the massive influx of impoverished patients.[45]

During the early 1960s, officials at the Children's Bureau and directors of adolescent clinics in inner-city areas joined forces to pressure Congress for increased federal funding for adolescent medical programs. Among the leaders in this endeavor were Heald; Arthur Lesser, who was the director of the Children's Bureau's Division of Health Services and a close associate of Heald's; and Robert Deisher, director of the Adolescent Unit at the University of Washington in Seattle, who served briefly as deputy Children's Bureau chief during the early 1960s. In June of 1961, Lesser chaired a conference on the special project grants, which discussed "a number of areas which need strengthening in the teaching of pediatrics which are directly related to the interests of the Children's Bureau." One of the major areas the conference addressed was the health needs of adolescents: conference participants pointed to studies of young men rejected for service in Korea as evidence that adolescents were not being served adequately by the medical profession.[46]

Evidence about the poor health of American "manpower" was not new: studies of military recruits during the Second World War helped justify increased medical attention directed toward the problems of adolescents. What had changed by the early 1960s was the political climate: although the 1950s did not witness a destruction of the liberal programs of the Roosevelt-Truman era, President Eisenhower was generally opposed to increasing federal spending on domestic programs. The election of President John F. Kennedy in 1960 symbolized the return to a more activist federal government that was willing to make a financial investment in preserving the health of the nation's youth.[47] In a special "Youth Message" delivered to Congress on February 14, 1963, President Kennedy outlined his commitment to the health and welfare of American children and adolescents. Kennedy observed that despite phenomenal advances in medical therapeutics and technology during and after the Second World War, data from a National Health Survey in 1958 indicated that the health of many children and youth, particularly those from minority groups and impoverished economic conditions, was still far from optimal. Alarmed that the nation's "most important asset and resource" was going "so largely undeveloped," Kennedy requested that the Congress place a high priority on preserving the health of the nation's children and youth, and increase funding for projects that would help extend the benefits of modern health care systems to all Americans, regardless of ability to pay.[48]

Kennedy's interest in the health of children and youth was prompted by a combination of old and new thinking on the problems of adolescents in American society: on the one hand, cold war interests in preserving "manpower" continued to play a role in both Kennedy's and Johnson's pronouncements about the health of the nation's youth. Concerns about the social dangers posed by adolescents were also at the forefront of Kennedy's interest in the future of American young people. Like his predecessors, Kennedy was alarmed by what appeared to be growing rates of juvenile delinquency, particularly among young men, and quoted statistics that indicated that juvenile delinquency rates had more than doubled in the previous decade. Kennedy was also concerned about the high incidence of nervous and mental disorders among military recruits: among the most prevalent reasons for rejection were psychiatric conditions, which were second only to orthopedic disorders in the medical grounds for disqualification for military service. Finally, Kennedy expressed concern about increased sexual activity among teenagers, which had resulted in a rapid rise in the incidence of venereal disease and out-of-wedlock pregnancy.[49]

The main difference between the "manpower" concerns of the late 1940s and 1950s, and those of the 1960s and 1970s, was the increased focus on racial minorities and disadvantaged socioeconomic groups. Prompted by the demands of civil rights leaders and the discovery of an "other America" that lacked access to adequate health care, Kennedy and his successor President Lyndon Baines Johnson directed increasing attention to the health needs of children and adolescents who had been left out of the so-called affluent society of the 1950s.[50]

At the end of his Youth Message to Congress in 1963, Kennedy authorized the secretary of health, education, and welfare to prepare a study of health programs and "to make recommendations regarding any action which may be required." The result of Kennedy's request was a study, written by the Children's Bureau's Arthur Lesser, entitled *Health of Children of School Age* (1964). The report disclosed large inequalities within the American health care system. Although the growth in medical services during the postwar era had dramatically improved the health of middle-class Americans, the report indicated that both the quantity and the quality of medical care received by children and adolescents in low-income families was grossly inadequate, and pointed to "the need for new approaches and for concentrating our community resources where they are most needed." Once again, Lesser underscored the alarming number of young men rejected for military service because of preventable illnesses and defects, and used this evidence to call for improved health services for adolescents.[51]

Lesser's report and similar testimonies on the health problems of the poor provided the impetus for a variety of Great Society programs aimed at addressing the health care needs of impoverished children and youth. The best-known health care program for the poor established by Great Society reforms was Title XIX of the Social Security Act, which authorized the Medicaid program of health insurance for low-income families. The Medicaid program was able to eliminate some of the financial barriers to health care by giving health care providers reimbursement for some, but not all, medical procedures. Unlike the Medicare program for the elderly, Medicaid was administered by the individual states, which determined who was eligible for medical reimbursement and what medical procedures would be covered by the program. Coverage by Medicaid varied considerably from state to state, and there were some concerns during the early years of the program that the absence of federal guidelines allowed southern states to deny or severely limit coverage of African Americans. In all states, eligibility for Medicaid was closely tied to qualifications for other welfare benefits, and was restricted to the aged, the blind, the disabled, and one-parent families. This policy therefore excluded large numbers of the working poor.[52]

Moreover, Medicaid did not address a much broader cause of the maldistribution of health care in the United States, namely, the small number of health professionals and medical services available in impoverished inner-city and rural areas. As Lesser noted, although Medicaid provided a way to pay for medical services, it did not "in itself create clinical resources where they are in short supply."[53] Many impoverished rural and inner-city areas had few if any health care providers, and those that existed tended to be fragmentary and crowded. Inner-city residents typically relied on emergency rooms affiliated with university hospitals for most of their health care; rural families were forced to travel great distances to see a physician.[54] The House Ways and Means Committee in its report on the Social Security Amendments of 1965 acknowledged the drawbacks of Medicaid, remarking that many communities did not have "adequate resources to which children can be referred for diagnosis and treatment," thereby making the issue of reimbursement for medical services moot.[55]

To make up for the shortcomings of Medicaid, Congress in 1965 approved revisions to Title V of the Social Security Act that created new programs for funding maternal and child health programs. The most significant programs for adolescents were the Children and Youth (C & Y) projects, which provided matching funds to state health departments and to medical schools and affiliated hospitals to create new health care services for children and adolescents of school age, "particularly in areas with concentrations of low-income families."[56] The C & Y projects differed markedly from earlier child health programs funded by the Children's Bureau, which had focused on specific health problems such as rheumatic fever, hearing impairments, or the plight of crippled children. The C & Y projects, in contrast, were comprehensive in scope, that is, they covered the full range of health services for children and adolescents up to the age of twenty one. In other words, the C & Y projects attempted to address the problem of fragmentary health care by providing one-stop service for all child and adolescent health problems.[57]

The C & Y projects significantly increased the availability of health services for children and youth from impoverished families: by 1972 there were fifty-nine C & Y projects in twenty-eight states, the District of Columbia, the Virgin Islands, and Puerto Rico, serving approximately a half a million children. During the early years of the grants, the projects tended to see a larger percentage of young children rather than older children and adolescents: over two-thirds of patients seen in the clinics funded under C & Y grants were nine years old or younger, while 20 percent were aged ten to fourteen and 9 percent were aged fifteen to twenty. Nevertheless, the C & Y projects did make a conscious effort to include as many adolescents as possible: most projects accepted patients up to the age of eighteen or nineteen, with some going as high as age twenty-one. By the early 1970s, 120,000 of the approximately half-million children enrolled in the C & Y projects were between the ages of ten and twenty-one.[58]

Two related Title V programs that indirectly benefited adolescents were the Maternity and Infant (M & I) Care Projects Grants, authorized by Congress in 1963; and Family Planning Services, which were created by amendments to Title V approved by Congress in 1967 and 1972. The M & I projects grew out of Kennedy's interest in preventing mental retardation, an interest that was related to his concern about manpower issues since a significant number of young men were rejected for military service because of low intelligence. Indeed the 1963 amendments were originally intended to simply increase the amount of funding for crippled children programs that also served mentally handicapped children and adolescents, and to create special projects for mentally retarded children.[59]

Growing medical evidence about the close relationship between poor prenatal and childhood medical care convinced Congress to approve appropriations for the M & I program, which would provide comprehensive

medical services to pregnant women and young children, thereby addressing the problem of mental retardation at its source.[60] Because they were
comprehensive, the M & I projects differed substantially from many state
and local programs, providing a broad range of medical and social services—not just ob/gyn care—both before and after delivery.[61]

The Family Planning programs were an extension of the M & I projects,
and were designed to provide contraceptive services and more long-term
postpartum medical care to women involved in the M & I projects. One of
the motivating factors behind the Family Planning amendments was to
reduce the number of children supported by AFDC by reducing the birthrate among women who were dependent upon public assistance. Consequently, annual federal expenditures for family planning increased from 11
million dollars in 1967 to 149 million dollars by 1973.[62]

Neither the M & I nor the Family Planning program were intended
specifically for adolescents. As Constance Nathanson observes in her history of the social control of adolescent female sexuality, the issue of using
public funds to support prenatal care and birth control for teenagers was so
controversial that the amendments would not have passed had they been
justified primarily on the basis of preventing or at least alleviating the
negative consequences of adolescent pregnancies.[63] Nevertheless, approximately 30 percent of the more than two million women seeking the services of these programs were under nineteen years of age.[64]

Like Medicaid, the projects funded by Title V of the Social Security Act
were only a partial solution to the health needs of impoverished adolescents, since they only reached a small proportion of the teenagers living in
poverty. A potentially more far-reaching Great Society program that affected the health needs of impoverished youth was the Economic Opportunity Act of 1964, which created the Office of Economic Opportunity
(OEO). The most important branches of the OEO that addressed adolescent health issues were the Job Corps; the Neighborhood Youth Corps; and
the Neighborhood Health Centers, which were part of the community
action programs set up by the OEO. The health programs created by the
OEO differed substantially from Medicaid and the Title V programs in
their vision of what constituted health and disease and who should be
included in health care decision making. Whereas Medicaid and the Title V
projects primarily funded medical schools and university-based medical
centers, and therefore tended to focus on the concerns of health care pro-

fessionals, the OEO programs were based on the principle of "maximum feasible participation" by the poor in decisions affecting their own health. Moreover, the OEO programs went beyond issues of health care delivery and examined nonmedical influences on health caused by the social and economic environment.[65]

Initially the OEO's commitment to health care was small: when the OEO was first established in 1965, the agency funded only eight neighborhood health centers. The demands of community action groups, however, compelled the OEO to increase its commitment to issues of health care delivery. Community members and civil rights leaders involved with the OEO programs saw health care as one of the great unmet needs of the poor, as well as a contributing factor in the cycle of poverty, and therefore lobbied for more neighborhood health centers. This prompted amendments to the Economic Opportunity Act in 1966 that helped support the "development and implementation of comprehensive health services programs focused upon the needs of persons residing in urban or rural areas having high concentrations of poverty and a marked inadequacy of health services." In 1967 the Department of Health, Education, and Welfare published an ambitious plan to expand the number of neighborhood health centers to 1,000, serving a patient population of 25 million.[66] Unfortunately, budgetary constraints forced the OEO to scale back the program considerably. Nevertheless, by the early 1970s, the total number of neighborhood health centers had expanded to 125, which served a total of 1.5 million people.[67]

The Job Corps and the Neighborhood Youth Corps were originally aimed at providing job skills for adolescents and young adults, not at providing medical care for low-income youth. The professionals who worked with youth enrolled in these programs, however, quickly realized that poor health was as much a barrier to full employment as was lack of education and marketable job skills. In response to these findings, Job Corps and Neighborhood Youth Corps personnel created the Office for Health Affairs and established relationships with local physicians and hospitals to help address the unmet health needs of corps members. Among the most serious needs of corps enlistees was assistance with the emotional problems that grew out of their isolation from friends and family during their participation in the job training programs.[68]

Physicians involved in adolescent medicine saw the Great Society programs as something of a godsend, a way to provide financial security for struggling programs and create new adolescent programs in hospitals where none had existed before. Dale Garell, for example, pointed out the "natural fit" between adolescent medicine and the Great Society programs. Garell observed that "since its very inception, the concept of medical care for the adolescent has been comprehensive in its scope providing total care for the adolescent age patient" rather than dividing the patient among various subspecialties. Because many of the Great Society programs for health care were also "comprehensive in scope," and "since our approach in adolescent clinics already is patterned after these principles," Garell argued, "it seems only natural to assume that physicians who are involved in the care of the adolescent age patient might also take a personal interest in the development of these comprehensive services for all ages."[69]

Medicaid solved some of the income problems of adolescent clinics by providing reimbursement for certain procedures and coverage for inpatient services, thereby permitting adolescent facilities to see a greater number of medically indigent patients without worrying about budgetary problems. Officials at the National Children's Hospital, for example, reported that the Medicaid program had a "decent effect" on the chronic budget deficits faced by the hospital, allowing them to expand the variety and quantity of services that the hospital offered to the local community, especially those for adolescents.[70]

Grants from the Title V programs administered by the Children's Bureau also allowed some clinics to appoint additional personnel and thereby expand their hours of service. Mt. Zion Hospital in San Francisco and Roosevelt Hospital and Jewish Hospital in New York City all reported to the *Adolescent Medicine* newsletter that funding from the Children's Bureau programs gave them the ability to hire additional staff and to remain open more hours per week than they had done before.[71] Grants from maternal and child health projects also gave numerous medical schools and hospitals the ability to start new adolescent programs, as was the case of those affiliated with the University of Alabama; the University of Texas in Dallas; the Children's Hospital of Omaha, Nebraska; and Beth Israel, Mt. Sinai, and Montefiore Hospitals in New York City.[72]

The Adolescent Unit at the University of Alabama is a good example of the way in which Title V funding could benefit an adolescent service. According to the clinic's founder, William Daniel, "Had it not been for C & Y funds there would not have been an adolescent unit" at the University of

Alabama. The C & Y project allowed Alabama to bring in Daniel as head of the adolescent service and to hire nurses, psychologists, social workers, nutritionists, and other professionals to staff the outpatient clinic and the inpatient ward. Several years after the clinic started in 1966, Daniel received a training grant from the Children's Bureau, also funded under Title V, which allowed him to expand the staff of the adolescent division even further.[73]

Many adolescent clinics also became involved with the various health programs created under the Economic Opportunity Act. Clinics did not benefit from OEO funds directly: instead, they served as sponsors to neighborhood health centers and used these centers to train medical students and residents as well as justify adding additional staff to the parent institution. Some adolescent units that originally served a predominantly middle-class clientele, such as those at Columbus and Boston Children's Hospitals, set up satellite clinics at neighborhood health centers in low-income areas.[74] Adolescent Units that were already located in low-income areas, such as those at Mt. Sinai (East Harlem), Los Angeles Children's Hospital (South Central), and Montefiore (Bronx), made links with nearby neighborhood health centers as well as setting up additional clinics at other centers throughout their respective cities. Several adolescent clinics, most notably those at Los Angeles Children's Hospital, Montefiore Hospital, Cincinnati Children's Hospital, and the University of Washington in Seattle, became involved in providing medical and dental care to adolescents involved in the Job Corps and the Neighborhood Youth Corps.[75]

Financial assistance from Great Society programs not only helped adolescent clinics economically: participation in the various programs brought the field of adolescent medicine in contact with populations that were vastly different from the white, middle- and upper-class adolescents who frequented the Adolescent Unit in Boston during its early years. By the late 1960s, even that facility began to see a more racially and socioeconomically diverse patient population as a result of conscious efforts to reach impoverished minority clients around the city. Since its inception, the Adolescent Unit had provided consultative services to several local child welfare institutions, including the Hayden Goodwill Inn for delinquent boys, the Industrial School for Crippled Children, and the Boys' and Girls' Clubs of Boston. When he assumed the directorship of the Adolescent Unit in 1967, Robert P. Masland found that these activities did not begin to serve the needs of minority youth. A generation younger than Gallagher, Masland had a broader vision of the myriad problems faced by youth around the city, not just those from Boston's wealthy suburbs. During his first year as director of the Adolescent Unit, Masland invited Dr. Robert Coles from the Harvard University Health Services to give a lecture on contemporary problems in the black community entitled "Children of the Ghetto—Children of the Suburbs" for the unit's postgraduate course. Masland observed that response to Coles's talk was "enthusiastic," and added that "now we must transfer our desire to help underprivileged adolescents into action." To aid the clinic in this endeavor, Masland gladly accepted Coles's offer to serve as a consultant to the unit and began setting up satellite services for adolescents in low-income neighborhoods around the city.[76]

Although at first the majority of problems treated and research projects pursued by the newer clinics tended to follow earlier patterns established by the Boston unit, the newer facilities began to treat and conduct research on sexually transmitted diseases, substance abuse, and teenage pregnancy as early as the mid-1960s. By the late 1960s and early 1970s, these issues dominated the daily business of most adolescent clinics, including the one in Boston. The adolescent problems encountered by physicians in the 1960s made it even more imperative for them to listen to the voices of their young patients and to design health services to meet their rapidly changing needs.

"More than Hippie Window Dressing"

One of the major discoveries made by physicians in adolescent clinics was that growing numbers of teenagers felt "alienated" from traditional centers of medical care because of racism, poverty, or lifestyle choice. Teenagers from low-income and/or minority backgrounds frequently complained of blatantly racist attitudes among the doctors and nurses they encountered, and consequently tended to distrust most health care professionals and institutions.[77]

The changing lifestyle choices of adolescents from middle- and upper-class backgrounds also put them in conflict with traditional forms of health care delivery. These teenagers had run away or been thrown out of their parents' homes because of conflicts over drug use, sexual behavior, differences of opinion over political and social issues such as the Vietnam War and the civil rights movement, or rejection of their parents' middle-class social ambitions. Many of these young people had grown disillusioned with their parents' demands for educational and occupational achievement and embraced an alternative, hippie subculture based on values of noncompetition and mutual support.[78] Members of this new counterculture tended to shun institutions like hospitals and medical clinics, which they associated with the mainstream establishment they were trying to escape. Often these teenagers' avoidance of the medical system grew out of the fear that they would be arrested and unwillingly returned to their parents' homes. They were also fed up with the condescending attitudes of conservative medical personnel, who either refused to treat them or subjected them to "long judgmental and moralistic harangues on their habits and lifestyle." As a result, even the most basic health needs of these adolescents and young adults did not receive adequate attention.[79]

During the mid- to late sixties, therefore, physicians in adolescent medicine debated how to create new systems of medical care that did not "turn off" teenagers. One of the sources of inspiration for adolescent medicine was the free clinic movement, which began to flourish in major cities around the United States and Canada during the late 1960s. The first free clinic was founded by David Smith and Richard Seymour in the Haight-Ashbury section of San Francisco to care for the thousands of teenagers and young adults who had flocked to the city during the "Summer of Love" in 1967. The Haight-Ashbury Free Clinic was originally intended to be a "calm center" for young people experiencing adverse drug reactions. Smith soon realized that "a general medical clinic was also necessary because many of these people felt alienated from society to such a degree, or were so fearful of legal complications, that they would not use the standard city facilities for their general health problems." The hippie subculture had not created alternatives to replace establishment health care institutions, and the Haight-Ashbury clinic was intended to fill this void. Smith was inspired in part by the model of health care adopted by the neighborhood health centers created by the OEO, and received much guidance from a black nurse named Florence Martin who worked at the neighborhood health center in the Watts section of Los Angeles. Like the health professionals who worked with the various OEO programs, Smith and his colleagues believed that health care was "a right and not a privilege" and that the clinic clientele should have maximum input into how health care was delivered. The word "free" implied not only the absence of fees for service, but also freedom from the rigidity and formality of hospitals and medical clinics. Smith's strategies for getting young people to come to the clinic included "informality of both decor and manner" at the clinic, and "strictest regard for the confidential character of personal records and problems. Patient-doctor relationships were relaxed, and the greatest possible use was made of hippie volunteers," many of whom were former patients. To further allow young people themselves to have a central role in determining how the facility was run, staff members consulted regularly with young people from the area in an effort to tailor their services to local needs.[80]

Like San Francisco, Boston had its own share of alienated teenagers and young adults who because of their distrust of mainstream medical institutions did not receive adequate medical care. At least 50,000 young people between the ages of twelve and twenty-five were believed to be living on the streets during the summers of 1968 and 1969.[81] Between 1968 and 1970, two health services were created to handle the health problems of alienated youth. The first was the Cambridgeport Medical Clinic founded in 1968 by Dr. Joseph Brenner, a psychiatrist affiliated with the University Health Services at the Massachusetts Institute of Technology. Brenner was prompted to create the clinic after an experience in the autumn of 1967, when a student came to him urgently seeking advice for a friend of his who was suffering from the aftermath of a septic abortion but adamantly refused to see a doctor. She had originally sought help at a municipal hospital, but the nurse who took the young woman's history was so openly hostile, saying that she "deserved what she got, living the way she did, sleeping around, getting pregnant, having an abortion," that the girl and her friends left before receiving treatment. Brenner noticed similar cases where young people "were getting less than adequate medical care from established medical facilities, whether public or private, especially if their dress was strange or different and their style of living appeared to be such that hospital staffs could characterize them as hippies." Moreover, Brenner noticed that a fair number of those who were on the streets were too young to seek medical treatment at established medical institutions without parental consent. These experiences convinced Brenner that a new kind of medical service was needed. Looking to the Haight-Ashbury clinic for guidance, Brenner established the Cambridgeport Medical Clinic, which was intended to give young people "hassle-free" medical care without the threat of parental knowledge or legal retribution.[82]

Another medical service for alienated youth in the Boston area during this period was a medical van service founded in 1970 by Dr. Andrew D. Guthrie, Jr., a former trainee at the Adolescent Unit at Boston Children's Hospital and director of the Ambulatory Division of the Massachusetts General Hospital Children's Service. Guthrie's interest in the problems of Boston street youth grew out of his involvement with Bridge Over Troubled Waters, a multiservice organization for street youth established by a group of priests and nuns from the local Order of St. Joseph. The Bridge, as it was commonly called, was originally founded to provide a link between street youths and "establishment" institutions such as the legal system, welfare and social services, and counseling services. During the winter of 1969–70, Guthrie suggested that the organization begin to create a medical "bridge" for these youngsters as well. Guthrie's concerns about the health and welfare of these young people prompted him to enlist the help of a group of interns, residents, staff physicians, nurses, and other medical personnel from Mass General and other local hospitals, including the Children's Hospital, to organize a mobile medical van that would make regular daily stops at Harvard Square, the Boston Common, and other local spots where young people were known to hang out. Like the Cambridgeport and Haight-Ashbury clinics, the mobile medical service did not require parental consent for medical treatment, although staffers would, at the patient's request, attempt to reestablish channels of communication between the patient and his or her family. The van service obviously went further than the free clinics in its outreach to local youth, believing that the best way to care for Boston area teens was to meet them "on their own terms wherever they congregate."[83]

Other cities followed the example of San Francisco and Boston by establishing free clinics of their own, and within a few years there were more than 175 such facilities around the country.[84] By 1970 the free clinic movement had become so large that clinic directors and personnel formed their own professional organization—the National Free Clinic Council (NFCC). The NFCC served as a national clearinghouse to collect and disseminate information to free clinics around the country and as a major lobbying organization to obtain funding for free clinics from federal, state, and local agencies.[85]

The guiding philosophy of all the free clinics was that they would include young people in medical decision making. The clinics therefore posed a formidable challenge to traditional models of medical care, in which the physician was the unquestioned authority and the patient was dependent on her, or more likely his, judgment. As respondents to a survey of free clinics conducted in the early 1970s observed, "to work exclusively in the medical model, without in turn raising the consciousness of their own professional staff, [free clinics] might in time act as a deterrent to the community members continuing to come to a clinic for help."[86] Free clinics were often staffed by a "new breed" of "socially conscious" medical personnel, who believed patients should be equals rather than subordinates in the clinical setting. Surveys indicated that medical personnel involved with the free clinic movement were "for the most part liberal in their political philosophies," although time constraints prevented many of them from becoming as active as they would like in political causes.[87]

Challenging the medical model also meant dissolving established hierarchies among health care professionals. Although most free clinics were directed by physicians, the nonhierarchical structure of the clinics extended to nonphysicians as well as to patients. Nurses, social workers, nutritionists, and other allied health personnel played a more substantial role in decision making at the free clinics than they did in traditional hospital settings.[88]

Some of the free clinics adopted a broad definition of health services that encompassed all aspects of the social environment affecting youth. These facilities offered not only medical treatment but also vocational training, legal advice, counseling, and delinquency prevention services. The best known of these "multiservice" clinics was The Door: A Center of Alternatives in Greenwich Village, which was founded in January of 1972 "by a group of volunteers who believed in cutting through the bureaucracy surrounding youth services, and treating adolescents as whole individuals with a variety of needs and hopes." The organizers of the Door were particularly concerned with reaching "disadvantaged and troubled urban youth" who were "vulnerable to but have not as yet engaged in self-destructive or antisocial activities" such as substance abuse or delinquent activities. One of the cofounders, Loraine Henricks, was a child psychiatrist who had grown disillusioned with the shortcomings of traditional psychotherapy, which focused on the individual and ignored the impact of the social environment on mental and physical health. The Door offered help with the "many pressing reality problems" such as legal, housing, educational, and vocational difficulties that might impede a young person's psychological well-being.[89] The Haight-Ashbury Free Clinic also eventually evolved into a multiservice facility, and by the early 1970s was offering legal, housing, and educational advice in addition to medical and drug treatment.[90]

Among the socially conscious physicians and allied health professionals who volunteered at and offered advice to the free clinics were those who worked in the adolescent clinics of nearby hospitals and medical centers. To them, the youth-centered environment of the free clinics was a logical extension of Gallagher's belief in making the adolescent the primary focus of medical care. Masland, for example, was friends with many of the physicians who worked for free clinics in the Boston area. He was particularly close to his former student Andrew Guthrie, and encouraged medical students and residents who did rotations at the Adolescent Unit to volunteer for both the medical van service and the free clinic.[91] Similarly, staff members of adolescent clinics in Cincinnati, Washington, D.C., Seattle, Los Angeles, San Francisco, and other major cities were enthusiastic about volunteering their advice and time to free clinics in their area. The Door was particularly attractive to physicians from adolescent units in New York City, who were "aware that these adolescent services are not being used by many young people in need of health care who simply will not go to hospitals or existing health clinics out of fear, alienation, lack of money or out of inadequate knowledge of how to use existing health facilities." Physicians who worked at the Door shared the center's belief that urban hospital clinics were often impersonal and did not always address "the variety of psycho-social problems which are often intertwined with their medical problems."[92]

Hospital-based adolescent outpatient clinics and inpatient units also served as referral centers for teenagers and young adults who had serious medical complaints that could not be met by the relatively meager medical resources of the free clinics. Most of the free clinics operated on shoestring budgets. Frequently they relied on donations of supplies and equipment from local hospitals and private practices, and therefore only had the most basic medical equipment. Because the staff of adolescent units were typically sympathetic to the political outlook and goals of free clinics, the units quickly gained a reputation for being "safe" places to bring teenagers who needed X-rays, lab tests, surgery, or other sophisticated treatments unavailable at the free clinics.

Participation in the free clinics often helped to raise the consciousness of adolescent medicine personnel, causing them to reexamine some of the practices at their own hospitals. Adolescent clinics became especially concerned with soliciting the advice of their young patients on how to make their services more accessible and accommodating to local youth. Catering to teenage tastes had been a centerpiece of the field of adolescent medicine since Gallagher's early days at Boston, of course, and many of the changes in adolescent units during the late 1960s and 1970s were a logical extension of his ideas. There were probably some economic incentives behind the changes in adolescent clinics during this period: directors may have been concerned that free clinics were drawing patients away from their facilities. Physicians at adolescent units did interviews for articles in popular magazines for teenagers and their parents, and went out of their way to describe the "hip" decor, "cool" environment, and liberal political views of their staff members.[93]

Adolescent clinic staff also realized, however, that they needed more than "hippie window dressing" if they were going to reach the full spectrum of youth in their communities: physicians had to incorporate the political views of their young patients and revise their model of health care delivery to make it less threatening to young people who distrusted establishment institutions. Emulating the free clinics, adolescent clinics relied on teenage volunteers and peer counselors to help attract reluctant patients and to give advice on how to make clinic services less intimidating to local teenagers. Some adolescent clinic directors, most notably Dale Garell at Children's Hospital of Los Angeles, began experimenting with emergency telephone hotlines in an effort to reach youth who were too frightened to come to the clinic. The hotline was staffed by teenagers (some of whom were former patients) who had been trained in crisis counseling, and was designed to draw on teenagers' natural affinity for the telephone. The hotline at Los Angeles was established in April of 1968, and in the first two months alone handled over 900 telephone calls. By the early 1970s, the hotline was handling more than 150,000 calls per year.[94]

Hotline services had limited applications, since the teenage volunteers who staffed them could not make diagnoses or administer treatments over the telephone. Adolescent clinics therefore explored other forms of community outreach. The history of the adolescent clinic at the Montefiore Hospital in the Bronx illustrates some of the ways in which hospital-based adolescent clinics tried to adapt their services to their local communities. The Montefiore program began in 1967 as a twenty-bed inpatient unit for adolescent medical and gynecological patients. Gradually the program expanded into follow-up care for discharged inpatients, and by 1971 had become a general outpatient clinic for adolescents. In 1968 adolescent clinic staff members extended themselves "far beyond the confines of the parent institution" by setting up services at local juvenile detention centers, high schools, and college health services.[95] Other clinics around the country created similar forms of community outreach: the Adolescent Unit at Children's Hospital of Los Angeles, for example, set up a "traveling adolescent clinic" to provide on-site health care in local housing projects and to train Neighborhood Youth Corps members in first aid.[96] Likewise, the Adolescent Unit in Boston began to set up satellite clinics in impoverished areas around the city during the late 1960s and early 1970s.[97]

To further incorporate the views of adolescents themselves, physicians invited teenagers to professional meetings in order to get their perspective on how to improve adolescent medical services. The culmination of these efforts was a series of conferences on "Youth, Health, and Social Systems," the first of which was held in Breckenridge, Colorado, in 1973. One of the high points of the meeting was a brutally frank interview with a young black male referred to as "Minority Youth," who complained bitterly about the "institutional paternalism and racism" of many health care professionals and institutions. Making a direct analogy to the civil rights movement, "Minority Youth" claimed that to be an adolescent "means to be politically, socially, and humanly powerless" because of "legal, social and economic restraints on choice and responsibility for youth." Although "Minority Youth" agreed that some of the restrictions on teenagers were designed for their own protection, he argued that "we should have some say in that protection."[98]

The Breckenridge conference made it clear that this sentiment was not confined to teenagers from minority or economically disadvantaged backgrounds: a "significant segment" of white, middle-class youth also found social services in general, and the medical system in particular, to be "unpalatable and unresponsive" to their needs, as well as "depersonalizing" in offering "factory-like" care designed to treat large numbers of patients in as short a time as possible.[99]

"Minority Youth" also observed that there were marked differences in the kinds of treatments offered white and minority adolescents. For white teenagers, "at least the institutional parent or agency . . . can identify with the white youth in a protective, positive manner." For minority teenagers, "the parenting becomes less protective of a positive future and more impersonal and controlling toward the minority's future in society." As an example, "Minority Youth" outlined the treatment of two fifteen-year-old girls, one white and one black, who went to a birth control clinic for advice. In the case of the white girl, agency adults were "concerned about her 'early' sexuality and how it relates to her 'communication with her parents and what this behavior means to her 'self-concept' and future." In the case of the black girl, in contrast, "the agency staff considers this normal and acceptable behavior for her with very little inquiry as to her parent 'communication' or 'self-concept.'" Instead of immediately assuming the worst of nonwhite teenagers, health care professionals had to recognize that "minority youth are America's children too" and treat them with the same level of respect and dignity as they did middle-class "hippie white kids." [100] Statements like those of "Minority Youth" would force adolescent health care workers to take a hard look at some of the unquestioned assumptions about race and gender that the field had inherited from Gallagher.

"Lost Souls Medically"

Gender and racial biases in adolescent medicine were most glaring in the area of adolescent female sexuality. During the early years of the Adolescent Unit at Boston Children's Hospital, as already noted, Gallagher's views on adolescent female sexuality prohibited examination of female genitals except when disease was suspected, and even then this was permitted only under anesthesia. Although the unit did treat some gynecological problems in adolescent girls, most notably menstrual difficulties, Gallagher did not consider routine gynecological examinations to be appropriate for teenage girls because it could traumatize them psychologically. Gallagher and his associates agreed that too much caution could result in undetected disease.

Somers Sturgis, for example, observed that the adolescent girl was a "lost soul medically," since neither pediatricians nor gynecologists were willing or prepared to take care of her gynecological needs. Sturgis concluded that many of the problems he saw in adult women "might have been reversed if they had been approached early enough."[101] Nevertheless, Sturgis shared Gallagher's opposition to performing pelvic examinations on adolescents unless absolutely necessary, warning that "an attempt to explore the vagina digitally will generally stir up extreme resentment and hostility" in the teenage patient.[102]

More important, Gallagher and other physicians who treated adolescents feared that gynecological examinations would prematurely awaken sexual passions in young girls. Most physicians during this period viewed premarital adolescent sexuality and unwed pregnancy in pathological terms, and their views on adolescent sexuality were heavily shaped by racial biases. Physicians attributed unwed pregnancy among black teenagers to either the innate "moral incapacities" of black women or to an allegedly greater tolerance of illegitimacy among African Americans. White girls who became pregnant out of wedlock, in contrast, were depicted as neurotic or maladjusted, particularly if they insisted on keeping their babies without marrying the father. The "cure" for a white unwed mother's maladjustment, therefore, was to convince her to either legitimize her pregnancy by marrying the child's father or to give up the baby for adoption and prepare for a "normal" path to marriage and motherhood.[103]

During the early 1960s some health care professionals and social workers attempted to extend this therapeutic approach to black teenagers. Interest in black teenage pregnancy arose partly out of concerns about the growing number of unwed, young women who were dependent on the Aid to Families with Dependent Children (AFDC) program. Some of this anxiety was based on unfounded and racist stereotypes of illegitimacy and welfare dependency as a "black problem." As Rickie Solinger argues in her history of unwed pregnancy and race, despite the fact that by the 1960s, a growing percentage of AFDC recipients were Caucasian, white politicians and taxpayers tended to portray AFDC as a "black-identified program" and claimed that "black women used their bodies in ways that were morally and fiscally destructive to the nation."[104]

In 1963 growing interest in finding ways to cut back the AFDC rolls prompted the Children's Bureau to begin funding the Webster School Project, a demonstration-research project on pregnant school-aged girls in Washington, D.C. Although the project was aimed at "pregnant school girls" as a whole, because the project drew on a predominantly African-American, inner-city population, 99 percent were black and over 70 percent were from families on public assistance.[105] The first full-time public school for pregnant adolescents in the country, the Webster School was based on the premise that "pregnant teenagers would want to attend school with their peers, and could be easily reached for health care and instruction and counseling for personal problems if they were brought together in one program." The Webster School represented a movement away from older solutions to the problem of pregnant schoolgirls, which usually involved expulsion of the young mother—but not the father—from school, thereby reducing the adolescent girl's career opportunities and social mobility. Researchers associated with the Webster School demonstrated that their approach "was highly successful in motivating students to continue in school thus increasing their life chances." The success of the Webster project led to the creation of similar projects around the country: by the mid-1960s there were nearly forty projects for pregnant school girls, which served over 8,000 pregnant teenagers nationwide. Since these projects were located in impoverished inner-city areas, the race and class components of these projects were similar to those of the Webster School: over 90 percent were black, and over 70 percent came from families on some form of public assistance.[106]

Although the Webster School and similar programs were less punitive than earlier, moralistic solutions to black teenage pregnancy, they did represent what Solinger calls a "white, middle-class approach" to black clients. The main goal of these programs was to persuade black teenage girls to accept white, middle-class social standards and norms regarding "sexual discipline." As in the case of white teenage pregnancy, these programs tended to frame the problem of black teenage pregnancy in terms of individual psychology, focusing on the girl's "mentality" rather than on factors in the social environment that might contribute to unwed pregnancy.[107]

By the mid-1960s imposing white, middle-class standards of conduct on black teenagers became increasingly problematic, since the sexual behavior of white, middle-class girls and young women was rapidly changing during the 1950s and 1960s.[108] As early as 1953, Alfred Kinsey's study *Sexual Behavior in the Human Female* disclosed that over 50 percent of the women in his sample had engaged in premarital sex, a figure that was particularly shocking given that the average age of marriage at the time was the late teens.[109] Obstetricians and gynecologists also found that growing numbers of "nice" girls, that is, those from white middle-class backgrounds, were becoming sexually active—and pregnant—at increasingly younger ages, much to the dismay and embarrassment of their status-conscious parents. Jerome S. Menaker, an obstetrician from Wichita, Kansas, observed in 1958 a "marked shift of early unmarried pregnancies into the more privileged classes," a phenomenon he attributed to "the lessening of parental supervision plus the increased availability of privacy provided by the automobile." Rather than viewing teenage pregnancy as a problem limited to impoverished ghetto youth, physicians like Menaker found alarming incidence of "promiscuity in the youngsters of even the most privileged and well-to-do."[110]

Physicians at adolescent clinics observed similar trends in sexual behavior among white females and consequently started to view Gallagher's conservative attitude toward adolescent pelvic examinations as unrealistic. Clinic directors found that a significant number of their female patients, both black and white, sought their services because of pregnancy, a sexually transmitted disease, or because they desired advice on contraception. The experiences of Joseph L. Rauh, director of the Adolescent Clinic at Children's Hospital Medical Center of Cincinnati, were typical of many adolescent clinic heads at this time. In his first annual report, Rauh noted that of the 67 female patients seen in 1960, 5 had been pregnant, and several others had asked for advice on how to prevent pregnancy. Although the number of patients seeking reproductive health care was small, the fact that there were such patients at all challenged Gallagher's policy on adolescent female sexuality. Rauh concluded that he needed to quickly adapt his services to meet the needs of these female patients, since he believed that these pregnancies could have been avoided if contraceptive advice were part of his clinic's program.[111]

Physicians observed that even girls who were virgins were quite knowledgeable about reproductive anatomy and therefore would not be traumatized by physical examination of the vagina and genitalia. Anna Southam, a gynecologist who treated adolescents at a clinic affiliated with Columbia University College of Physicians and Surgeons, observed that "girls these days are taught something about menstrual function and reproductive physiology in the *7th* and *8th* grade." Southam also noted that "many girls these days use Tampax" and were therefore unlikely to be traumatized by a "gentle one-finger examination." Therefore, Southam argued, a girl who came to an adolescent service with a menstrual complaint will "wonder how you can know if there's anything wrong with her uterus or her ovaries if you don't examine that system as well as her heart and lungs and her breasts."[112]

The growing presence of women in adolescent medicine prompted further changes in the treatment of adolescent girls. In 1965 women made up less than 20 percent of the physicians involved in adolescent medicine: by the late 1970s, this number had grown to 25 percent, and by the mid-1980s nearly one-third of all physicians in adolescent medicine were women.[113] Feminist-oriented physicians and allied health professionals followed the example of the women's health movement of the early 1970s and abandoned the notion that gynecological examinations would hinder young women's feminine development. The popular book *Our Bodies, Our Selves* (1973) and other feminist health care publications promoted self-determination in women's health care and challenged traditional ideas about femininity. In the area of adolescent medicine, feminist practitioners claimed that young women themselves, not their parents, should have the final say over what happened to their bodies.[114]

These changing attitudes toward adolescent female sexuality are symbolized by the new vocabulary that was used to describe teenage sexual behavior. Until at least the mid-1960s, most physicians used morally charged terms such as "promiscuity" and "sexual delinquency" to describe sexual activity among teenagers. By the early 1970s, physicians were increasingly using the more neutral term "sexually active" to describe girls who engaged in extramarital sexual intercourse. Joan Jacobs Brumberg observes in her history of adolescent girls and their bodies that the term "sexually active" was "an important semantic innovation because it described a social state without reference to morality." There were economic motives behind this change in vocabulary: physicians did not want to drive adolescent girls away from their practices by using morally laden language. But Brumberg also demonstrates that this semantic shift represented physicians' recognition that the "family claim" to a daughter's virginity was no longer appropriate.[115]

A similar transition occurred in the health care of minority and economically disadvantaged youth. Charges of racism among health care professionals made by minority youth, combined with the growing presence of minorities in the health care professions, forced medical practitioners to become more sensitive to the cultural and social differences among teenagers and to try and eliminate some of the stereotypical thinking that inhibited medical care of minority underprivileged adolescents. Health care professionals pointed out that the health care needs of these patients "did not differ greatly in kind from those of their more affluent peers." More energy should therefore be invested in creating comprehensive health services for these groups, rather than simply addressing specific behaviors such as drug abuse, delinquency, and sexually transmitted disease. Most important, these teenagers needed personnel who were "sensitive to their cultural backgrounds and beliefs" and who avoided an air of cultural superiority and condescension in dealing with nonwhite teenagers.[116]

Creating greater sensitivity to issues of gender, race, and class among medical professionals could not erase another formidable barrier to health care faced by many adolescents: the need to obtain parental consent for medical treatment. Many of the problems for which young people sought medical attention in the 1960s and 1970s were at odds with parental values, and they were reluctant to seek medical care if it entailed informing their parents. To resolve this problem, physicians in adolescent medicine began pushing for changes in state and federal regulations that would give adolescents access to medical care without parental consent or knowledge.

"My Parents Just Can't Know": Consent and Confidentiality in Adolescent Medical Care

On December, 1969, Robert P. Masland of the Adolescent Unit at Boston Children's Hospital received an anguished letter from a young woman who had read about the Adolescent Unit in an article in the *New York Times*. Seventeen-year-old "Sally" wrote that she had "read about your clinic yesterday and I felt kind of excited because I thought you might be able to help me. I want to come there and see somebody but I can't. My parents would have a fit. They don't even know about my problems." At age thirteen, Sally had been sexually abused by a neighbor, and her mother had refused to believe her. Two years later, Sally had an affair with an older man who she eventually found out was married. "I kept seeing him," she wrote, "but I couldn't stop feeling guilty . . . If I want to have sex with someone, why does it have to be wrong?" Sally pleaded with Masland to allow her to come to the clinic so she could talk about her problems with someone, but added, "you understand of course that I can't come if its necessary for you to meet my parents . . . I want to trust you but I'm afraid. My parents just can't know."[117]

Cases like Sally's were not unique and reflected an increasingly troubling dilemma faced by many adolescent health care practitioners during the late 1960s and early 1970s. Like Sally, many young patients needed medical advice for sexually transmitted diseases, pregnancy, and substance abuse, but were reluctant to seek medical care for these kinds of problems if doing so entailed informing their parents. Laws regulating medical care of patients under twenty-one years of age put medical professionals in an awkward position: most states had laws that made it illegal to administer medical treatment to minors without parental consent under nearly all circumstances. Exceptions to parental consent guidelines included cases of emergencies, parental neglect, or when the minor could prove legal emancipation from his or her parents because of marriage, military service, attendance at college, or economic self-sufficiency. The final and most ambiguous exception to the general rule requiring parental consent was the "mature-minor" concept, which gave unemancipated minors the ability to consent to medical care provided they were of "sufficient intelligence and maturity" to understand the nature and consequences of such treatment. The terms "sufficient intelligence and maturity" were exceedingly difficult to define in any precise manner, and most physicians chose to circumvent this issue by simply refusing to treat minors altogether unless they had the consent of their parents.[118]

Faced with the dilemma of either treating young people without parental permission or having them forgo medical care altogether out of fears of parental retribution, physicians in adolescent medicine began pushing for changes in state and federal regulations that would give adolescents access to medical care without parental consent or knowledge. Indeed, there is evidence that some physicians had already begun to treat some adolescents without consent or knowledge of their parents even in the absence of legal authorization to do so. At Boston, Masland noted in a letter to one of his former trainees in 1971 that "for some time" he and his staff had been treating adolescents with sexually transmitted diseases, who were pregnant, or who had problems with substance abuse "and not always with the consent or knowledge of the parents. Our legal friends in the hospital tell us that we are acting in an ethical fashion and I am happy that we have their support. Fortunately we do not have to make this decision on a daily basis but when we do make it, it is after considerable thought and with the help of numerous medical people as well as administrative people in the hospital." [119]

Physicians often employed creative interpretations of existing laws to get around legal restrictions on the health care of minors. For example, Adele Hofmann, whose experiences directing the adolescent clinic at Beth Israel Hospital in New York City's Lower East Side brought her in contact with numerous adolescents who were alienated from their parents, recalled that she and other medical workers frequently employed an "emergency" designation to get around parental consent requirements, even if an adolescent's condition was not life-threatening. In the case of girls who wanted contraception, Hofmann stated that it was not uncommon to circumvent legal restrictions by recording the diagnosis of "dysmenorrhea" on the charts of female patients requesting birth control pills. [120] The Haight-Ashbury clinic avoided the legal barriers to the health care of minors by allowing patients to use aliases on their admission forms and to lie about their ages, even when it was obvious that a patient was underage. [121]

Other physicians used the mature-minor provisions of state laws regulating the medical treatment of minors. Yet this strategy was difficult given the ambiguity of the mature-minor category. Moreover, all of the court cases employing the mature-minor rule involved medical treatment that was beneficial and relatively uncomplicated in nature. Finally, the fact that the mature-minor doctrine was based on a case-by-case appraisal of a particular minor's competency raised fears that future court cases would result in unfavorable decisions against physicians. [122]

The legal complications associated with the treatment of minors prompted many physicians and health care professionals to begin lobbying for legislation granting adolescents access to confidential medical services on their own consent. One of the leaders in this endeavor was Adele Hofmann, who along with other leaders in the field pointed to recent efforts to expand the legal rights of minors—most notably the *In re Gault* Supreme Court decision in 1967, which recognized minors' rights to due process in juvenile court proceedings; and *Tinker v. Des Moines Independent School*

District (1969), which recognized minors' rights to free speech.[123] Physicians claimed that these decisions should be used as a foundation for extending the medical rights of adolescents as well. In an article for *Adolescent Medicine,* Dale Garell argued that legal rights for minors were a logical extension of adolescent medicine's concern with the special needs of the adolescent patient, and observed that legislators "must begin to talk about the legal rights of adolescents and adolescent law much in the same way that we in medicine have recently begun to take a look intensively at the medical problems of the adolescent age group."[124]

During the early 1970s Hofmann and other members of the Society for Adolescent Medicine, in conjunction with the Committee on Youth of the American Academy of Pediatrics, drafted a model bill that would allow minors to receive health care without parental consent or knowledge. The activism of leaders in adolescent medicine helped precipitate a flurry of legal activity on the state and national levels. By the late 1970s virtually all states had passed statutes permitting minors to consent to diagnosis and treatment of sensitive health issues like sexually transmitted diseases and substance abuse. A few states had also enacted comprehensive statutes that allowed minors to consent to the full range of medical services. Finally, three landmark Supreme Court decisions, *Planned Parenthood of Central Missouri v. Danforth* (1976), *Bellotti v. Baird* (1979), and *Carey v. Population Services International* (1977) clearly established adolescent women's right to obtain contraceptive services—including abortion—without parental consent.[125]

In many ways, these legal developments were the culmination of Gallagher's treatment philosophy. As early as 1960 Gallagher had suggested that "adolescents have reached the point in their development where they not only can profit from a confidential relationship with a physician whom they consider to be their own but also may require such a relationship if their health needs are to be best served."[126] Gallagher himself frequently had to compromise on this principle, however, partly because he did not have the legal mandate to follow through on the issue of confidentiality. Those who fought for consent and confidentiality in adolescent health care in the 1960s and 1970s ensured that Gallagher's outlook was written into American law.

Yet the struggle for minors' rights to medical care was far from over. Legal policies regarding minors' access to medical care remain inconsistent to this day, mainly because many Americans remain deeply ambiguous about how much freedom and independence from parental control adolescents should be permitted. These cultural assumptions are so powerful that they even pervade the legislation that grants teenagers access to medical care without parental consent. Although the legal policies that regulate adolescent reproductive health services were created in response to the "sexual revolution" of the late 1960s, the language used to justify such legislation avoided using terminology that condoned sexual freedom among teenagers. Instead, the legislation was framed in terms of a "least harm" perspective, which justified removing parental consent barriers because doing so would protect young people from the consequences of their sexual behavior. The more fundamental issue of whether young people in general, and young women in particular, had the right to make reproductive decisions independently of their parents was carefully avoided, possibly because advocates feared that using a "reproductive rights" argument would make their cause even more controversial than it already was. For example, statutes permitting minors to obtain treatment for sexually transmitted diseases without parental consent were aimed at preserving the public health and protecting the minor from the health risks associated with sexual intercourse, not at increasing the minor's self-determination. Similarly the decision in *Carey v. Population Services International* (1977), which justified giving sexually active adolescents independent access to birth control, did so on the grounds that it would prevent pregnancy, not on the basis of a young woman's maturity or right to be sexually expressive.[127]

Federal support for adolescent medical care also waned during the 1970s. Indeed, popular enthusiasm and federal spending for child and adolescent health programs had begun to diminish as early as 1967, as military intervention in Vietnam drew money and attention away from the War on Poverty, and rioting and militancy in the inner cities appeared to demonstrate to many white, middle-class voters the futility of increased government spending on the poor. This dissatisfaction led to funding cutbacks and/or financial restructuring of many federally funded health programs during the 1970s, as Johnson's Great Society gave way to Nixon's New Federalism. By 1974 most of the Title V funds for maternal and child health had been converted into block grants to individual states rather than grants to particular maternal and child health programs. This allowed states greater leeway in deciding which health programs to fund, although each state had to have at least one program in each of the five areas of maternal and infant care: health care for high-risk infants, dental care, family planning, and child and preschool health care. Under this new funding structure, programs that did not fall within these five categories were often the first to be eliminated. The C & Y projects, for example, frequently compensated for funding cuts by excluding children over the age of fifteen from their programs. Female adolescents continued to receive comprehensive medical and dental care through the M & I and Family Planning programs, but obviously the recipients of this aid were limited to a narrow category within this age group. Although 15 percent of the Title V funds continued to be reserved for "special projects of regional and national significance"—including projects on adolescent health care—they were too small in number to reach all adolescents.[128]

The programs sponsored by the OEO suffered a similar fate. OEO programs were particularly unpopular among the voters from Nixon's "silent majority," most of whom never really bought the idea of "maximum feasible participation" of the poor in antipoverty programs, especially when the poor were nonwhite and militant. The desire to streamline the federal bureaucracy during the Nixon administration shifted control of the neighborhood health centers from the OEO to the Department of Health, Education, and Welfare. This transition cut funds for environmental and nonmedical activities and shifted the focus of the neighborhood health centers from the broad goal of community action to more narrow issues of medical care. Congress successfully blocked funding cuts to the neighborhood health centers during the Nixon and Ford administrations, but funding was kept constant despite tremendous increases in the cost of health care delivery. Although some of this was made up by Medicaid coverage, not all procedures were covered, and many neighborhood health centers were forced to admit patients who were not poor and to begin charging fees for medical care, thereby arousing much resentment among community activists who believed the centers should continue to offer services free of charge.[129]

The decline in federal support for adolescent health programs could not have come at a worse time for the field of adolescent medicine. During the 1970s and 1980s, physicians in adolescent medicine were engaged in a struggle to more clearly define the nature of their field and to carve out a unique space for themselves within the medical profession. Waning federal dollars, combined with continued ambivalence about the status of teenagers in American society, would only complicate this process.

"We Can't Be All Things to Everyone"

The movement to increase the availability of health care services for teenagers and the number of health care professionals trained to treat them created professional problems for the field of adolescent medicine. Physicians worried that by encouraging other medical specialists and allied health care professionals to move into adolescent health care, they would soon drive themselves out of business. Dale Garell expressed this dilemma best in a 1969 editorial for *Adolescent Medicine* entitled "On Being Relevant," in which he described the observations of an "overseas visitor" who praised the accomplishments of adolescent medicine in expanding the variety and availability of health services for adolescents, particularly those from underprivileged backgrounds. This foreign visitor also remarked that adolescent medicine had "a limited future" in that most of what the field did "would be incorporated into family medicine and comprehensive health care for all ages, and, having served that purpose, would quietly disappear."[130]

Throughout the next two decades, therefore, physicians in adolescent medicine found themselves working for two, often contradictory goals: increasing the number of health care professionals who were trained to take care of teenagers, while at the same time maintaining a special professional position for the field of adolescent *medicine*. To accomplish the first of these goals, the Society for Adolescent Medicine began forming alliances with other medical organizations and allied health groups during the early 1970s. The society was especially interested in convincing general pediatricians in private practice and in ambulatory pediatric clinics in inner-city medical centers to include adolescent health care in their service offerings. To facilitate the involvement of general pediatricians in SAM, society members decided to hold their annual conference separately from the Washington postgraduate seminars, preferably in conjunction with the American Academy of Pediatrics (AAP), which was the main national forum for pediatricians in private practice.[131] In the fall of 1970, SAM held its first meeting with the AAP, and in 1971, the academy decided to provide the society with space at its annual meeting each year.[132]

SAM members found that one of the main obstacles to recruiting pediatricians into adolescent medical care was lack of training: a survey conducted by Adele Hofmann in 1971 indicated that there were only twenty-eight fellowship programs in the country for physicians interested in adolescent medicine, and that most pediatric departments did not consider adolescence important enough to include in pediatric residency training.[133] To combat this problem, SAM formed a Committee on Education in 1972, which was intended to establish a core curriculum for medical students and residents interested in the health care of adolescents. SAM members hoped that the Committee on Education would not only help to make adolescence part of all pediatric training programs, but it would also enhance the prominence of the field "by developing a core curriculum in adolescent medicine."[134]

Incorporating adolescent medicine into pediatric education was hastened by the cooperation of the American Academy of Pediatrics, which established a Section on Adolescence within the Academy in 1978. The AAP Section on Adolescence was prompted by concerns within the pediatric profession that medical education was increasingly out of step with the kinds of problems that pediatricians encountered in everyday practice. The AAP noted that pediatricians in private practice and in outpatient clinics in major university hospitals were increasingly encountering adolescent patients, but did not have adequate preparation in their medical school or residency training to deal with teenagers. The purpose of the Section on Adolescence was to help establish educational criteria for pediatricians interested in practicing adolescent medicine, and to integrate at least some exposure to adolescent health problems into all pediatric residency programs.[135]

Efforts to integrate adolescent medicine into medical school and residency training received an additional boost when members of SAM became a part of the Task Force on Pediatric Education in 1976. Formed in January of 1976, the task force was a response to the "recognition that many of the important health needs of infants, children, and adolescents are not being met as effectively and as fully as they should be." The primary goal of the task force, therefore, was "to identify those health needs and to point out the educational strategies that are required to prepare the pediatrician of the future to meet them."[136] One of the unmet needs the task force uncovered was the health care of adolescents, particularly those with health problems that had their basis in psychological and social causes. The task force members therefore recommended that the health needs of adolescents "should be explicitly considered in planning the educational program. There should be increased emphasis on the biosocial aspects of pediatrics and adolescent health."[137]

During the late 1970s and early 1980s, this collaboration between SAM and the AAP paid off. The establishment of the AAP Section on Adolescence and the recommendations of the Task Force on Pediatric Education in 1978 helped adolescent medicine gain a stronger foothold in medical school and pediatric residency training. For many members of SAM, these developments were signs that adolescent medicine was finally receiving the recognition it deserved. Michael I. Cohen observed in his report on the Task Force for Pediatric Education that the AAP's recommendations on adolescent health care represented "the first time that pediatrics as a discipline acknowledged that adolescent health needs are inadequately met . . . the first time that the whole of pediatrics stated it will assume responsibility for this area of care . . . [and] the first time a statement calling for inclusion of adolescent health issues has been made in a document dealing with the content of the pediatric curriculum."[138]

SAM made similar overtures to the fields of internal medicine, family practice, and obstetrics and gynecology. In October of 1976, the executive council noted the necessity of fostering vigorous liaison activities with the American Academy of Family Practice, the American College of Physicians, and the American College of Obstetricians and Gynecologists in order to encourage these physicians to take more of an interest in the health needs of adolescents.[139]

At the same time that SAM was encouraging more pediatricians, internists, and ob/gyns to become trained in the health care of adolescents, some members began looking for ways to attract nonphysicians who were interested in teenage health care into the organization. It is probably no coincidence that this outreach to allied health professionals, most of whom were female, occurred during the term of SAM's first female president, Adele Hofmann. Since the early 1960s Hofmann had worked to increase the reproductive rights of young women. During her presidency of SAM, Hofmann continued her advocacy on behalf of youth, but also focused increased attention on the needs of female health care professionals. Believing that the complex health problems facing adolescents in the 1970s could "only be successfully mediated through an interdisciplinary approach," Hofmann and other members of the executive council sponsored several initiatives to make SAM more attractive to nonphysicians. The executive council helped incorporate more sessions of interest to nonphysicians in the annual conference, provided nonphysicians with opportunities to serve on the SAM's various committees, and encouraged them "to contribute their perspectives and commentary on various issues to the president and council." [140] Hofmann further underscored the society's commitment to nonphysicians by issuing a statement of purpose that reaffirmed SAM's interdisciplinary nature and its desire to promote and improve adolescent health "wherever and by whomever it is rendered." Therefore, wrote Hofmann, the organization gave "equal weight and merit to the membership of any health professional with a significant commitment to adolescent health," including "psychologists, nurses, social workers, nutritionists, and lawyers, as well as physicians." [141]

These developments did not please all members of SAM, however. To some, meeting with the American Academy of Pediatrics and encouraging nonphysicians to join the society reinforced their identity as a primarily clinically oriented, and thus inferior, medical field. The fact that SAM held its main annual meeting jointly with the American Academy of Pediatrics set adolescent medicine apart from the research-oriented pediatric subspecialties such as pediatric endocrinology, neonatology, and cardiology, which held their professional meetings with the joint conference of the American Pediatric Society (APS) and the Society for Pediatric Research (SPR), which was the main national forum for pediatricians in academic and research posts. Although the American Academy of Pediatrics did hold scientific sessions on pediatric subspecialties, they were oriented mainly around the interests of subspecialists in private practice, rather than those of academic researchers. [142] Furthermore, by encouraging nurses, psychologists, and other nonphysicians engaged in adolescent health care to join SAM, the society moved even further from its roots in academic medicine.

Felix Heald was particularly concerned about this problem, since his original goal in starting the Washington meetings for adolescent clinic directors was to increase the research component and academic standards of the field. When Heald assumed the presidency of the society in 1970, he attempted to move SAM even further in this direction by adding a more research-oriented component to the society's annual meetings. Together with Michael Cohen, Heald helped establish the first research sessions at the society's annual meeting in 1973. Heald and Cohen also successfully worked toward incorporating research on adolescence into the joint conferences of the APS and SPR, which held their first sessions on adolescence in 1976.[143]

During the late 1970s Heald tried to move the Society even further toward a research emphasis by making a clear demarcation between SAM and the AAP Section on Adolescence. Although Heald admired SAM's success in increasing interest in adolescence within the AAP and the society's efforts to reach out to nonphysicians, he was also concerned that in trying to be "all things to all people," SAM no longer had a unique sense of mission that was distinct from other areas of the medical profession. Furthermore, noted Heald, the development of the Section on Adolescence within the AAP forced "the Society for Adolescent Medicine to clarify its goals and identity" in order to persuade practitioners to join SAM rather than the AAP Section on Adolescence. Heald concluded that since the AAP Section on Adolescence was intended primarily as a forum for physicians in private practice, the best way for the society to justify its continued existence was to "become a more academic society" by focusing primarily on physicians involved in education and research.[144] After several hours of intense discussion over what the society's new identity should be at a 1979 retreat, the executive council eventually agreed with Heald's suggestions: they decided that the best way to distinguish themselves from the AAP Section on Adolescence was to shift their focus toward a more academically and research-oriented educational mission. In 1979 the society's executive council issued a statement that argued that the major emphasis of SAM should be "to promote the development, synthesis, and dissemination of scientific and scholarly knowledge unique to the developmental and health care needs of adolescents."[145] In other words, the society's new emphasis would be to oversee the training of academic physicians who would head divisions of adolescent medicine in medical schools and teaching hospitals, who would in turn train allied health professionals and physicians going into private practice and social service agencies.

The reaction of the membership at large to the executive council's decision to change the focus of SAM was mixed. Although most members thought it was a good idea to reevaluate the society's mission in light of developments within the AAP, some were afraid that the new emphasis on academic medicine and research would discourage a significant number of adolescent health care providers, particularly nonphysicians, from joining SAM. Even members of the executive council were ambivalent about SAM's change in emphasis. John Edlin of Southwestern Medical School in Dallas, for example, believed the society's new emphasis on research would compromise the training of community practitioners, as well as discouraging nonacademics from joining the society.[146] The most outspoken on this issue were the nonphysician members of the society, who felt that the new emphasis on research was an elitist attempt to exclude allied health professionals, many of whom were female. Jackie Ficht, RN, from the Ad Hoc Committee on Inter-Disciplines, even suggested that rather than emphasize research and teaching, SAM should become even more interdisciplinary and change its name to "Society for Adolescent Health Care" to reflect its commitment to nonphysicians.[147]

Others, however, felt that by finding a distinct mission for SAM that was separate from that of the AAP Section on Adolescence, SAM would encourage more internists, general practitioners, and ob-gyn specialists to participate in the society.[148] Still others felt that redefining the goals of the society was not sufficient to establish the independent identity of adolescent medicine. Instead, they saw SAM's new focus as the first logical step toward their larger objective: board certification in adolescent medicine.

"Sitting at the Table": The Debate over Board Certification

SAM members first began to consider the issue of board certification in the early 1970s as part of the revisions in pediatric residency programs sponsored by the society's Committee on Education. Members of the Committee on Education believed that reforming pediatric residencies to include more material on adolescent health care was the first "step towards defining and identifying Adolescent Medicine as a subspecialty." The next step would be to obtain board certification for adolescent medicine, which would put the field on the same level as other pediatric subspecialties.[149]

The goal of board certification in adolescent medicine turned out to be much more difficult to attain than reforms in pediatric education. At first, the Committee on Education attempted to obtain an independent board for adolescent medicine. This proved to be impractical, however, mainly because of the American Board of Medical Specialties' reluctance to institute boards for medical disciplines that were not already subdisciplines within existing medical specialties. During the early 1940s, the ABMS began to limit the number of new specialties that were emerging, since there seemed to be much overlap and little coordination among the existing medical specialties. As Rosemary Stevens observes in her history of medical specialization, the emergence of new specialties seemed to many to be more a product of professional self-interest than a means of better serving the public's broader health needs. In 1972 the ABMS passed a moratorium on the creation of new specialty boards, stating that from hence forth it would only allow subboards within existing medical specialties. Although the ABMS made an exception to this rule in 1979 and allowed emergency medicine to institute its own independent board, for most aspiring specialists creating a board that was independent of an existing specialty was nearly impossible.[150]

Instead of pursuing an autonomous board, the SAM Committee on Education decided that the most practical route was to establish a subspecialty board within pediatrics or some other primary specialty board. In October of 1975, the executive council of SAM decided to petition the American Board of Pediatrics (ABP) to establish subspecialty certification in adolescent medicine. The resolution included the provision that the society would encourage other specialty groups that were represented in the society's membership, such as family practice, obstetrics and gynecology, and internal medicine, to pursue similar ends if they so desired.[151]

Obtaining subspecialty accreditation for adolescent medicine proved to be an arduous and controversial process. Not the least of the society's problems were the stringent objections of a significant number of the society's own members. When the executive council's resolution was put to a vote at the business meeting of the general membership in 1975, it was defeated 24 to 23. Adele Hofmann, head of the Committee on Education, then moved that the entire membership of the society be polled regarding their opinions on board certification. Out of the 353 ballots that were returned, 192 voted "yes," 22 voted "yes, with reservations," and a 139 voted "no."[152] Those in favor of the resolution believed that board certification would make adolescent medicine more competitive in the medical marketplace and help ensure that specialists in this field would receive adequate reimbursement from health insurers and other third-party payment plans.[153] Members' reasons for opposing the resolution were more varied. Some were not opposed to the idea of board certification altogether, but feared that if certification was obtained through the American Board of Pediatrics, adolescent medicine would soon be swallowed up by pediatrics and lose its independent identity as a medical field. They therefore suggested that adolescent medicine should pursue board certification on its own initiative, despite the cost and inconvenience.[154] Others argued that financial considerations were a poor reason for seeking board certification, and claimed that it was more important to ensure that physicians were qualified to take care of adolescents than to obtain board certification.[155]

By far the most prevalent objection to board certification was the risk it would pose to the multidisciplinary nature of the society and of adolescent health care more generally. Opponents argued that board certification through the American Board of Pediatrics would not only estrange nonpediatricians within the SAM, but would also alienate nonphysicians who were involved in adolescent health care. Underlying many of these objections was a philosophical objection to specialization. Opponents maintained that there were already too many medical specialties, that overspecialization was one of the main causes of the fragmentation and inaccessibility of adolescent health care, and that adolescents would be better served by improving the quality of care and method of health care delivery than by giving physicians a specialty title.[156]

Among the more prominent individuals who were opposed to using board certification to set adolescent medicine apart from other medical disciplines were Gallagher and Masland. Gallagher founded the Adolescent Unit on the principle that physicians should treat the patient as a whole rather than only addressing a particular disease or organ. The purpose of an adolescent clinic, Gallagher believed, was to provide a centralized facility for addressing the totality of a particular youngster's medical, psychological, educational, and social needs rather than dividing his or her care among a plethora of specialists and health care workers.[157] When Masland assumed the directorship of the Adolescent Unit in the late 1960s, he continued Gallagher's philosophy on specialization. Thus, when the Society for Adolescent Medicine began discussing the possibility of obtaining board certification in the mid-1970s, Masland opposed it. Like Gallagher, Masland believed that if board certification in adolescent medicine were attained, then the field would subsequently splinter into a series of subspecialties, thereby defeating the original purpose of adolescent medicine. Although Masland agreed that there should be some sort of educational standards for practicing adolescent medicine, he believed that such training should be made available to all physicians and allied health professionals who wanted to add adolescents to their practices, rather than limiting training simply to those who wished to become board certified. Finally, Masland argued, board certification would actually reduce the number of qualified practitioners in adolescent medicine. Young physicians would be unwilling to undergo the extra years of training required to become eligible for board certification, especially since the financial rewards in adolescent medicine were much lower than more lucrative specialties such as surgery.[158]

In 1977, developments within the American Medical Association made the issue of board certification in adolescent medicine even more critical: that year, the board of trustees of the AMA officially recognized adolescent medicine as a medical subspecialty.[159] To some members of SAM, particularly those involved in private practice, approval by the AMA rendered the whole issue of board certification irrelevant: since AMA designation allowed physicians to list themselves as adolescent specialists in the AMA directory, and to seek third party reimbursement under the specialty designation, board certification appeared redundant.[160] President-elect Verdain Barnes was confident enough to declare in 1977 that "the struggle for legitimacy is behind us" and that the SAM should focus on improving availability and access to adolescent health care more broadly.[161]

For others, however, AMA recognition created a new problem: how to decide who was actually qualified to practice adolescent medicine. Members of SAM's executive council, many of whom were in academic adolescent medicine posts, were especially worried about reports that "individuals who have had very little prior, if any, training in adolescent medicine have claimed expertise in this area through membership in the Society." However, opposition to board certification was still strong among the membership at large, most of whom were physicians in private practice who did not want to undergo extra training in order to be certified to treat adolescents. As a stop-gap measure, Verdain Barnes proposed a strategy that had been used by medical societies earlier in the twentieth century, before specialty certification was common: creating a special designation of "Fellow of the Society for Adolescent Medicine" which "would certify that the named individuals would be recognized by the Society for Adolescent Medicine as having expertise in their field and as having satisfied defined qualifications for attainment of same." Other members of the executive council, however, wondered "how the Society would validate these qualifications, accredit training programs, and, in general, implement 'watch-dog' procedures," given the SAM's limited financial resources. In the end, the executive council decided to bring the issue before the full membership before deciding to establish Fellow status within the society.[162]

Executive council members realized that they needed to be careful in presenting the idea of Fellow status to avoid alienating members who might view the measure as a precursor to board certification. In his President's Message to the membership in 1980, Richard MacKenzie wrote that Fellow status should "not to be construed as moving toward specialty status, but more as an effort to establish recognition for that individual who has a special set of skills to offer the teenager." MacKenzie was particularly reassuring toward nonphysicians, noting that the concept of adolescent medicine "not only operates within the medical model, but by definition, includes an equal status for the creative involvement of nonphysician health professionals."[163] The multidisciplinary nature of SAM was further underscored by the new journal for the society that began publication in 1980, and which was purposely called *Journal of Adolescent Health Care* rather than *Journal of Adolescent Medicine* in order to provide a vehicle for "new information and insight about the adolescent from a variety of disciplines," not just medicine.[164]

Therefore, when Fellow status was approved by the executive council and a vote of the SAM membership in 1983, nonphysicians were allowed to become Fellows of the society, provided they had the appropriate terminal degree and were licensed to practice in their field. Physicians were required to have an M.D. or equivalent from an accredited university; psychologists had to have a doctoral degree from a graduate program approved by the American Psychological Association; nurses had to have an approved degree or certificate in nursing; and all other professionals had to be certified or licensed "when appropriate and/or available." In addition to the degree and licensing requirements, applicants for Fellow status had to be "individuals of high professional standing with a commitment and dedication to adolescent health care."[165]

Although the Fellow designation gave some recognition to outstanding members within SAM, it did not resolve the issue of adolescent medicine's status within the medical profession as a whole. The Fellow status still did not specify a required training period or body of knowledge that Fellows had to master. Moreover, by permitting nonphysicians to become Fellows, some physicians in the society, most notably Heald, felt they had done little to improve their image among other medical specialists.

By the mid-1980s the field of adolescent medicine had entered into what Victor Strasburger of the University of New Mexico School of Medicine appropriately called a "mid-life crisis." Despite three decades of "advertising" and official recognition by the American Academy of Pediatrics and the American Medical Association, observed Strasburger, adolescent medicine's status in the medical professional as a whole was still rather low.[166] Adolescent medicine's standing was particularly tenuous in academic pediatric departments. Although the number of training programs had grown impressively beginning in the late 1960s, by the mid-1980s the number of adolescent divisions in medical schools and major medical centers in the United States was declining. Despite the recommendation of the Task Force on Pediatric Education that adolescent medicine was an essential part of both undergraduate and graduate medical training, a sharp decline in the number of teenagers in the general population during the 1980s suggested that the market for such services was shrinking.[167] Some states had no adolescent medical facilities, despite the presence of several medical schools. Furthermore, existing adolescent medicine divisions seldom received the same kind of respect or priority from pediatric department chairs that the other pediatric subdivisions received. As Strasburger bitterly noted in an account of his experiences searching for an academic job, "adolescent medicine is viewed as an academic luxury, not a necessity." Adolescent division directors, observed Strasburger, were typically treated as "second-class citizens" within their home institutions: they were usually relegated to junior-level clinical appointments rather than being offered the more prestigious academic appointments within medical school pediatric departments, seldom received tenure, and even those with tenure were often the first to be fired when financial pressures necessitated staff cutbacks.[168]

Other studies conducted in the 1980s indicated that even in institutions with relatively strong adolescent divisions, adolescent medicine was frequently accorded a lower priority than other pediatric departments. For example, a survey conducted by the SAM Ad Hoc Committee on Pediatric Residency indicated that residents in over half the pediatric programs with adolescent divisions spent less than 15 percent of their time working with teenagers.[169] Similarly, several surveys of pediatric and internal medicine residents about their preparedness to practice adolescent medicine indicated that many felt they were underskilled in such critical areas of adolescent health care as contraceptive advice-giving, adolescent history-taking, counseling, evaluation of psychopathology, and treatment of dysmenorrhea and hypertension.[170]

These disclosures of adolescent medicine's low status within academic medicine led some members of SAM to raise the board certification issue once again. Supporters of board certification argued that this measure would instantly raise the standing of adolescent medicine within pediatric departments. Strasburger remarked that board certification would do what the Task Force on Pediatric Education failed to do, that is, give adolescent medicine the same standing as other pediatric subspecialties. "Instituting board certification would be expensive, time-consuming, and politically bothersome," Strasburger wrote, "[b]ut it would give the field instant credibility—credibility that has slowly built up over 35 years but is now threatened with erosion. No department chair, Residency Review Committee, or Dean would be able to ignore the fundamental need for adolescent medicine in a pediatric training program," if there was board certification. "Boards would accomplish what the Task Force on Pediatric Education failed to accomplish in 1978 through good faith and common sense," concluded Strasburger, since they "would inject renewed self-esteem and pride into specialists who are tired of fighting for recognition against cardiologists, neonatologists, and others."[171]

Strasburger's colleagues in SAM shared his belief that board certification would improve the visibility and credibility of adolescent medicine: in the late 1980s the society's executive council once again began to discuss the pros and cons of board certification. In 1986 the executive council appointed an Ad Hoc Committee to explore the feasibility of subspecialty boards in adolescent medicine, which was composed of Charles E. Irwin, H. Verdain Barnes, Donald Greydanus, Sherrel L. Hammar, Iris F. Litt, Donald P. Orr, and Joseph L. Rauh. Once again, they decided it was economically unfeasible to pursue an independent board in adolescent medicine. They also decided that since 90 percent of the physicians in SAM were pediatricians, and 95 percent of the adolescent medicine programs in the United States and Canada were based in Departments of Pediatrics, it would be most practical to petition the American Board of Pediatrics to grant subspecialty status to adolescent medicine. They were careful not to exclude nonpediatricians, however, and asked the American Board of Internal Medicine and the American Board of Family Practice whether they would like to join the American Board of Pediatrics in a combined specialty application to the American Board of Medical Specialties. The Internal Medicine Board was enthusiastic about the proposal, and agreed to go along with the ABP's plans. The Family Practice Board, however, declined to become involved in the board certification process because it believed that subspecialization in any field would undermine its identity as a primary-care specialty.

In 1987, after having explored the feasibility of board certification, SAM president Joe Sanders appointed a subspecialty committee to write up a proposal for the American Board of Pediatrics. After receiving the approval of SAM's executive council in the Fall of 1988, the subspecialty committee of SAM submitted the proposal to the subspecialty approval committee of the ABP. In 1989 the subspecialty committee of the American Board of Pediatrics recommended to the entire board that it approve the application process, and in October of 1989, the ABP decided to go ahead and submit the application to the American Board of Medical Specialties (ABMS) for final approval.[172]

The subspecialization committees of SAM and the ABP encountered some difficulties in persuading the ABMS to approve granting adolescent medicine subspecialty status. The ABMS initially rejected the proposal for three reasons: first, it believed it would be detrimental to the field of pediatrics; second, it did not feel it was appropriate to grant subspecialty status to adolescent medicine without the involvement of the American Board of Family Practice; and finally, it believed that the three-year training period required before an individual could take the board certification exam was too lengthy, despite the fact that the American Board of Pediatrics required three years of fellowship training in order to sit for boards in other pediatric subspecialties.[173]

Another important obstacle was the opposition of significant numbers of SAM members to board certification. Shortly before the proposal was sent to the ABMS for a final decision, the society held an open panel on the board certification issue at its annual business meeting in March of 1990, during which a number of concerns about the impending decision on board certification were raised. Tony Dekker feared that board certification would destroy the society's identity as a "congress of multi-disciplines." Barry Lachman worried that board certification would be limited to members of SAM, and would thus leave out the large majority of physicians who treated adolescents in private practice and other nonacademic medical settings. Michael Brady expressed a similar concern, arguing that unless the society made a greater effort to gain the support of the American Board of Family Practice, family practitioners, who provided a substantial portion of adolescent health care in the country, would be left out of the board certification process. Even Victor Strasburger argued that while he agreed in theory with the idea of board certification and the credibility it would lend to the field of adolescent medicine, the mandatory three-year training period required for board eligibility in adolescent medicine "would do more harm than good." Strasburger pointed out that the number of residents going into pediatrics was extremely shaky at best. To ask young physicians to undertake three additional years of training in adolescent medicine, without the remuneration or status accorded other pediatric subspecialists, concluded Strasburger, would simply turn them off of the field completely.[174]

Despite these objections, the American Board of Medical Specialties finally granted approval to the American Board of Pediatrics to initiate subcertification in adolescent medicine during its March 1991 meeting. At the same meeting, the American Board of Internal Medicine announced that it would also make an application to the ABMS for subcertification in adolescent medicine. The first board examination for subcertification in adolescent medicine took place in the fall of 1993.[175]

Opinions vary on how board certification will affect the field of adolescent medicine. For some members of SAM, board certification has finally given adolescent medicine the recognition and status they feel it deserves.

As Charles Irwin, director of the Adolescent Division at Children's Hospital of San Francisco and member of the subspecialty board for adolescent medicine noted, "we [adolescent specialists] sit at the table now," and enjoy the same privileges as the organ- and disease-based pediatric subspecialists.[176]

Others, however, are worried that the mandatory three-year fellowship for adolescent medicine will decrease the number of physicians in adolescent medicine. Strasburger, formerly an avid supporter of board certification, observed in an interview conducted in 1993 that "we're shooting ourselves in the foot with boards." Although he agrees with Irwin that board certification has given adolescent medicine more credibility among other pediatric subspecialists, the lengthy training period will discourage young physicians from entering the field, since they can become pediatric cardiologists or endocrinologists in the same amount of time while reaping substantially larger financial rewards. Strasburger's fear is that the training period will be so discouraging that the numbers of young physicians going into adolescent medicine "will diminish so severely that [in a generation] we will have a field that's dying out."[177]

Furthermore, there is some concern that board certification will discourage nonphysicians from joining the society and pursuing adolescent health care. SAM members seem to have anticipated the potential problems that board certification could cause, and have worked hard to project a nonelitist image to the public and to other medical professionals. SAM's commitment to multidisciplinary approaches to adolescent health care is particularly apparent in the society's policy toward nonphysicians. Several executive council meetings in the 1980s addressed the problem of getting more nonphysicians to join the society and making them feel welcome at annual meetings and other SAM functions. Although some argued that the low percentage of nonphysicians in the society was a reflection of the small numbers of nonphysicians actively involved in adolescent health care, others argued that the society leadership was not doing enough to recruit nonphysicians into SAM. After an executive council retreat in 1984, the society resolved to do more to publicize SAM among nonphysicians and to improve its methods of detecting and recruiting talented nonphysicians involved in adolescent health care. Yet there is some indication that nonphysicians, and even nonpediatricians, do not feel welcome at society functions. In 1986 approximately 90 percent of SAM's membership were physicians, and 75 percent of the physicians were pediatricians, a proportion that has remained constant over the past decade despite the outreach efforts of SAM's members.[178] Informal discussions with nonphysicians at the society's annual meetings suggest that many nonphysicians feel like they do not "fit in," and that the society could do a better job of seeing that nonphysicians' professional needs are met.

Will board certification make adolescent medicine more credible, and therefore more attractive to medical students and residents? Or will board certification discourage young physicians from entering adolescent medicine, and alienate nonphysicians from adolescent health care? Is there even a need for a special field known as adolescent medicine, or will the subspecialty disappear as more nonphysicians take over the health care of adolescents? These are only some of the many dilemmas that adolescent medicine must face in the years ahead as it enters its own middle age.

Conclusion

When I was a teenager in the late 1970s, I needed a sports physical in order to participate on the cross-country team. I remember telling my mother that I did not want to go to the "baby doctor," nor did I want to share a waiting room with infants and toddlers. Since our local hospital did not have an adolescent clinic at this time, my mother decided to take me to her internist. I remember being mortified because my mother stayed in the room and because the doctor did a breast exam, asked me questions about my periods and other sensitive subjects, all the while telling me to "stop giggling and pretending to be embarrassed."

When I started this project, and learned there was a medical specialty dedicated to teenagers, at first I thought it would have been wonderful if there had been an adolescent unit at my local hospital, a place where I could see a doctor who was sensitive to teenagers' self-consciousness about their bodies. As I continued my work, however, I began to wonder if there had been an adolescent clinic, would I have known about it? Would I have had the courage or resources to go by myself? Would I have even cared about having a "doctor of my own"?

Various studies on laypersons' views of adolescent medical services raise similar questions about the success of adolescent medicine as a medical field. Despite nearly five decades of advertising, many contemporary teenagers and adults alike are unaware that there is a medical specialty devoted exclusively to adolescents. The most frequent response from fellow historians when I tell them I am working on a history of adolescent medicine is "I didn't know there was such a thing." Even when teenagers are aware of the existence of adolescent clinics, they tend not to use them because they are afraid that health care providers will inform their parents; because these facilities seem unapproachable or unsympathetic to adolescent patients; or because of inconvenient hours and/or remote geographic location.[1]

Furthermore, having a "doctor of their own" has not led to a greater degree of health among American teenagers: if anything the health of contemporary teenagers is worse than when the field began in the early 1950s. Adolescents are the only age group in the United States whose mortality rate has actually increased over the past thirty years. One out of five adolescents have at least one serious health problem. As in the past, those who are most at risk are adolescents who are both poor and members of racial or ethnic minorities, mainly because these individuals do not have access to adequate health care and because they lack the familial and community support systems that help more privileged youngsters deal with the emotional turmoil often associated with adolescence. Yet white, middle-class teenagers also face excessive health risks, despite their greater access to health care facilities and social support networks.[2]

Some would argue that the high rate of ill-health among American teenagers, combined with the fact that few people of any age know about the specialty, are evidence that adolescent medicine has failed in its mission as a medical discipline. Yet this view overlooks one of the major points of this book, which is that adolescent medicine has been and continues to be shaped by adult attitudes toward adolescents and their proper place in American society. The field of adolescent medicine grew out of profound changes in theories about adolescence that emerged during the 1930s and 1940s. Experts in adolescent development, most notably Lawrence Frank, claimed that rebellion against parental values was a normal sign of growing maturity within the individual, a way of enabling youth to meet the demands of the future. Gallagher incorporated the notion of normalized teenage rebellion into his treatment style at the Boston Children's Hospital Adolescent Unit, often to the dismay of parents. Gallagher and his staff created a teen-centered environment and fostered a doctor-patient relationship that valued the views of the teenage patient more than those of parents.

My description of the new doctor-patient relationship developed by adolescent medicine modifies a point often raised by radical historians, most notably Christopher Lasch, about the way in which medicine has been used as an agent of social control. According to Lasch, medicine and other helping professions such as social work have not worked to promote social good: instead these fields have "invaded" the family in order to promote their own professional self-interests. In the process, helping professionals have reinforced the regulatory powers of the state by assuming functions once provided by family members themselves.[3] This book has demonstrated that at times, medicine has been used to reinforce prevailing ideas about race, gender, and class. This tendency was particularly true during the early years of adolescent medicine. However, this book has also shown that in the case of adolescent medicine, professional intervention affected parents and teenagers in different ways.[4] There is no doubt that physicians' therapeutic style ultimately served to weaken parental authority. Rather than permit parents to use the clinic as a means of social control of their teenage children, doctors posed themselves as intergenerational mediators who tried to work out solutions that would benefit adolescent patients as well as parents. This clinical approach implied that parents and children could not resolve generational conflicts without expert intervention. Moreover, by selling their services to teenagers as well as their parents, physicians socialized young people to turn to medical professionals rather than to family members, peers, or other experts for guidance along the difficult path to adulthood. The treatment style at the Adolescent Unit, however, did give teenagers a much greater role in medical decisions than they had enjoyed before. Although his views on adolescence were constrained by prevailing views about race, gender, and class during the postwar period, Gallagher was the first to recognize that teenagers needed a "doctor of their own" who considered their needs and opinions paramount.

Doctors continued to listen to the voices of adolescent patients as the field of adolescent medicine expanded during the 1960s and 1970s, but the things teenagers told their physicians changed dramatically: adolescents began to engage in behaviors that were increasingly at odds with parental values, and which placed them at risk for new health problems such as sexually transmitted diseases, drug addiction, and pregnancy. In fact, many teenagers refused to seek medical attention at all, since laws governing medical treatment of minors required parental consent. The new behavior of American teenagers prompted physicians to help change the laws governing adolescent health care.

New views about gender, race, and class also helped revise the model of patient care employed by adolescent medicine. Civil rights activists and advocates for the poor drew increasing attention to the inequalities in the American health care system, particularly those based on racism and sexism. The entry of growing numbers of women and minorities into the medical profession helped increase awareness of racist and sexist practices within medicine. Professionals in adolescent medicine worked hard to eliminate gender and racial biases in medical theory and practice, thereby making their services more acceptable and accessible to teenagers from a variety of racial, ethnic, and socioeconomic backgrounds.[5]

Despite the efforts of adolescent medicine experts over the past half-century, our society still remains deeply ambivalent toward teenagers and their proper roles and responsibilities. Although American popular culture caters to teenage tastes and glorifies a youthful appearance, adults often see real adolescents as disruptive, unruly, and in need of adult supervision and management. Even baby boomers, whose experience provided much of the framework for adolescent medicine, tend to overlook their own youthful behavior and view modern teenagers with high degree of distrust and anxiety. In the words of one eighteen-year-old interviewed for a recent oral history of teenagers, most adults "look at teenagers like we're a totally alien life-form."[6]

These contradictory views of teenagers are part of a larger reaction against the alleged "excesses" of the sixties during the past two decades: conservative politicians have called for a return to the "traditional" family values of the 1950s, when sex was reserved for marriage, mothers stayed at home to raise their children, parents prevented their teenagers from having premarital sex or abusing drugs, and children received information about sexual issues from their parents rather than at school or in other institutions outside of the home. Even parents who consider themselves politically liberal nevertheless often believe that the changes of the past thirty years have gone too far and long to return to a period when extramarital sex, drugs, AIDS, gangs, and other social dangers of modern American society did not exist.[7]

Using teenagers as surrogates for broader sociocultural disruptions is not new: this book has demonstrated that discussions about youth and their problems have been one of the major ways that adults have expressed their anxieties about unsettling and disruptive social change. During the Progressive Era, many individuals were anxious about the rise of urban-industrial society, and saw adolescence as the embodiment of a simpler, more primitive period in human history. Likewise, during the middle years of the twentieth century, fears about fascism, communism, and nuclear war focused increasing attention on the mental hygiene of American youth, who were seen as strategic players in defending American institutions from contaminating foreign ideologies. Finally, the social unrest of the 1960s and early 1970s, in which teenagers and young adults played a prominent role, heightened adult anxieties about the potentially disruptive force of American youth.

The reaction against recent social change has undermined much of the optimism about young people and their role as agents of strategic social change that emerged during the 1930s and 1940s. Society has lost sight of the fact that teenagers are not only a trope for the social dangers of modern life, but also can be our link to the future. Instead, adults tend to demonize teenagers, blaming them for the consequences of their own poor choices rather than seeing adolescent health problems as symptoms of larger inequities within American society. The same notions of risk and blame have also been applied to adult health problems as part of a broader shift over the past three decades toward individualistic approaches to health and disease. The historian of medicine Allan Brandt has convincingly argued that "theories of causality of disease may reflect powerful social and political ideologies concerning risk and responsibility." In the case of the modern health care system, disease theories are heavily shaped by conservative political desires to reduce spending on health care for elderly and indigent populations. According to Brandt, over the past thirty years modern bio medicine has linked many diseases like heart disease and cancer to individual "risk-taking behaviors" such as smoking and poor eating habits. This model holds "victims of disease socially accountable for their illness, disability, or even, death." Rather than having a "right" to health care and to a social environment that promotes good health for all Americans, as was the case in the 1960s, individuals now have a "duty" to be healthy by avoiding disease-producing forms of behavior. Infants and young children are an exception to this conceptualization of individual risk and blame for disease because they are usually considered innocent victims of maternal irresponsibility in regards to health.[8]

The place of teenagers on this spectrum of personal responsibility for disease and disability is more equivocal. On the one hand, adults believe that adolescents lack the cognitive ability and maturity needed to make decisions regarding their own welfare. Therefore, teenagers need protection from their own recklessness until they reach an age when they are capable of making more responsible choices. This view is not entirely unfounded given what is known about adolescent developmental psychology. Even those who are sympathetic toward adolescents recognize that cultivating healthy behaviors in youth is often an uphill struggle against teenagers' "personal fables" of invulnerability, invincibility, and denial.[9] On the other hand, adolescents are not viewed in the same way that younger children are and are more likely to encounter adult condemnation when they persist in unhealthy and self-destructive behaviors.

The degree to which an adolescent is blamed for the consequences of his or her behavior also continues to be heavily shaped by stereotypes about race, class, and gender. For example, discussions of inner-city violence and substance abuse among youth of color are frequently edged with a certain degree of fatalism, a sense that these problems are rooted in the alleged depravity of inner-city life and culture. Within this viewpoint, all attempts to remedy the situation of inner-city youth are considered futile. This pessimistic attitude leads many adults to favor highly punitive solutions to the seemingly intractable problems of inner-city minority youth. Rather than addressing factors in the social environment that may be contributing to teenage health problems, sensationalistic stories about an underclass of "super predators" have led to increasing demands that uncontrollable, violent youth be locked up before their behavior threatens the rest of the body politic. Consequently minority youth in general, but black males in particular, are overrepresented in the juvenile justice system.[10]

Solutions for the problems of white middle-class youth can also be harsh. For example, white teenagers are just as likely to be involuntarily committed to state mental health facilities for conduct disorders as are blacks and Hispanics of the same age. White youth, however, particularly those who have private health insurance, are also more likely to get psychiatric treatment for emotional and behavioral disorders, while black, Hispanic, Asian, and Native American adolescents tend to be sent to juvenile correctional facilities for the same kinds of problems. The overrepresentation of lower-class youth of color in the juvenile justice system suggests that white, middle-class Americans are reluctant to apply the same punitive strategies to their own children.[11]

Unwed teenage mothers, especially those who are nonwhite and poor, are similarly depicted as threats to traditional family values and drains on the taxpayers' dollars. Although unwed motherhood does not carry the social stigma it once did, reports about "babies having babies" are still tinged with social fears about the uncontrolled sexuality of young women.[12] Studies of parent-child communication about sexual matters indicates that both boys and girls tend to be poorly informed about sexual issues. However, adolescent girls are much more likely than boys to receive control messages that indicate they should abstain from sexual intercourse and "save themselves for marriage."[13]

Negative stereotypes about adolescents and the alleged threat of uncontrolled teenage behavior to American society have thwarted programs that are designed to help adolescents deal with the many pressures of modern American life in a healthy manner. Politically charged issues like teen pregnancy, sexually transmitted disease, and drug abuse have overshadowed other areas of adolescent health care. As a result, adolescent health care professionals have had a hard time building public and governmental support for teenage health programs.[14]

Hostile views of American teenagers have also hindered the development of adolescent medicine as a field. Because teenagers are considered to be a difficult age group with which to work, adolescent medicine is not a particularly attractive medical specialty for many young physicians. Although professional developments over the past two decades have improved the standing of adolescent medicine, it is still not considered to be as prestigious as organ- or technology-based pediatric subspecialties. Consequently, less than 1 percent of pediatric residents choose to pursue subspecialty training in adolescent medicine.[15]

Depicting young people as "problems" who are responsible for all the ills facing modern society not only is counterproductive, it also fails to recognize the role that adults play in creating the problems and pressures faced by contemporary teenagers. There is strong evidence that physical and sexual abuse of adolescents by adults is the major cause of many of the allegedly "pathological" behaviors exhibited by inner-city teenagers. Adult culpability is particularly high in the area of female teenage sexuality, and those who have done research on this subject have found that rape, incest, and other exploitive adult-teen sexual relationships are responsible for a large percentage of the so-called epidemic of teenage pregnancy and sexually transmitted diseases.[16]

Even when adults are not directly involved, unhealthy teenage behaviors do not exist in a vacuum: instead, they are a mirror of adult attitudes and actions. Teenagers are told to "just say no" to drugs, drinking, and sex, but are constantly bombarded with media images that encourage them to "just say yes" by depicting smoking, drinking, and sexual intercourse as "cool" and "grown-up" behaviors. Rather than seeing teenage behavior as a product of mixed messages within popular culture, adults tend to condemn teenagers for failing to resist larger cultural pressures that affect everyone.

By showing how ambivalent attitudes toward teenagers have shaped adolescent health care, I do not mean to suggest that adolescent health problems are totally manufactured by oppressive adults and have no basis in reality. Teenagers today do encounter serious threats to their health. High-risk behaviors like drug abuse and sexual activity are more dangerous than they were in the past because of the appearance of new diseases like AIDS and because the illegal drugs available today are much more potent than those taken by young people in the 1960s.[17]

As in the past, many modern adolescent health problems are resistant to the "magic bullet" model of treatment used for infectious diseases like measles or chicken pox. Instead, many of the health risks facing adolescents today grow out of a combination of biological, psychological, and social factors, including poverty, peer pressure, street culture, and conflicts with parents. Treating these problems successfully often entails lengthy, multiple sessions with a health care provider with whom the adolescent has developed a confidential, trusting relationship. Even with diseases such as juvenile diabetes or cystic fibrosis, which are caused by a specific biomedical factor, medical therapy can be complicated by the psychological and social pressures of adolescence itself. Research on adolescents' compliance with medical advice indicates that teenagers often reject prescriptions or other therapeutic regimens when treatment is inconvenient, painful, or makes them appear different from their peers.[18]

Finally, there are recent changes in the adolescent life stage that society must address. Americans are currently living in an era where adolescence as a social category appears to be both disappearing and expanding. On the one hand, there is what the child psychologist David Elkind refers to as the "hurried child" syndrome, which is caused by increased exposure to sex, violence, and other adult themes in the mass media and by time-starved, socially ambitious parents who insist that their children become autono-

mous and assume adult responsibilities at ever earlier ages. There have even
been changes in the biological features of adolescence: children are literally
"growing up" faster than ever before, as the average age of sexual maturity
continues to decline.[19] On the other hand, there is the phenomenon of
"boomerang kids," that is, adult children who return to live with parents
because of job loss, divorce, graduate education, loneliness, or the high cost
of housing. Since the late 1960s, the number of adult children living with
parents has more than doubled from 2 million to 5 million, and it is
estimated that nearly 40 percent of all young adults have returned to their
parents' home at least once.[20] Therefore, it appears that the period of economic dependency usually associated with adolescence is expanding into
the twenties, and for some individuals, the thirties and forties. The Society
for Adolescent Medicine responded to these changes in both the biological
and the social features of adolescence by recently adopting a position statement that declared that adolescent medicine covered the ages of ten to
twenty-five, with some members even arguing that the field should be
extended to cover the late twenties and early thirties.[21]

The gravity of contemporary adolescent health problems, the changing
biological and social features of adolescence, and the persistence of stereotypes about race, gender, and class in our society's views about teenagers do
not demonstrate that adolescent medicine has failed. Rather, these facts
indicate that teenagers need a medical field dedicated to their unique needs
now more than ever. Unfortunately, there are not enough trained professionals to meet the needs of America's nation's young people. Currently,
there are approximately 38 million teenagers, with the number expected to
rise as the baby "boomlet" of the 1980s reaches adolescence early in the
next century. Yet there are only 1,400 physicians who are subspecialists in
adolescent medicine, most of whom are pediatricians.[22] Critics of the board
certification movement argue that this number will actually shrink given
the extended period of training (a minimum of three years of fellowship
beyond residency) required before an individual can sit for boards. Furthermore, there are only thirty-eight fellowship programs in the United
States and Canada that train subspecialists in adolescent medicine, each of
which accepts only one or two fellows per year. Critics also argue that
relying solely on subspecialists in adolescent medicine is unrealistic and
impractical, since there are not enough trained subspecialists to serve all of
the teenagers who need care. Even the most ardent supporters of board

certification in adolescent medicine admit that most adolescent problems do not require an adolescent subspecialists' care, and can be handled by a primary health care professional who has had adolescent health care as a component of his or her training program. Therefore, most of those involved in adolescent health care agree that "the vast majority of U.S. teenagers" will not be served by subspecialists in adolescent medicine, but instead will be cared for by family practitioners, pediatricians, internists, nurse practitioners, psychologists, and other health care professionals who, it is hoped, will have been exposed to the health care needs of teenagers during their training.[23]

Unfortunately, many training programs for primary care providers fall short in the area of adolescent health care. Only 50 percent of the medical schools in the United States and Canada have a division of adolescent medicine, and there is evidence that many training institutions are attempting to streamline budgets by phasing out existing adolescent divisions or combining them with other departments. Even schools with adolescent divisions usually treat adolescent health care as a "luxury" rather than an essential part of training all health care providers.[24] This means that many of the primary health care providers in the United States—including pediatricians, family practitioners, internists, and nurse practitioners—have not had adequate exposure to the concepts of adolescent health care, and are therefore poorly equipped to diagnose and treat adolescent health problems. Research exploring health care professionals' competence in diagnosing and treating adolescent health problems indicates that many primary care providers have trouble identifying children and adolescents who have behavioral and emotional problems; are not effective in diagnosing and treating substance abuse problems; and consider themselves poorly trained in important areas of adolescent health such as sexuality, handicaps, endocrine problems, contraception, and psychosocial concerns.[25]

Recent trends in American health care may threaten the future of adolescent medicine even further. It is particularly unclear how adolescent medicine as a specialty will fare under the recent trend to transfer much of the American health care system to managed care. It is likely that individual health care providers will fare well under managed care. Currently, all five clinical disciplines that provide adolescent health care—medicine, nursing, psychology, nutrition, and social work—are considered both primary care providers and specialists under the guidelines of managed care. Adolescent health care providers argue that by delivering both primary and specialty care to teenagers, adolescent medicine can actually help to contain health care costs by avoiding referral to other specialists.[26]

However, managed care may threaten the future of adolescent medicine as a field. Managed care facilities draw patients away from adolescent health divisions in teaching hospitals, thereby eliminating a major source of income for these divisions and with it their ability to train health care providers and conduct research. Directors of hospital-based adolescent divisions are particularly disturbed by the movement toward managed care for Medicaid patients, who make up the bulk of the clientele of inner-city teaching hospitals. The financial stability of adolescent divisions in teaching hospitals will be further weakened if budget cuts are made to the Maternal and Child Health Bureau, one of the major funding sources for research and teaching in adolescent health care. If adolescent divisions are eliminated, it will be less likely that physicians and other health care professionals will be exposed to adolescent health care issues during their training.[27]

Adolescent medicine still has a valuable role to play in American health care and society, and should not be allowed to die out. Professionals in adolescent medicine have been more sensitive than other adults to the voices of young people, and have worked hard to make health care acceptable and accessible to teenagers from a variety of racial and socioeconomic backgrounds. Adolescent medicine has consistently served as an advocate for youth, and has helped to expand the legal rights of minors even in controversial areas such as reproductive health care and substance abuse. Finally, unlike many other medical disciplines, adolescent medicine provides an approach to the teenage patient that recognizes the particular psychological and sociological features of this life stage. Until all adults are willing to assume these responsibilities, those who care about the health and welfare of our nation's youth should recognize and support a medical discipline dedicated to giving young people a "doctor of their own."

Notes

Introduction

1. Marnie Chandler case record (1965), Adolescent/Young Adult Collection, Children's Hospital Archives, Children's Hospital Medical Center, Boston, Massachusetts, hereafter referred to as Children's Hospital Archives. The names of all patients and their families have been changed to protect their privacy. The number in parentheses indicates the year of the patient's first visit to the Unit.

2. Marnie Chandler to Robert P. Masland, 10 January 1966, Marnie Chandler case record.

3. My emphasis on capturing the voice of the teenage patient is modeled after recent scholarship on the social history of medical specialization, which examines how the clients of medical care contributed to the development of new medical disciplines. For an overview of this literature see Judith Walzer Leavitt, "Medicine in Context: A Review Essay of the History of Medicine," *American Historical Review* 95/5 (1990): 1471–1484; Susan Reverby and David Rosner, "Beyond the Great Doctors" in *Health Care in America: Essays in Social History,* ed. Reverby and Rosner (Philadelphia: Temple University Press, 1979), pp. 3–16; and Gerald Grob, "The Social History of Medicine and Disease in American: Problems and Possibilities," *Journal of Social History* 10(1977): 391–409.

4. Halpern, *American Pediatrics: The Social Dynamics of Professionalism, 1880–1980* (Berkeley: University of California Press, 1988), p. 147. Although I disagree with Halpern about the factors that contributed to the emergence of adolescent medicine, I have found her work on the emergence of pediatrics to be very useful.

5. Joseph M. Hawes and N. Ray Hiner, *American Childhood: A Research Guide and Historical Handbook* (Westport, Conn.: Greenwood Press, 1985); David Nasaw, *Children of the City: At Work and at Play* (New York: Oxford University Press, 1985); and Eliott West and Paula Petrik, eds., *Small Worlds: Children and Adolescents in America, 1850–1950* (Lawrence: University of Kansas Press, 1992).

6. For more on the history of American youth culture, see Paula Fass, *The*

Damned and the Beautiful: American Youth in the 1920s (New York: Basic Books, 1977); Joseph Kett, *Rites of Passage: Adolescence in America 1790 to the Present* (New York: Basic Books, 1977); James Gilbert, *A Cycle of Outrage: America's Reaction to the Juvenile Delinquent in the 1950s* (New York: Oxford University Press, 1986); and William Graebner, *Coming of Age in Buffalo: Youth and Authority in the Postwar Era* (Philadelphia: Temple University Press, 1990).

7. Important works on the history and sociology of professionalization include Burton Bledstein, *The Culture of Professionalism* (New York: Norton, 1976); Rosemary Stevens, *American Medicine and the Public Interest* (New Haven: Yale University Press, 1971); Jeffrey L. Berlant, *Profession and Monopoly: A Study of Medicine in the United States and Great Britain* (Berkeley: University of California Press, 1975); Magali Sarfatti Larson, *Rise of Professionalism: A Sociological Analysis* (Berkeley: University of California Press, 1977); Eliot Friedson, *Professional Powers: A Study of the Institutionalization of Formal Knowledge* (Chicago: University of Chicago Press, 1986); and Andrew Abbott, *The System of Professions* (Chicago: University of Chicago Press, 1988).

8. The most comprehensive history of pediatrics in the United States is Halpern, *American Pediatrics*. See also Rima Apple, *Mothers and Medicine: A Social History of Infant Feeding, 1850–1950* (Madison: University of Wisconsin Press, 1988); Richard Meckel, *Save the Babies: American Public Health Reform and the Prevention of Infant Mortality* (Baltimore: Johns Hopkins University Press, 1990); Kathleen W. Jones, "Sentiment and Science: The Late Nineteenth Century Pediatrician as Mother's Advisor," *Journal of Social History* 17 (1983): 85–89; and Dorothy Pawluch, "Transitions in Pediatrics: A Segmental Analysis," *Social Problems* 30/4 (April 1983): 449–465.

9. The other subspecialty areas in pediatrics are cardiology, hematology and oncology, nephrology, neonatal and perinatal medicine, endocrinology, diagnostic laboratory immunology, critical care medicine, and pulmonary disease.

10. Shortell, "Occupational Prestige Differences within the Medical and Allied Health Professions," *Social Science and Medicine* 8 (1974): 2.

11. Apple, *Mothers and Medicine*, pp. 35–36; Halpern, *American Pediatrics*, pp. 48, 51; Meckel, *Save the Babies*, pp. 48–49.

12. Abbott, *The System of Professions;* Charles Bosk, *Forgive and Remember: Managing Medical Failure* (Chicago: University of Chicago Press, 1979); and Allan M. Schwarzbaum, John B. McGrath, and Robert A. Rothman, "The Perception of Prestige Differences among Medical Specialties," *Social Science and Medicine* 7 (1973): 365–371.

13. Information on this clinic is scarce, a further reflection of its marginality in the California medical community. The only article on the clinic is Amelia E. Gates, "The Work of the Adolescent Clinic of Stanford University Medical School," *Archives of Pediatrics* 35 (1918): 236–243. There is also passing reference to the clinic

in the Annual Reports of the Children's Clinic of Lane Hospital, which are located in the University Archives, Lane Medical Library, Stanford University Medical Center, Stanford, Calif.

14. For more on the training program in adolescent medicine at Boston Children's Hospital and its impact on the growth in the number of adolescent units during the 1960s, see *Annual Reports of the Adolescent Unit,* Children's Hospital Archives; and J. Roswell Gallagher, "The Origins, Development, and Goals of Adolescent Medicine," *Journal of Adolescent Health Care* 3 (1982): 57–63.

15. A notable exception is the Adolescent Unit at Children's Hospital Medical Center in Cincinnati, which was directed by Dr. Joseph L. Rauh from its creation in 1960 until 1997. Continuity of leadership, combined with Rauh's sensitivity to historical issues and service as historian for the Society for Adolescent Medicine, has ensured the preservation of historical materials related to not only the Adolescent Unit in Cincinnati but also the Society for Adolescent Medicine. I am grateful to Dr. Rauh for allowing me to examine these documents. Even the Cincinnati records are not as rich as those at Boston, however, and since Rauh modeled his work in Cincinnati after that of Gallagher, it made sense to focus on the Boston clinic. To help compensate for this lack of written primary documents outside Gallagher's clinic, I have conducted oral histories with Rauh and other physicians who trained with Gallagher and his associates at Boston Children's Hospital and created clinics of their own in other areas of the country.

16. This was the only clinic at which it was possible to do such an in-depth study of patient case records. The Adolescent Unit at Boston Children's Hospital was the only adolescent clinic that filed patient records within the clinic itself, rather than interfiling them with other pediatric records. Since other adolescent clinics have not kept lists of the names of patients that are no longer current, it has been impossible to retrieve adolescent patient records. Nevertheless, because the Adolescent Unit at the Boston Children's Hospital was the first such facility in North America, and served as a fountainhead for similar programs, the records are a good source of evaluating how adolescent medicine was initially sold to parents and teenagers.

17. For more information on the current state of adolescent health in the United States, see U.S. Congress, Office of Technology Assessment, *Adolescent Health— Volume I: Summary and Policy Options,* OTA-H-468 (Washington, D.C.: U.S. Government Printing Office, April 1991); and Janet E. Gans, *America's Adolescents: How Healthy Are They?* (Chicago: American Medical Association, 1990).

1. The Professional and Social Roots of a Medical Discipline

1. G. Stanley Hall, *Adolescence: Its Psychology and Its Relation to Physiology, Anthropology, Sociology, Sex, Crime, Religion, and Education* (New York: D. Appleton and Co., 1904).

2. Dorothy Ross, *G. Stanley Hall: The Psychologist as Prophet* (Chicago and London: The University of Chicago Press, 1972), p. 336n48.

3. Joseph Kett, *Rites of Passage: Adolescence in America, 1790 to the Present* (New York: Basic Books, 1977), pp. 215–244.

4. G. Stanley Hall, "Adolescence: The Need of a New Field of Medical Practice," *Monthly Cyclopædia of Practical Medicine* n.s. 8/6 (June 1905): 242.

5. William P. Dewees, cited in Richard Meckel, *Save the Babies: American Public Health Reform and the Prevention of Infant Mortality, 1850–1929* (Baltimore and London: Johns Hopkins University Press, 1990), pp. 45–46.

6. Arthur Tenney Holbrook, " quoted in Charlotte G. Borst, *Catching Babies: The Professionalization of Childbirth, 1870–1920* (Cambridge, Mass.: Harvard University Press, 1995), p. 139. Borst adds that the image of the specialist as professionally suspect persisted well into the twentieth century. For example, as late as the 1920s, L. H. Preston, former president of the Wisconsin Medical Society, argued that "medical graduates who took up specialties directly after graduation were untrustworthy." Pelton, quoted in Borst, *Catching Babies*, p. 139.

7. U.S. President's Commission on the Health Needs of the Nation, *Building America's Health*, cited in Sydney Halpern, *American Pediatrics: The Social Dynamics of Professionalism, 1880–1980* (Berkeley, Calif.: University of California Press, 1988), p. 2.

8. Jacobi, "An Address on the Claims of Pediatric Medicine," *Transactions of the American Medical Association* 31 (1880): 709–710. Twenty years later, Jacobi continued to lament rampant overspecialization "which has contributed much to narrow the scientific, mental, and moral horizon of many a young man who means to become a wealthy and famous specialist without ever having been a physician." Jacobi, quoted in Halpern, *American Pediatrics*, p. 53.

9. According to Halpern, infant feeding "lent pediatrics a scientific aura that helped justify specialists' claim to unique expertise." Halpern, *American Pediatrics*, pp. 63–65. See also Meckel, *Save the Babies*, pp. 48–49; Rima Apple, *Mothers and Medicine: A Social History of Infant Feeding, 1850-1950* (Madison: University of Wisconsin Press, 1987); and Kathleen W. Jones, "Sentiment and Science: The Late Nineteenth Century Pediatrician as Mother's Advisor," *Journal of Social History* 17 (1983): 85–89.

10. Meckel, *Save the Babies*, p. 103.

11. Robert Wiebe observes in his classic book on the history of progressivism that protection of children was *the* central theme that united the various strands of the Progressive movement. Wiebe, *The Search for Order, 1877–1920* (New York: Hill and Wang, 1967), p. 169. See also Meckel, *Save the Babies*, pp. 101–103; and Halpern, *American Pediatrics*, pp. 73–74.

12. Jacobi, quoted in Dorothy Pawluch, "Transitions in Pediatrics: A Segmental Analysis," *Social Problems* 30/4 (April 1983): 451. See also Meckel, *Save the Babies*,

pp. 46–47. The reformulation of childhood as a distinct life stage was part of a larger trend toward greater age consciousness during the late nineteenth century. See Kett, *Rites of Passage,* pp. 11–14; and Howard P. Chudacoff, *How Old Are You?: Age Consciousness in American Culture* (Princeton: Princeton University Press, 1989). Chudacoff demonstrates that similar arguments were used to justify the creation of geriatrics as a medical specialty during the early twentieth century.

13. Halpern, *American Pediatrics,* pp. 80–109. For more on the history of child development, see Milton J. E. Senn, "Insights on the Child Development Movement," *Monographs of the Society for Research in Child Development* 40/3–4 (August 1975): 1–99; Steven L. Schlossman, "Philanthropy and the Gospel of Child Development," *History of Education Quarterly* 21 (1981): 275–299; Hamilton Cravens, "Child-Saving in the Age of Professionalism, 1915–1930," in *American Childhood: A Research Guide and Historical Handbook,* ed. Joseph M. Hawes and N. Ray Hiner (Westport, Conn.: Greenwood Press, 1985), pp. 405–436; idem, *Before Home Start: The Iowa Station and America's Children* (Chapel Hill, N.C.: University of North Carolina Press, 1993); Alice Smuts, "Science Discovers the Child, 1893–1935: A History of the Early Scientific Study of Children" (Ph.D. diss., University of Michigan, 1995); and Julia Grant, *Raising Baby by the Book: The Education of American Mothers, 1800–1960* (New Haven: Yale University Press, 1998).

14. Harry F. Dowling, *Fighting Infection: Conquests of the Twentieth Century* (Cambridge: Cambridge University Press, 1977); and Paul B. Beeson, "Changes in Medical Therapy during the Past Half Century," *Medicine* 59 (1980): 79–85.

15. United States Bureau of the Census, *Historical Statistics of the United States: Colonial Times to the Present,* cited in Dorothy Pawluch, "Transitions in Pediatrics," p. 455.

16. For more on the history of federally funded medical research, see Stephen Strickland, *Politics, Science, and Dread Disease: A Short History of United States Medical Research* (Cambridge, Mass.: Harvard University Press, 1972); and Victoria Harden, *Inventing the NIH: Federal Biomedical Research Policy, 1887–1937* (Baltimore: Johns Hopkins University Press, 1986).

17. U.S. President's Commission on the Health Needs of the Nation, *Building America's Health,* cited in Halpern, *American Pediatrics,* p. 2.

18. Halpern, *American Pediatrics,* p. 82.

19. Pawluch, "Transitions in Pediatrics," pp. 456–457.

20. Ibid., p. 457.

21. Theodore M. Brown, "American Medicine and Primary Care: The Last Half-Century," in *The Training of Primary Physicians,* ed. Stephen J. Kunitz (Lanham, Md.: University Press of America, 1986), p. 9.

22. For more on popular images of physicians during the post–World War II era, see John C. Burnham, "American Medicine's Gold Age: What Happened to It?" *Science* 215 (March 19, 1982): 1474–1479; Marcel C. LaFollette, *Making Science Our*

Own: Public Images of Science, 1910–1955 (Chicago: University of Chicago Press, 1990), pp. 169–171; and Robert S. Alley, "The Medical Melodrama," in *TV Genres: A Handbook and Reference Guide,* ed. Brian G. Rose (Westport, Conn.: Greenwood Press, 1985), pp. 73–90. Surveys of patients' opinions on medical care include Ernest Dichter, *A Psychological Study of the Doctor-Patient Relationship* (California Medical Association, 1950); idem, "Do Your Patients Really Like You?" *New York State Journal of Medicine* 54 (1954): 222–226; and Eliot Friedson, *Patients' Views of Medical Practice* (New York: Russell Sage Foundation, 1961).

23. Halpern, *American Pediatrics,* pp. 110–127.

24. Ibid., pp. 118–121.

25. Pawluch, "Transitions in Pediatrics," p. 459; and Halpern, *American Pediatrics,* pp. 128–148.

26. Charles D. May, quoted in Halpern, *American Pediatrics,* pp. 140–141.

27. Pawluch, "Transitions in Pediatrics," p. 459.

28. For more on the history of the Commonwealth Fund, see A. McGehee Harvey and Susan L. Abrams, *"For the Welfare of Mankind": The Commonwealth Fund and American Medicine* (Baltimore: Johns Hopkins University Press, 1986).

29. Joan Jacobs Brumberg, *The Body Project: An Intimate History of American Girls* (New York: Random House, 1997), pp. 3–25.

30. Susan M. Juster and Maris A. Vinovskis, "Adolescence in Nineteenth-Century America," in *Encyclopedia of Adolescence,* 2 vols., ed. Richard Lerner, Anne C. Petersen, and Jeanne Brooks-Gunn (New York: Garland, 1991), p. 699. In fact, age classifications for all life stages were rather vague until the early twentieth century. See Chudacoff, *How Old Are You.* There were similar trends in the history of European youth. See John R. Gillis, *Youth and History: Tradition and Change in European Age Relations, 1770–Present* (New York: Academic Press, 1974), Michael Mitterauer, *A History of Youth,* trans. Graeme Dunphy (Oxford and Cambridge: Blackwell, 1992); and John Neubauer, *The Fin-de-Siècle Culture of Youth* (New Haven: Yale University Press, 1992).

31. The description of adolescence as a "psychosocial moratorium" comes from Erik Erikson's classic work in adolescent developmental psychology. Erik Erikson, *Identity: Youth and Crisis* (New York: Norton, 1968), p. 156.

32. For more on middle-class identity and gender roles, see Barbara Welter, "The Cult of True Womanhood," *American Quarterly* 18 (Summer 1966): 151–174; Nancy F. Cott, *The Bonds of Womanhood: "Woman's Sphere" in New England, 1780–1835* (New Haven: Yale University Press, 1977); Carroll Smith-Rosenberg, *Disorderly Conduct: Visions of Gender in Victorian America* (New York: Oxford University Press, 1985); Mary Ryan, *Cradle of the Middle Class: The Family in Oneida County, New York, 1790–1865* (Cambridge: Cambridge University Press, 1981); and Christine Stansell, *City of Women: Sex and Class in New York, 1789–1860* (Urbana and Chicago: University of Illinois Press, 1987).

33. For examples of this perspective, see Issac Ray, quoted in Kett, *Rites of Passage*; and Orson Fowler, quoted in Kett, *Rites of Passage*, pp. 134–135.

34. Brumberg, *The Body Project*, pp. 3–25.

35. Kett, *Rites of Passage*, p. 138; Joseph M. Hawes, "The Strange History of Female Adolescence in the United States," *Journal of Psychohistory* 13/1 (Summer 1985): 51–63; and Anne M. Boylan, "Growing up Female in Young America," in *American Childhood*, ed. Hawes and Hiner, p. 164.

36. Kett, *Rites of Passage*, chap. 5; Stansell, *City of Women*, pp. 193–216.

37. Hall, *Adolescence*, 2:428.

38. Jackson Lears, *No Place of Grace: Antimodernism and the Transformation of American Culture, 1890–1920* (New York: Pantheon Books, 1981).

39. Hall, *Adolescence*, 2:747; Lears, *No Place of Grace*, pp. 147–148, 247–251.

40. Stansell, *City of Women*, pp. 83–101; Kathy Peiss, *Cheap Amusements: Working Women and Leisure in Turn-of-the-Century New York* (Philadelphia: Temple University Press, 1986), pp. 11–33.

41. For more on the history of attempts to control working-class girls' sexuality, see Peiss, *Cheap Amusements*; Constance A. Nathanson, *Dangerous Passage: The Social Control of Sexuality in Women's Adolescence* (Philadelphia: Temple University Press, 1991); Regina G. Kunzel, *Fallen Women, Problem Girls: Unmarried Mothers and the Professionalization of Social Work, 1890–1945* (New Haven: Yale University Press, 1993); Mary E. Odem, *Delinquent Daughters: Protecting and Policing Adolescent Female Sexuality in the United States, 1885–1920* (Chapel Hill: University of North Carolina Press, 1995); and Ruth Alexander, *The "Girl Problem": Female Sexual Delinquency in New York, 1900–1930* (Ithaca: Cornell University Press, 1995).

42. Hall, *Adolescence*, 1:xiv, 342.

43. For more on Progressive-era reforms for adolescents, see Peiss, *Cheap Amusements*; Kett, *Rites of Passage*, pp. 215–244; and Paul Boyer, *Urban Masses and Moral Order in America, 1820–1920* (Cambridge, Mass.: Harvard University Press, 1978).

44. U.S. Bureau of the Census, *Fourteenth Census of the United States*, rev. ed., cited in Chudacoff, *How Old Are You*, pp. 72, 108–109. See also Grace Palladino, *Teenagers: An American History* (New York: Basic Books, 1996), pp. 34–46.

45. Peiss, *Cheap Amusements*; Alexander, *The "Girl Problem."*

46. Peiss, *Cheap Amusements*, p. 184. James R. McGovern was the first to observe that the "revolution in manners and morals began before World War I, not in the 1920s." McGovern, "The American Woman's Pre–World War I Freedom in Manners and Morals," *Journal of American History* 55 (September 1968): 315–333.

47. Winthrop D. Lane, quoted in Allan Brandt, *No Magic Bullet: A Social History of Venereal Disease in the United States since 1880* (New York: Oxford University Press, 1985, 1987), p. 80. See also Alexander, *The "Girl Problem,"* p. 21.

48. For more on the youth culture of the 1920s, see Paula Fass, *The Damned and the Beautiful: American Youth in the 1920s* (New York: Oxford University Press, 1977); and Beth Bailey, *From Front Porch to Back Seat: Courtship in Twentieth-Century America* (Baltimore: Johns Hopkins University Press, 1988).

49. For more on the history of high schools and the rise of peer culture, see Chudacoff, *How Old Are You*, pp. 98–108; Palladino, *Teenagers*, pp. 2–15; Reed Ueda, *Avenues to Adulthood: The Origins of the High School and Social Mobility in an American Suburb* (Cambridge: Cambridge University Press, 1987); and John Modell, *Into One's Own: From Youth to Adulthood in the United States, 1920–1975* (Berkeley: University of California Press, 1989). William Graebner points out that even in the post–World War II era, when high school became a nearly universal experience for most adolescents, high school students divided themselves into a number of different subcultures based on race, ethnicity, and social class. Nevertheless, Graebner observes that these various teen subcultures "were also bound by certain universal stories" and therefore it is possible to speak of a more general youth culture at this time. Graebner, *Coming of Age in Buffalo: Youth and Authority in the Postwar Era* (Philadelphia: Temple University Press, 1990), pp. 6–7.

50. Alexander, *The Girl Problem*, p. 20; Peiss, *Cheap Amusements*, p. 184.

51. McAdoo, "The Frightful Pace of Modern Jazz," *Ladies Home Journal* 44 (October 19, 1927), pp. 22–23; Alexander, *The "Girl Problem,"* pp. 59–60. For more on the Klan's attempts to regulate youth culture at this time, see Kenneth T. Jackson, *The Ku Klux Klan in the City* (New York: Oxford University Press, 1967); and Kathleen M. Blee, *Women of the Klan: Racism and Gender in the 1920s* (Berkeley: University of California Press, 1991).

52. United States Children's Bureau, *Some Facts about Juvenile Delinquency*, quoted in James Gilbert, *A Cycle of Outrage: America's Reaction to the Juvenile Delinquent in the 1950s* (New York: Oxford University Press, 1986), pp. 66–67.

53. Leroy Ashby, "Partial Promises and Semi-Visible Youths: The Depression and World War II," in *American Childhood*, ed. Hawes and Hiner, p. 508.

54. Richard A. Reiman, *The New Deal and American Youth: Ideas and Ideals in a Depression Decade* (Athens: University of Georgia Press, 1992), pp. 34–35.

55. Erik Erikson, "Hitler's Imagery and German Youth," *Psychiatry* 5 (November 1942): 475–493.

56. J. Edgar Hoover, quoted in Gilbert, *A Cycle of Outrage*, p. 72.

57. Quoted in Reiman, *The New Deal and American Youth*, p. 29. Geoffrey Smith demonstrates that the use of disease metaphors to describe threats to national security posed by immigrants, women, homosexuals, and other "outsiders" was common during this period. See Smith, "National Security and Personal Isolation: Sex, Gender, and Disease in the Cold-War United States," *International History Review* 14/2 (May 1992): 307–337.

58. Sol Cohen, "The Mental Hygiene Movement, The Development of Personal-

ity, and the School: The Medicalization of American Education," *History of Education Quarterly* 23/2 (1983): 126. For more on American mental hygienists' reaction to Freud, see Nathan G. Hale's two-volume history: *Freud and the Americans: The Beginnings of Psychoanalysis in the United States, 1876–1917* (New York: Oxford University Press, 1971); and *The Rise and Crisis of Psychoanalysis in the United States: Freud and the Americans, 1917–1985* (New York: Oxford University Press, 1995).

59. William A. White, quoted in Kathleen W. Jones, *Taming the Troublesome Child: American Families, Child Guidance, and the Limits of Psychiatric Authority* (Cambridge: Harvard University Press, forthcoming).

60. Jones, *Taming the Troublesome Child*. See also Smuts, "Science Discovers the Child"; and Margo Horn, *Before It's Too Late: The Child Guidance Movement in the United States, 1922–1945* (Philadelphia: Temple University Press, 1989).

61. For more on the history of parent education, see Grant, *Raising Baby by the Book;* Smuts, "Science Discovers the Child"; Roberta Lyn Wollons, "Women Educating Women: The Child Study Association as Women's Culture," in *Changing Education: Women as Radicals and Conservators,* ed. Joyce Antler and Sari Knopp Biklen (Albany: State University of New York Press, 1990), pp. 51–67; Steven L. Schlossman, "Before Home Start: Notes toward a History of Parent Education in America, 1897–1929," *Harvard Educational Review* 46/3 (August, 1976): 436–467; and idem, "Perils of Popularization: The Founding of *Parents Magazine*," *Monographs of the Society for Research in Child Development* 50/4–5 (1985): 65–77.

62. Stephen J. Cross's biography of Frank points to "a substantial body of tributes by professional colleagues—notably child development researchers, gerontologists, and anthropologists, psychiatrists, and social psychologists in the interdisciplinary field of 'culture and personality'" that clearly demonstrate that "Frank played an instrumental role in shaping the fields with which his work as a foundation officer brought him in contact." Cross, "Designs for Living: Lawrence K. Frank and the Progressive Legacy in American Social Science" (Ph.D. diss., Johns Hopkins University, 1994), p. vii. William Graebner also describes Frank as "perhaps the most influential figure" in the child development and parent education movements. Graebner, *The Engineering of Consent: Democracy and Authority in Twentieth-Century America* (Madison: University of Wisconsin Press, 1987), p. 130. Frank's influence is also apparent from personal testimonies of child development researchers, collected in the Milton J. E. Senn Oral History Interviews in Child Development, History of Medicine Division, National Library of Medicine, National Institutes of Health, Bethesda, Md. See also Senn, "Insights on the Child Development Movement."

63. Lawrence K. Frank, "Society as the Patient," *American Journal of Sociology* 42 (1936): 335–344.

64. Lawrence K. Frank, "Introduction: Adolescence as a Period of Transition,"

in *Forty-third Yearbook of the National Society for the Study of Education, Part I: Adolescence* (Chicago, Ill.: Department of Education, University of Chicago, 1944) [hereafter referred to as *Forty-third Yearbook*], p. 7.

65. William Fielding Ogburn, *Social Change: With Respect to Culture and Original Nature* (1922; New York: Viking, 1952).

66. Margaret Mead, "Social Change and Cultural Surrogates," *Journal of Educational Sociology* 14 (1940): 92–110; and idem, "Problems of the Atomic Age," *The Survey* 85 (July, 1949): 385.

67. Lawrence K. Frank, "The Reorientation of Education," *Mental Hygiene* 23 (1939), reprinted in Frank, *Society as the Patient: Essays on Culture and Personality* (New Brunswick, N.J.: Rutgers University Press, 1948), pp. 250–251.

68. Frank, "The Adolescent and the Family," in *Forty-third Yearbook*, p. 240.

69. Erikson, *Childhood and Society*, pp. 227–229. Frank's professional interaction with Erikson is described by Graebner, *The Engineering of Consent*, pp. 131–132; and Cravens, *Before Home Start*, pp. 164–165, 244–245.

70. Graebner, *The Engineering of Consent*.

71. Frank, quoted in Graebner, *The Engineering of Consent*, pp. 134–135.

72. Adler's work on the inferiority complex is best expressed in Adler, *The Neurotic Constitution: Outlines of a Comparative Individualistic Psychology and Psychotherapy*, trans. Bernard Glueck and John E. Lind (Salem, N.H.: Ayer Co., 1983, 1926); and idem, *The Practice and Theory of Individual Psychology*, trans. P. Radin (New York: Harcourt, Brace; London: K. Paul, Trench, Trubner, 1932). American psychiatrists' reaction to Adler are described in Hale, *The Rise and Crisis of Psychoanalysis*, pp. 75, 79.

73. Lawrence K. Frank, "Certain Problems of Puberty and Adolescence," *Journal of Pediatrics* 19/3 (September 1941): 298–299.

74. Grant, *Raising Baby by the Book*; Smuts, "Science Discovers the Child." Both Grant and Smuts look at parents' letters to Gesell, which describe parents' dismay when their children did not develop according to developmental norms. These letters are deposited in the Arnold Gesell Papers, Library of Congress, Washington, D.C.

75. Lawrence K. Frank, "Adolescence and Public Health," *American Journal of Public Health* 31 (1941): 1144.

76. The psychoanalyst Hilde Bruch was the first to suggest that Frölich's syndrome was extremely rare, and argued that obesity in boys and girls was usually due to psychodynamic conflicts rather than to hormonal disturbances. Bruch, "The Constructive Use of Ignorance," in E. James Anthony, *Explorations in Child Psychiatry* (New York, 1975), pp. 247–264. For more on the history of endocrinology during this period, see Joan Jacobs Brumberg, *Fasting Girls: The Emergence of Anorexia Nervosa as a Modern Disease* (Cambridge, Mass.: Harvard University Press, 1988), pp. 205-230; Diana Long Hall, "Biology, Sex Hormones, and Sexism

in the 1920s," *Philosophical Forum* 5 (1974): 81–96; Merriley Borell, "Organo-therapy and the Emergence of Reproductive Endocrinology," *Journal of the History of Biology* 18 (1986): 1–30; and Nelly Oudshoorn, *Beyond the Natural Body: An Archaeology of Sex Hormones* (London and New York: Routledge, 1994).

77. Frank, "Certain Problems of Puberty and Adolescence," p. 296.

78. Ibid., p. 297; Frank, "Psycho-cultural Approaches to Medical Care," *Journal of Social Issues* 13 (1952): 31–44.

79. Frank, "The Reorientation of Education," p. 251; Frank, "Psychocultural Approaches to Medical Care," pp. 53–54.

80. For more on the history of research in child development funded by the LSRM and other private foundations during this period, see Senn, "Insights on the Child Development Movement in the United States"; Grant, *Raising Baby by the Book*; Schlossman, "Philanthropy and the Gospel of Child Development"; Cravens, *Before Head Start*; idem, "Child-Saving in the Age of Professionalism, 1915–1930," pp. 405–436; and Smuts, "Science Discovers the Child."

81. Glen Elder has noted the predominance of white middle-class subjects in adolescent growth and development studies during this period, but does not comment on the significance of this fact. Glen H. Elder, Jr., *Children of the Great Depression: Social Change in Life Experience* (Chicago: University of Chicago Press, 1974). Alice Smuts notes the problems of using white, middle-class children as the norm for child and adolescent growth and development. See Smuts, "Science Discovers the Child."

82. For more on this "crisis of masculinity" during the 1930s, see Barbara Melosh, *Engendering Culture: Manhood and Womanhood in New Deal Public Art and Theater* (Washington, D.C.: Smithsonian Institution Press, 1991); Robert McElvaine, *The Great Depression* (New York: Times Press, 1984); and Susan Ware, *Holding Their Own: American Women in the 1930s* (Boston: Twayne Publishers, 1982).

83. For concerns about gender roles during World War II, see Smith, "National Security," pp. 312–313; Allan Bérubé, *Coming Out under Fire: The History of Gay Men and Women in World War II* (New York: Free Press, 1990); Elaine Tyler May, *Homeward Bound: American Families in the Cold War Era* (New York: Basic Books, 1988); Sonya Michel, "American Women and the Discourse of the Democratic Family in World War II," in *Behind the Lines: Gender and the Two World Wars*, ed. Margaret Randolph Higonnet et al. (New Haven: Yale University Press, 1987).

84. The findings of these studies are summarized in Elder, *Children of the Great Depression*. However, Elder is as uncritical of gender assumptions in child and adolescent development research as he is of the slant toward white, middle-class subjects. Grace Palladino demonstrates how these concerns were translated into advice literature for parents in *Teenagers*, pp. 17–33.

85. Studies in this area include Frank Shuttleworth, "Sexual Maturation and the

Physical Growth of Girls Aged Six to Nineteen," *Monographs of the Society for Research in Child Development* 2/5 (1937); William Greulich and Frank Shuttleworth, "A Handbook of Methods for the Study of Adolescent Children," *Monographs of the Society for Research in Child Development* 3/2 (1938); Greulich, "Somatic and Endocrine Studies of Pubertal and Adolescent Boys," *Monographs of the Society for Research in Child Development* 7/3 (1942); idem, "Physical Changes in Adolescence," in *Forty-third Yearbook*, pp. 8–32; Greulich and H. Thoms, "The Growth and Development of the Pelvis in Individual Girls before, during, and after Puberty," *Yale Journal of Biology and Medicine* 17 (1944): 91–97; P. E. Kubitschek, "Sexual Development of Boys with Special Reference to Appearance of Secondary Sexual Characters and Their Relationship to Structural and Personality Types," *Journal of Nervous and Mental Disease* 76 (November 1932): 425–451; Herbert Stolz, *Somatic Development of Adolescent Boys* (New York: Macmillan, 1951); Herbert and Lois Meek Stolz, "Adolescent Problems Related to Somatic Variations," in *Forty-third Yearbook*, pp. 80–99; Nancy Bayley and Read D. Tuddenbaum, "Adolescent Changes in Body Build," in *Forty-third Yearbook*, pp. 33–55; and Nathan Shock, "Physiological Changes in Adolescence," in *Forty-third Yearbook*, pp. 56–79.

86. Paul H. Mussen and Mary Cover Jones, "Self-conceptions, Motivations, and Interpersonal Attitudes of Late- and Early-Maturing Boys," *Child Development* 28 (1957): 243–256; idem, "The Behavior-Inferred Motivations of Late- and Early-Maturing boys," *Child Development* 29 (1958): 61–67; Nancy Bayley and Mary Cover Jones, "Some Personality Characteristics of Boys with Retarded Skeletal Maturity," *Psychological Bulletin* 38 (1941): 603; F. J. Curran and J. Frosch, "Body Image in Boys," *Journal of Genetic Psychology* 60 (March 1942): 37–60; W. A. Schonfeld, "Deficient Development of Masculinity; Psychosomatic Problem of Adolescence," *American Journal of Diseases of Children* 79 (January 1950): 17–29; and idem, "Inadequate Masculine Physique as Factor in Personality Development of Adolescent Boys," *Psychosomatic Medicine* 12 (January-February 1950): 49–54.

87. Stolz and Stolz, "Adolescent Problems Related to Somatic Variations"; and George E. Gardner, "Sex Behavior of Adolescents in Wartime," *Annals of the American Academy of Political and Social Science: Adolescents in Wartime* 236 (1944): 60–66.

88. George J. Mohr, "Sexual Education of the Adolescent," *Journal of Pediatrics* 19 (1941): 387–391; and Douglas A. Thom, "Psychologic Aspects of Adolescence," *Journal of Pediatrics* 19 (1941): 392–402.

89. Shock, "Physiological Changes at Puberty," p. 57; Stolz and Stolz, "Adolescent Problems Related to Somatic Variations," pp. 84–89; P. Blos, *The Adolescent Personality* (New York: Appleton-Century, 1941); H. R. Stolz, "Shorty Comes to Terms with Himself," *Progressive Education* 17 (1940): 405–411; C. P. Stone and R. G. Barker, "Aspects of Personality and Intelligence in Postmenarcheal and Pre-

menarcheal Girls of the Same Chronological Age," *Journal of Comparative Psychology* 23 (1937): 439–445; C. B. Zachry and M. Lightly, *Emotion and Conduct in Adolescence* (New York: Appleton-Century, 1940); L. M. Bayer and S. Reichard, "Androgyny, Weight, and Personality," *Psychosomatic Medicine* 13 (1951): 358–374; Hilda Bruch, "The Psychology of Obesity," *Cincinnati Journal of Medicine* 31 (1950): 273–281; Nancy Bayley and Mary Cover Jones, "Some Personality Characteristics of Boys with Retarded Skeletal Maturity," *Psychological Bulletin* 38 (1941): 603; F. J. Curran and J. Frosch, "Body Image in Boys," *Journal of Genetic Psychology* 60 (March 1942): 37–60; Schonfeld, "Deficient Development of Masculinity"; idem, "Inadequate Masculine Physique."

90. Bayley and Tuddenbaum, "Adolescent Changes in Body Build," p. 53.

91. Stolz, *Somatic Development of Adolescent Boys,* chap. 18.

92. Stolz and Stolz, "Adolescent Problems Related to Somatic Variations."

93. Leonard G. Rowntree, Kenneth H. McGill, and Thomas I. Edwards, "Causes of Rejection and Incidence of Defects among 18 and 19 year old Selective Service Registrants," *JAMA* 123/4 (September 25, 1943): 181–185; Norman R. Ingraham, "Health Problems of the Adolescent Period," *Annals of the American Academy of Political and Social Science: Adolescents in Wartime* 236 (1944): 117–127; Thomas K. Cureton, "The Unfitness of Young Men in Motor Fitness," *JAMA* 123/2 (September 11, 1943): 69–74; J. Roswell Gallagher and Lucien Brouha, "Physical Fitness: Its Evaluation and Significance," *JAMA* 125/12 (July 22, 1944): 834–838; and E. Allen, "Problems in Adolescence," *Western Journal of Surgery* 50 (September 1942): 476–478.

94. Lawrence K. Frank, "Physiological and Emotional Problems of Adolescence," *American Journal of Public Health* 35 (1945): 578.

95. Lillian Cottrell, "Understanding the Adolescent: The Adolescent and His Emotional Reaction to Illness," *American Journal of Nursing* 45 (1946): 181–183; S. Gibson, "Athletic Activity at Puberty, with Special Reference to Cardiac and Tuberculosis Patients," *Journal of Pediatrics* 19 (Sept. 1941): 382–386; S. Benjamin, "Psychosomatic Phase in Management of Diabetes Mellitus," *Medical Annals of the District of Columbia* 16 (July 1945): 361–365; H. Bruch, "Physiologic and Psychologic Interrelationships in Diabetes in Children," *Psychosomatic Medicine* 11 (1949): 200–210; Ephraim Shorr, "Endocrine Problems in Adolescence," *Journal of Pediatrics* 19 (September 1941): 327–346; H. C. Stuart, "Symposium on Clinical Advances: The Adolescent," *Pediatric Clinics of North America* 1 (May 1954): 467–481; N. Arnold, "Adjustments of Adolescents to Poliomyelitis," *Journal of Pediatrics* 45 (September 1954): 347–361; L. H. Taboroff and W. H. Brown, "Study of Personality Patterns of Children and Adolescents with Peptic Ulcer Syndrome," *American Journal of Orthopsychiatry* 24 (July 1954): 602–610; and J. Roswell Gallagher, "Rest and Restriction: Conflict with Adolescent's Development," *American Journal of Public Health* 46 (November 1956): 1424–1428.

96. Gibson, "Athletic Activity at Puberty."

97. Shorr, "Endocrine Problems in Adolescence."

98. Brumberg, *The Body Project,* pp. 59–94.

2. J. Roswell Gallagher and the Origins of Adolescent Medicine

1. J. Roswell Gallagher, oral history interview by Heather Munro Prescott, 28 December 1989, tape recording deposited in Boston Children's Hospital Archives; "J. Roswell Gallagher, M.D.: Reminiscences," videotape interview with J. Roswell Gallagher, Robert P. Masland, Jr., Esterann Grace, and Jean Emans by Prescott and Joseph L. Rauh, 25 October 1993. Tape deposited in Children's Hospital Archives and available from JLR. See also Heather Munro Prescott, Joseph L. Rauh, and Robert P. Masland, Jr., "In Memoriam: James Roswell Gallagher, 1903–1995," *Journal of Adolescent Health* 18/1 (January 1996): 2–3.

2. J. Roswell Gallagher, "Pediatrics and the Adolescent: Remarks on Receiving the C. Anderson Aldrich Award," *Pediatrics* 51/3 (March, 1973): 458.

3. "J. Roswell Gallagher, M.D.: Reminiscences."

4. Charles A. Janeway, "Pediatrics and the Adolescent. Presentation of the C. Anderson Aldrich Award to J. Roswell Gallagher," *Pediatrics* 51/3 (March 1973): 455.

5. Claude Moore Fuess, *Independent Schoolmaster* (Boston: Little, Brown, 1952), p. 177.

6. Claude Moore Fuess, "Peirson Sterling Page," *Phillips Bulletin* (July, 1939): 12; Frederick S. Allis, *Youth from Every Quarter: A Bicentennial History of Phillips Academy, Andover* (Hanover, N.H.: University Press of New England, 1979), p. 466.

7. Gallagher, "The Academy's Department of Health," *Phillips Bulletin* 31 (1936): 9.

8. Gallagher, "The Health Examination of Adolescents," *New England Journal of Medicine* 229 (1943): 316. For more on infection and mortality rates from tuberculosis during this period, and the link between class and infection rates, see Barbara Bates, *Bargaining for Life: A Social History of Tuberculosis, 1876–1938* (Philadelphia: University of Pennsylvania Press, 1992); and Georgina D. Feldberg, *Disease and Class: Tuberculosis and the Shaping of North American Society* (New Brunswick, N.J.: Rutgers University Press, 1995).

9. Gallagher, "The Academy's Department of Health," p. 9.

10. Gallagher, *Understanding Your Son's Adolescence* (Boston: Little, Brown, 1951), pp. 30–33. Although this book was published in 1951, it was based on Gallagher's research at Phillips Academy during the 1930s and 1940s.

11. Gallagher, "The Academy's Department of Health," p. 12.

12. E. Anthony Rotundo, *American Manhood: Transformations in Masculinity from the Revolution to the Modern Era* (New York: Basic Books, 1993), pp. 257–258.

13. Gallagher, "The Academy's Department of Health," pp. 9–10.

14. Ibid., pp. 7–11; Reports of the Department of Health, Phillips Academy,

1935–1940, located in the Medical Department Files, Headmaster's Office, Oliver Wendell Holmes Library, Phillips Academy, Andover, Massachusetts (hereafter referred to as Medical Department Files).

15. Gallagher, "Pediatrics and the Adolescent," p. 458.

16. Ibid., p. 458.

17. I examined histories of Andover's main competitors during this time and found that while most of them had diagnostic and treatment facilities comparable to that of Andover, there is no evidence that they were conducting research on adolescent development. In fact, in 1940, Gallagher held a conference for school physicians to "bring them up to speed" on issues of adolescent development. See "Conference of the Adolescent Study Unit of the Department of Health, Phillips Academy, Andover, Massachusetts, 12 April 1940," Medical Department Files. In a memorandum discussing Gallagher's support by the Carnegie Corporation, Carnegie's president Charles Dollard noted that "to my knowledge, Gallagher is the one school medical officer in the country who is concerned with something more than patching up his boys and curing their measles." "Office of the President, Record of Interview, Charles Dollard and Dr. Roswell Gallagher," 11 December 1947, Carnegie Corporation Papers, Rare Book and Manuscript Library, Columbia University, New York, hereafter referred to as Carnegie Corporation Papers.

18. Gallagher, "Foreword" to Grant Proposal to the Carnegie Corporation, 1938, p. 2, Medical Department Files.

19. Gallagher, untitled medical report dated March 25, 1946, Medical Department Files.

20. Gallagher to Fuess, 10 December, 1946; and Gallagher to Fuess, April 1, 1947, Medical Department Files. These letters were written when Fuess was considering cutting funding for the Adolescent Study Unit, and Gallagher referred back to conversations they had during the late 1930s about why such a facility was important to maintaining the prestige of the health services offered at Phillips Academy.

21. In his autobiography, Headmaster Claude Moore Fuess observed that prominent Andover alumni included a "Mayor of Denver, a Governor of Wisconsin, a Bishop of Minnesota, author of *The White Tower*, the producer of *Oklahoma!*, the President of Oberlin College, the Director of the Detroit Symphony Orchestra, the Director of the Yale Art School, the President of Boston's largest bank, the Headmaster of Lawrenceville School, the Managing Editor of *Fortune*, the Sports Editor of *Newsweek*, a foreign correspondent of the *New York Times*, the Chairman of the New York Federal Reserve Board, two of the greatest of American surgeons, the toughest of motion picture actors and the most benign of clergymen, as well as heroes, alive and dead, on many a battlefield around the world." Fuess, *Independent Schoolmaster*, p. 186.

22. Gallagher, "Foreword," to Grant Proposal to the Carnegie Corporation, p. 1, Medical Department Files.

23. "J. Roswell Gallagher, M.D.: Reminiscences."

24. Claude Moore Fuess described this conversation in "Report of Progress of the Phillips Academy Program of Physical and Mental Hygiene," 1939–1940, Medical Department Files.

25. Claude Moore Fuess, *Creed of a Schoolmaster* (Boston: Little, Brown, and Co., 1939), pp. 117–124.

26. Fuess, *Independent Schoolmaster*, pp. 189–190.

27. Fuess, *Creed of a Schoolmaster*, pp. 47–48.

28. For more on the history of progressive education, see Lawrence Cremin, *The Transformation of the School: Progressivism in American Education, 1876–1957* (New York: Alfred A. Knopf, 1961; Vintage Books, 1964); and Steven L. Schlossman, "G. Stanley Hall and the Boys' Club: Conservative Applications of Recapitulation Theory," *Journal of the History of the Behavioral Sciences* 9 (1973): 140–147. The term "meritocracy of the mind" comes from the work of Lewis M. Terman, one of the leading designers of mental tests for children and adults. See Paul Davis Chapman, *Schools as Sorters: Lewis M. Terman, Applied Psychology, and the Intelligence Testing Movement, 1890–1930* (New York: New York University Press, 1988).

29. Sol Cohen, "The Mental Hygiene Movement, The Development of Personality, and the School: The Medicalization of American Education," *History of Education Quarterly* 23/2 (1983): 136–137.

30. For example, Fuess called Dewey's *My Pedagogic Creed* "a document of extraordinary vagueness," and found some progressive schools "completely unstabilized and unsystematic." Fuess, *Creed of a Schoolmaster*, pp. 120, 123.

31. Fuess, *Independent Schoolmaster*, p. 176.

32. Stephen B. Levine, "The Rise of American Boarding Schools and the Development of a National Upper Class," *Social Problems* 28/1 (October 1980): 74–76; Fuess, *Independent Schoolmaster*, pp. 187–188.

33. Fuess, quoted in Allis, *Youth from Every Quarter*, p. 616.

34. Levine, "The Rise of American Boarding Schools," p. 76.

35. Gallagher, "Conference on the Adolescent Study Unit of the Department of Health, Phillips Academy, Andover, Massachusetts, April 12, 1940"; Claude Moore Fuess, "Report of Progress of the Phillips Academy Program on Physical and Mental Hygiene," 1940, Medical Department Files.

36. Health Department Reports for 1939 and 1940 briefly mention Greulich's participation in the Phillips Adolescent Study Unit, Medical Department Files.

37. William Greulich et al., "Somatic and Endocrine Studies of Pubertal and Adolescent Boys," *Monographs of the Society for Research in Child Development* 7/3 (1942); Gallagher, "The Adolescent Study Unit at Phillips Academy, Andover," *Harvard Medical Alumni Bulletin* 14 (1940): 89.

38. Health Department Reports, 1939, 1940, Medical Department Files.

39. The Grant researchers always placed the term "normal" in quotation marks and I have followed this convention in discussing their work. For more on the

origins of the study, see Arlie V. Bock, "A Proposed Study of Unhappiness and Maladjustment, Using Young Men in Harvard University as a Laboratory," typescript dated September 1937, Grant Foundation Papers, Special Collections, Milbank Memorial Library, Teachers College, Columbia University, New York (hereafter referred to as Grant Foundation Papers), Box 81. Although this project is usually referred to as the "Grant Study" the term is something of a misnomer, since the Carnegie Corporation provided some of the funds for the Phillips Academy portion of the study. For more on the history of the Grant Study, see Prescott, "'Young Man, You Are Normal': Developmental Research and Theories of Masculinity at Harvard and Phillips Andover Academy, 1938–45," paper presented at the annual meeting of the History of Science Society, New Orleans, Louisiana, October 13–16, 1994.

40. Quoted in Emily Davis Cahan, *The William T. Grant Foundation: The First Fifty Years, 1936–1986* (New York: William T. Grant Foundation, 1986), pp. 10.

41. Quoted in Annual Report, Grant Foundation, 1992, pp. 8–9.

42. Eva Milofsky, "The Grant Study: A Panoramic View after Half a Century," unpublished typescript, Grant Foundation Papers, Box 77.

43. Earnest A. Hooton, *"Young Man, You Are Normal": Findings from a Study of Students* (New York: G. P. Putnam's Sons, 1945).

44. For more on Hooton's collaboration with Boas, see Elazar Barkan, "Mobilizing Scientists against Nazi Racism, 1933–1939," in *Bones, Bodies, Behavior: Essays on Biological Anthropology,* ed. George W. Stocking (Madison: University of Wisconsin Press, 1988), pp. 180–205.

45. Earnest A. Hooton, "Plain Statement about Race," *Journal of the American Association of University Women* (June 1936): 4. See also idem, "Why the Jew Grows Stronger," *Colliers* (May 6, 1939): 12–13, 71–72.

46. Earnest A. Hooton, "Morons into What?" *Woman's Home Companion* 70 (August 1943): 4.

47. Hooton, *Young Man, You Are Normal*, p. 8.

48. Selection criteria and information on the backgrounds of the participants are described in Clark Wright Heath, *What People Are: A Study of Normal Young Men* (Cambridge, Mass.: Harvard University Press, 1945), pp. 110–114; and John P. Monks, *College Men at War* (Boston: American Academy of Arts and Sciences, 1957), pp. 4–5.

49. Hooton, *Young Man, You Are Normal*, p. 111; Monks, *College Men at War*, pp. 4–5.

50. Carl C. Seltzer and J. Roswell Gallagher, "Somatotypes of an Adolescent Group," *American Journal of Physical Anthropology*, n.s., 4 (June 1946): 154–155.

51. Undated memo by Gallagher, ca. January 1941, Carnegie Corporation Papers.

52. Charles Dollard to J. Roswell Gallagher, 21 January 1941, Carnegie Corporation Papers.

53. Gallagher, "Foreword" to Grant Proposal to the Carnegie Corporation, p. 2, Medical Department Files.

54. See Gallagher and Lucien Brouha, "A Method of Testing the Physical Fitness of High School Girls," *Revue Canadienne de Biologie* 2 (1943): 395–406.

55. Heath, *What People Are,* pp. 12–13; Gallagher, "Adolescent Study Unit," pp. 89–91.

56. For more on Sheldon's somatotyping system, see Sheldon, *Varieties of Human Physique* (New York: Harper and Brothers, 1940). For a history of Sheldon's ideas and their relationship to other personality studies of this period, see Doris Webster Havice, *Personality Typing: Uses and Misuses* (Washington, D.C.: University Press of America, 1977); J. E. Lindsay Carter and Barbara Honeyman Heath, *Somatotyping: Development and Applications* (Cambridge and New York: Cambridge University Press, 1990); and Sarah W. Tracy, "An Evolving Science of Man: American Constitutional Medicine, 1920–1950," paper presented at the Conference on the Wholistic Turn in Western Biomedicine, McGill University, May 1995.

57. Hooton, *Young Man, You Are Normal,* pp. 95–96.

58. See Jennifer Terry, "Lesbians under the Medical Gaze: Scientists Search for Remarkable Differences," *Journal of Sex Research* 27/3 (August 1990): 317–339; idem, "Anxious Slippages between 'Us' and 'Them': A Brief History of the Scientific Search for Homosexual Bodies," in *Deviant Bodies: Critical Perspectives on Difference in Science and Popular Culture,* ed. Jennifer Terry and Jacqueline Urda (Bloomington and Indianapolis: Indiana University Press, 1995), pp. 129–169; idem, "Siting Homosexuality: A History of Surveillance and the Production of Deviant Subjects," (Ph.D. diss., University of California at Santa Cruz, 1992); and Allan Bérubé, *Coming Out under Fire: The History of Gay Men and Women in World War Two* (New York: Free Press, 1990).

59. William L. Woods, Arlie Bock et al. "Short Interview Method of Selection of Army Officers," April 14, 1942, Earnest A. Hooton Papers, Peabody Museum, Harvard University, Cambridge, Mass., hereafter referred to as Hooton Papers.

60. Monks, *College Men at War,* p. 181.

61. Hooton, *Young Man, You Are Normal,* pp. 82–83.

62. Arlie Bock, "A Short Method for Selecting Combat Officers," typescript, 1942, Grant Foundation Papers, Box 80.

63. William L. Woods, "Preliminary Study of Grant Co. Managers," typescript, September 1943, Grant Foundation Papers, Box 87.

64. Report by Charles Dollard on Conference on Andover Adolescent Study, 12 April 1940, Carnegie Corporation Papers.

65. Seltzer and Gallagher, "Somatotypes of an Adolescent Group," p. 163.

66. Gallagher, "Various Aspects of Adolescence," *Journal of Pediatrics* 39 (1951): 537–538.

67. The case Billy is described in a transcript of a faculty seminar on "Growth and Development in Adolescence," which Gallagher presented on November 9,

1948, Medical Department Files. The case was later published in "There Is No Average Boy," *Atlantic Monthly* 183 (March 1949): 42–45, which eventually became chapter 4 in *Understanding Your Son's Adolescence.*

68. Gallagher, "Growth and Development in Adolescence," p. 1.

69. Jerry's case is described in Gallagher, *Understanding Your Son's Adolescence,* pp. 161–165.

70. Gallagher, "The Adolescent Study Unit," p. 91.

71. Report to the Carnegie Corporation, May 1943, Medical Department Files.

72. Gallagher, faculty seminar on "Growth and Development in Adolescence," November 9, 1948, pp. 12–13, Medical Department Files.

73. Undated faculty seminar, circa 1948, Medical Department Files.

74. Ben's case is described in Gallagher, *Understanding Your Son's Adolescence,* pp. 137–139.

75. Report of the Department of Health, Spring 1941, Medical Department Files.

76. Report of the Department of Health, Spring 1949, Medical Department Files.

77. Report of the Department of Health, Spring 1941, Medical Department Files.

78. Report of the Department of Health, Fall 1942, Medical Department Files.

79. Report of the Department of Health Spring, 1949, Medical Department Files.

80. Those who have studied the social construction of learning disabilities have suggested that these categories have tended to reinforce power relationships in American society. The category of "dyslexia" or "learning disabled" typically was applied to children from white, upper- and middle-class homes, while low-income and minority children were diagnosed as either "mentally retarded" or "emotionally disturbed." See Gerald Coles, *The Learning Mystique: A Critical Look at "Learning Disabilities"* (New York: Pantheon Books, 1987); James G. Carrier, *Learning Disability: Social Class and the Construction of Inequality in American Education* (New York: Greenwood Press, 1986); Kenneth A. Kavale and Steven R. Forness, *The Science of Learning Disabilities* (San Diego: College-Hill, 1985); and Christine E. Sleeter, "Learning Disabilities: The Social Construction of a Special Education Category," *Exceptional Children* 53 (1986): 46–54.

81. Carl C. Seltzer and J. Roswell Gallagher, "Body Disproportions and Personality Ratings in a Group of Adolescent Males," *Growth* 23 (1959): 1–11.

82. For more on psychiatry during World War II, see Gerald Grob, *The Mad among Us: A History of the Care of America's Mentally Ill* (New York: Free Press, 1994), pp. 191–221.

83. For more on concerns about homosexuality during the war, see Bérubé, *Coming Out under Fire;* Geoffrey S. Smith, "National Security and Personal Isola-

tion: Sex, Gender, and Disease in the Cold-War United States," *International History Review* 14/2 (May 1992): 307–335; and Lawrence R. Murphy, "The House on Pacific Street: Homosexuality, Intrigue, and Politics during World War II," *Journal of Homosexuality* 12 (1985): 27–49.

84. Monk, *College Men at War,* pp. 181–183; Carl C. Selzer, "The Relationship between the Masculine Component and Personality," *American Journal of Physical Anthropology* 3 (1945): 41.

85. Gallagher, "Recommendations for Improvement. Department of Physical Education," memorandum to Claude Moore Fuess, 1 February 1942, Medical Department Files.

86. Gallagher, "Report to the Carnegie Corporation," May 1943, Medical Department Files.

87. Quoted in a letter to Headmaster Fuess from Gallagher, 9 August 1944, Medical Department Files.

88. Arthur H. Steinhaus to J. Roswell Gallagher, 11 May 1944, Medical Department Files.

89. Allis, *Youth from Every Quarter,* pp. 467–468; Gallagher, "The Adolescent Study Unit at Phillips Academy, Andover. Report to the Grant Foundation for the Period July 1, 1949 to August 1, 1950," Medical Department Files. Gallagher's article on learning disability is "Specific Language Disability: A Cause of Scholastic Failure," *New England Journal of Medicine* 242 (March 1950): 436–440.

90. Report of the Department of Health, Fall 1941, Medical Department Files. The proceedings of the symposium were published in the *Journal of Pediatrics* 19 (September 1941): 289–401.

91. Gallagher's articles for the *Atlantic* were "Can't Spell, Can't Read," 181 (June 1948): 35–39; "There Is No Average Boy," 183 (March 1949): 42–45; "Why Boys Fail," 185 (May 1950): 49–52; "Why Boys Steal," 188 (October 1951): 49–52; and "Why They Rebel," 191 (June 1953): 69–71. The article "There Is No Average Boy" was condensed and reprinted in *Reader's Digest* 59 (June 1949): 29–30, and all of the *Atlantic* essays were collected in *Understanding Your Son's Adolescence* along with additional material.

92. J. Roswell Gallagher, interview by Heather Munro Prescott, 9 February 1991, tape recording in the Children's Hospital Archives. Unfortunately Gallagher did not save any of these letters.

93. Gallagher's medical department reports for 1945–1950 mention that he occasionally would agree to see a possibly learning disabled patient who was not an Andover student. Usually these patients were friends or relatives of one of the students at the academy.

94. Allis, *Youth from Every Quarter,* p. 539; "J. Roswell Gallagher, M.D.: Reminiscences."

95. Gallagher, "The Health Examination of Adolescents," pp. 315–318.

96. Children's Hospital Medical Center, *Annual Report,* 1969, p. 20, Children's Hospital Archives.

97. Children's Hospital, *Annual Report,* 1944 and 1945, Children's Hospital Archives.

98. Clement A. Smith, *The Children's Hospital of Boston: "Built Better than They Knew"* (Boston: Little, Brown, 1983), pp. 222–228.

99. Janeway, "Annual Report of the Department of Medicine," 1950, Children's Hospital Archives.

100. Janeway, "Discussion," in Helen I. Witmer, ed., *Pediatrics and the Emotional Needs of the Child* (New York: The Commonwealth Fund, 1948), p. 51.

101. Information on Janeway's career comes from the Charles A. Janeway Papers, Countway Library of Medicine, Harvard Medical School, Boston, Massachusetts, hereafter referred to as Janeway Papers.

102. For more on the Mid-Century White House Conference, see Helen Leland Witmer and Ruth Kotinsky, *Personality in the Making: The Fact-Finding Report of the Mid-Century White House Conference on Children and Youth* (New York: Harper and Brothers, 1952); and Rochelle Beck, "The White House Conferences on Children: An Historical Perspective," *Harvard Educational Review* 43/4 (November 1973): 653–668.

103. Charles A. Janeway, "Discussion," in Joseph Weinreb, ed., *Recent Developments in Psychoanalytic Child Therapy* (New York: International Universities Press, 1960), pp. 66–68.

104. Dane Prugh, "Child Psychiatry and Pediatrics," in *Basic Handbook of Child Psychiatry,* vol. 4, Prevention and Current Issues, ed. Joseph D. Noshpitz (New York: Basic Books, 1979), p. 564.

105. Smith, *The Children's Hospital of Boston,* pp. 208–209.

106. Janeway, "Pediatrics and the Adolescent," p. 455; Janeway to Gallagher, 2 February 1947, Medical Department Files; Gallagher to Geddes Smith, 20 March 1947, Harvard University Program in Comprehensive Pediatric Medicine, Commonwealth Fund Collection, Box 134, Folder 1222, Rockefeller Archive Center, Pocantico Hills, New York, hereafter referred to as Harvard Program in Comp. Med., CF Collection.

107. Smith, *The Children's Hospital of Boston,* pp. 245–246.

108. Interview with Charles Janeway quoted in Arnold Nicolson, "The Adolescents Get a Doctor of Their Own," *Saturday Evening Post* 227 (July 10, 1954): 25.

109. Children's Hospital, *Annual Report,* 1942, p. 60, Children's Hospital Archives.

110. Children's Hospital, *Annual Report,* 1945, p. 29, Children's Hospital Archives; Smith, *The Children's Hospital of Boston,* pp. 221–224; Felix P. Heald, Jr., interview by Heather Munro Prescott, 24 March 1990, tape recording deposited in Children's Hospital Archives.

111. George P. Berry to Lester Evans, 30 December 1954, Harvard Program in

Comp. Med., CF Collection, Box 134, Folder 1225. Berry also instituted reforms in the basic science curriculum at the medical school. See Peter V. Lee, "Review of Commonwealth Fund Experiments in Medical Education" (memorandum), 8 October 1959, Harvard Program in Comp. Med., CF Collection, Box 134, Folder 1228.

112. Gallagher to Evans, 21 May 1952, Harvard Program in Comp. Med., CF Collection, Box 134, Folder 1222. The Grant Foundation did eventually award Gallagher a new two-year grant of $30,000 in 1954. See *Annual Report of the Adolescent Unit*, September 1954, Children's Hospital Archives.

113. Gallagher, "Prospectus on The Adolescent Unit at the Children's Medical Center," May 1952, Harvard Program in Comp. Med., CF Collection, Box 134, Folder 1222.

114. Evans, "Interview with Dr. J. Roswell Gallagher, Physician-in-Charge Adolescent Unit, The Children's Medical Center, Boston, April 30, 1952" (memorandum), 6 May 1952; "Adolescent Unit, Children's Medical Center, Boston, Comments by Geddes Smith," 9 May 1952; and "Adolescent Unit, Children's Medical Center, Boston, Comment by Dr. Charles O. Warren," 14 May 1952, Harvard Program in Comp. Med., CF Collection, Box 134, Folder 1222.

115. Mildred C. Scoville to Lester Evans 6 May 1952, Harvard Program in Comp. Med., CF Collection, Box 134, Folder 1222.

116. Charles O. Warren, "Harvard University Medical School. Program in Comprehensive Pediatric Medicine. Visit by Dr. Warren and Dr. Evans, December 15–17, 1954" (summary memorandum), 23 December 1954, Harvard Program in Comp. Med., CF Collection, Box 134, Folder 1225.

117. For statistics on the number of patient visits to the Adolescent Unit, see *Annual Reports of Adolescent Unit* for the years 1951–1954, Children's Hospital Archives.

118. *Annual Reports of the Adolescent Unit*, 1951, 1952, 1953; Geddes Smith, "Adolescent Unit, Children's Medical Center, Boston. Interview with Dr. J. Roswell Gallagher, 17 November 1952" (memorandum), Harvard Program in Comp. Med., CF Collection, Box 134, Folder 1222.

119. Information about Heald and Masland comes from interview with Felix P. Heald by Heather Munro Prescott, 24 March 1990, Atlanta, Georgia; interview with Heald by HMP, 21 September 1990, Baltimore, Md.; interviews with Robert Masland by HMP, 27 December 1989, 25 July 1990, and 19 February 1991, Boston, Mass.; and interview with Thomas Cone by HMP, 9 November 1990, Cambridge, Mass. Tape recordings of all these interviews are deposited in the Children's Hospital Archives. See also "J. Roswell Gallagher, M.D.: Reminiscences"; "Felix P. Heald, Jr.: Reminiscences," videotape interview by Prescott and Rauh 10 January 1994, tape available from Rauh; and entry on Heald in *American Men and Women of Science*, 14th ed. (1982), p. 2087.

120. Gallagher to Evans, 13 October 1953, Harvard Program in Comp. Med., CF Collection, Box 134, Folder 1223.

121. Gallagher to Evans, 2 February 1953, Harvard Program in Comp. Med., CF Collection, Box 134, Folder 1223.

122. Geddes Smith, "Children's Hospital Medical Center, Boston—Adolescent Unit. Interview with Dr. George Berry, February 20, 1953" (Memorandum), 24 February 1953, Harvard Program in Comp. Med., CF Collection, Box 134, Folder 1223.

123. Charles O. Warren, "Harvard University Medical School. Program in Comprehensive Pediatric Medicine. Visit by Dr. Warren and Dr. Evans, December 15–17, 1954" (summary memorandum), 23 December 1954, Harvard Program in Comp. Med., CF Collection, Box 134, Folder 1225.

124. Gallagher, "Adolescence: Summary of Round Table Discussion," *Pediatrics* 18/6 (1956): 1019; Gallagher, interview by Heather Munro Prescott, 28 December 1989, Lexington, Mass., tape recording, Children's Hospital Archives.

125. Margaret C. Scoville, "Children's Hospital (Boston)—Adolescent Clinic" (memorandum), 27 October 1953, Harvard Program in Comp. Med., CF Collection, Box 134, Folder 1223. Scoville was one of the most prominent women in the field of mental hygiene during this period. She obtained her degree from the Smith College School of Social Work. After serving with the Red Cross of Minneapolis for several years, she become assistant director of the National Committee for Mental Hygiene in 1921, and received the committee's Lasker Award in 1949. Scoville was also a key figure in the development of the Group for the Advancement of Psychiatry, which attempted to improve the place of psychiatry in the medical school curriculum. Scoville headed the American Association of Psychiatric Social Workers for a number of years and was the first woman appointed to the National Mental Health Advisory Council. A. McGehee Harvey and Susan L. Abrams, *"For the Welfare of Mankind": The Commonwealth Fund and American Medicine* (Baltimore: Johns Hopkins University Press, 1986), p. 628n4.

126. Evans, "Children's Hospital (Boston)—Adolescent Clinic" (memorandum), 2 November 1953, Harvard Program in Comp. Med., CF Collection, Box 134, Folder 1223.

127. Evans, "Children's Hospital (Boston)—Adolescent Clinic. Visit to Clinic by Dr. Evans, September 15, 1953" (memorandum), 15 October 1953, Harvard Program in Comp. Med., CF Collection, Box 134, Folder 1223.

128. Janeway to Evans, 20 March 1954, Harvard Program in Comp. Med., CF Collection, Box 134, Folder 1224.

129. Warren, "Harvard University Medical School. Program in Comprehensive Pediatric Medicine. Visit by Dr. Warren and Dr. Evans, December 15–17, 1954" (summary memorandum), 23 December 1954, Harvard Program in Comp. Med., CF Collection, Box 134, Folder 1225. See also John C. Eberhart, "Comments on Harvard University, Comprehensive Pediatric Medicine" (memorandum), 14 October 1954, Harvard Program in Comp. Med., CF Collection, Box 134, Folder 1225.

130. See the *Annual Reports of the Adolescent Unit* for 1955–1958, Children's Hospital Archives; Peter V. Lee, "Review of Commonwealth Fund Experiments in Medical Education" (memorandum), 8 October 1959, Harvard Program in Comp. Med., CF Collection, Box 134, Folder 1228.

131. Charles A. Janeway, "Report of the Commonwealth Fund on a Grant to Harvard Medical School to support a Program of Comprehensive Pediatric Medicine, July 1, 1955—June 30, 1958," Harvard Program in Comp. Med., CF Collection, Box 134, Folder 1226.

132. *Annual Report of the Adolescent Unit*, 1958, Children's Hospital Archives.

133. Harvey and Abrams, *"For the Welfare of Mankind,"* p. 242.

134. For example, see Lee, "Review of Commonwealth Fund Experiments in Medical Education," p. 26; and Warren, "Harvard University Medical School. Program in Comprehensive Pediatric Medicine. Visit by Dr. Warren and Dr. Evans, December 15–17, 1954" (summary memorandum), 23 December 1954, Harvard Program in Comp. Med., CF Collection, Box 134, Folder 1225.

3. The Adolescent Unit at Boston Children's Hospital

1. Gallagher, "Why We Feel Sick," *Seventeen* 19 (March 1960): 132–133, 191. For examples of other articles on the Adolescent Unit published by *Seventeen* magazine, see Gallagher, "Becoming a Woman," 16 (May 1957): 118–119, 192–194; and idem, "How Much Is It Worth to Win?" 23 (May, 1964): 152, 211. *Seventeen* continued to publish a series of articles on the Adolescent Unit and similar facilities throughout the 1960s. See Alice Lake, "Stick Out Your Tongue and Say Ah," 23 (November 1964): 130–132, idem, "Why You Need a Doctor of Your Own," 26 (February 1967): 146–147, 253; idem, "How You Can Beat Fatigue," 26 (June 1967): 113; idem, "What Happens behind the Doctor's Door," 26 (December 1967): 102–103, 137; and idem, "What Teen-Age Medicine Can Do for You," 29 (June 1970): 132–133, 185–187.

2. For examples of popular articles by or on Gallagher and the clinic, see Gallagher, "A Clinic for Adolescents," *Children* 1 (1954): 165–170; idem, "How to Understand the Adolescent Boy," *Parents' Magazine* 28 (September 1953): 40–41, 151–155; Vivian Cadden, "Their Specialty Is Teenagers," *Parents' Magazine* 31 (July 1956): 36–37, 83–87; and Arnold Nicolson, "The Adolescents Get a Doctor of Their Own," *Saturday Evening Post* 227 (July 10, 1954): 25–28.

3. Speaking engagements and television and radio appearances are listed at the end of each *Annual Report of the Adolescent Unit*.

4. Nicolson, "The Adolescents Get a Doctor of Their Own," p. 26.

5. Changes in the kinds of problems seen at the Adolescent Unit and other adolescent facilities during the late 1960s and 1970s will be examined further in

Chapter 4. Most of this chapter is based on cases from the 1950s. Historians of this period agree, however, that the mentalité of the 1950s did not end on New Year's Day in 1960. For example, Elaine Tyler May observes in her study of family life in the 1950s: "In the early 1960s, it was not immediately obvious that a unique historical era was coming to an end . . . Most cultural signs still pointed toward the cold war consensus at home and abroad, and the ideology of domesticity was still alive and well." May, *Homeward Bound: American Families in the Cold War Era* (New York: Basic Books, 1988), pp. 217–218. See also Arlene Skolnick, *Embattled Paradise: The American Family in an Age of Uncertainty* (New York: Basic Books, 1991), p. 2. The persistence of the 1950s mindset into the early 1960s is evident in the case records I examined from the early 1960s: school and behavioral problems continued to form the largest categories of patient visits. Furthermore, Gallagher's perspective on family relations and gender roles dominated the Adolescent Unit's approach until his retirement in 1967. Therefore this chapter includes a few cases from the early and mid-1960s.

6. Not surprisingly, the majority of private patients seen at the unit during the 1950s were from white, middle-class or upper middle-class backgrounds. Over 70 percent of the private patients were from Boston area preparatory schools and/or from well-to-do suburbs in Massachusetts and Rhode Island. A further examination of the social status of 54 patients (on the basis of parents' occupations and educational level) who visited the unit during the 1950s confirmed that these patients came from comfortable to privileged backgrounds. From this sample of 54, which was selected at random from my original sample of 191 case records from the 1950s, 22 fathers were doctors, lawyers, or some other professional requiring an advanced degree; 9 were employed in managerial or executive business positions; 10 owned their own businesses; 3 were in sales jobs; 2 were in well-paying skilled labor jobs; 1 was in the military; 1 was retired; 2 were deceased; and for 4 cases the father's occupation was unknown. Only two families in the sample could be classified as poor: in one case, the father was a physician who had abandoned his family and the wife had been forced to apply for AFDC; in the other, the father was an enlisted serviceman who did not earn enough to support the family in a middle-class lifestyle. Mothers' occupations tended to follow prescribed gender norms for this period; most indicated either that they were housewives (39 percent) or did not work outside the home (38 percent). Of those who were employed outside the home, most held a traditionally female service job such as teacher, nurse, or social worker. In terms of educational background, 57 percent ($N=31$) of the fathers sampled had at least some college education, and 77 percent ($N=24$) of these held a bachelor's degree or higher. The mothers showed a smaller but still impressive degree of educational success: 39 percent ($N=21$) had at least some college education, with 70 percent of these holding an associate's degree or higher, including one with a doctorate. Information on race and ethnic background is scant, since physi-

cians did not indicate this data in the patient record. Only one patient from the sample of 430 was referred to specifically as "Negro," and this case was from the early 1970s. Occasionally physicians would note religious background, but this was done so infrequently that it is impossible to make any generalizations about this characteristic.

7. I was unable to sample clinic patients because of the way patient case records were stored the Children's Hospital. The private patient records were and continue to be stored separately from other Children's Hospital records. The older private patient case records from 1951–1973 are now part of the Children's Hospital Archives. More recent private patient records are still stored in the Adolescent/Young Adult Unit. Nonprivate patient records, however, are interfiled with records from all the medical services at the Children's Hospital. Because none of these records was sorted by age or medical service, and the Adolescent Unit did not keep a list of nonprivate patients, it was impossible to get a sample of case records from this group. During the first two years that the unit was open, Gallagher did a "rough spot check" of diagnoses for his annual reports, but soon abandoned this policy as too time consuming. Even this, however, does not appear to have included all of the patients who were treated at the unit, since the number of diagnoses falls far short of the number of patient visits.

8. Roland Marchand, *Advertising the American Dream: Making Way for Modernity, 1920–1940* (Berkeley: University of California Press, 1985), pp. 250–252. For an example of market studies of adolescent spending behavior during the 1920s, see *The Age Factor in Selling and Advertising: A Study in a New Phase of Advertising* (Chicago: 1922), frontispiece and pp. 9, 43–44, 96.

9. Eugene Gilbert, *Advertising and Marketing to Young People* (Pleasantville, N.Y.: Printers' Ink Books, 1957), pp. 160–161. For more on the relationship between developmental psychology and youth marketing during this time, see James Gilbert, *A Cycle of Outrage: America's Reaction to the Juvenile Delinquent in the 1950s* (New York: Oxford University Press, 1986), pp. 198–211.

10. For the origins of the term "teenager" and its relationship to mass marketing, see Richard Maring Ugland, "The Adolescent Experience during World War II: Indianapolis as a Case Study" (Ph.D. diss, Indiana University, 1977); and Grace Palladino, *Teenagers: An American History* (New York: Basic Books, 1996).

11. Gallagher, *Medical Care of the Adolescent* (New York: Appleton-Century Crofts, 1960), pp. 10–11.

12. Joan Jacobs Brumberg, *Fasting Girls: The Emergence of Anorexia Nervosa as a Modern Disease* (Cambridge: Harvard University Press, 1988), pp. 166–167.

13. Kathleen W. Jones, *Taming the Troublesome Child: American Families, Child Guidance, and the Limits of Psychiatric Authority* (Cambridge, Mass.: Harvard University Press, forthcoming).

14. Betty Algers case record (1956). As noted in the Introduction, all patient

names have been changed to protect their privacy. The number in parentheses indicates the year of the patient's first visit to the clinic.

15. Steve Ellis case record (1956).

16. "The Adolescent Unit: A Significant New Venture." Promotional brochure issued by Children's Hospital Medical Center, Harvard University Medical School Program in Comprehensive Pediatric Medicine, Commonwealth Fund Collection, Rockefeller Archive Center, Pocantico Hills, New York (hereafter referred to as Harvard Program in Comp. Med., CF Collection), Box 134, Folder 1224. See also *Annual Reports of the Adolescent Unit,* 1950–1960, Children's Hospital Archives; and Nicolson, "The Adolescents Get a Doctor of Their Own," p. 25.

17. Gallagher, *Medical Care of the Adolescent,* pp. 12–13.

18. Ibid., p. 14.

19. Ibid., pp. 14–15.

20. Ibid., p. 24.

21. Ibid., p. 15.

22. For more on Piaget's work on cognitive development, see Piaget, *The Moral Judgment of the Child* (London: K. Paul, Trench, Trubner, 1932).

23. "The Adolescent Unit: A Significant New Venture."

24. Quoted in Cadden, "Their Specialty Is Teenagers," p. 85.

25. Gallagher, *Medical Care of the Adolescent,* p. 13.

26. Robert Black case record (1957).

27. Mike Gilman to Masland, 29 November 1955. Mike Gilman case record (1955).

28. Interview with Robert P. Masland, 27 December 1989, conducted by Heather Munro Prescott, tape recording deposited in Children's Hospital Archives.

29. Mrs. Jacobs to Masland, 6 July 1960, Ellen Jacobs case record (1960).

30. John Hurtz Sr. to Masland, 6 July 1965, Johnny Hurtz case record (1965).

31. Mother's testimony, Howard Dailey case record (1962).

32. Daniel Burg case record (1960); and Eddie Knight case record (1955).

33. Roseanne Bloom case record (1961).

34. Laura Chase to Masland, May 1960, Laura Chase case record (1958).

35. Kathy Barton case record (1961).

36. Mike Gilman to Masland, 29 November 1955, Mike Gilman case record (1955).

37. Quoted in Stanley Englebardt, "Now: Health Care Teenagers Can Believe In," *Today's Health* 51/6 (June 1973): 62.

38. Quoted in Cadden, "Their Specialty Is Teenagers," pp. 83–85. See also Gallagher and Herbert I. Harris, *Emotional Problems of Adolescents* (New York: Oxford University Press, 1958), pp. 5–7.

39. The best example of the popular stereotype of the 1950s is Joseph H. Satin, ed., *The 1950s: America's "Placid" Decade* (Boston: Houghton Mifflin, 1960). For a

critique of this view, see John Patrick Diggins, *The Proud Decades: American in War and Peace, 1941–1960* (New York, 1988). The term "other-directedness" comes from David Riesman, Nathan Glazer, and Reuel Denny, *The Lonely Crowd: A Study of the Changing American Character* (New Haven: Yale University Press, 1950). See also William Whyte, *The Organization Man* (New York: Simon and Schuster, 1956); and Talcott Parsons, "The Social Structure of the Family," in *The Family: Its Functions and Destiny,* ed. Ruth Anshen (New York: Harper and Row, 1949), pp. 241–273. For more on American social scientists' ambivalence about conformity during this time, see Gilbert, *A Cycle of Outrage,* pp. 109–126; and Wini Breines, *Young, White, and Miserable: Growing Up Female in the Fifties* (Boston: Beacon Press, 1992), pp. 25–46.

40. Learned Hand, quoted in J. Roswell Gallagher and Constance D. Gallagher, "Some Comments on Growth and Development in Adolescents," *Yale Journal of Biology and Medicine* 25 (1953): 348.

41. Cindy Wilson case record (1958).

42. Pamela Cartwright case record (1957).

43. Ron Houston case record (1958).

44. Annette Miller case record (1954).

45. Brian Defoe to Masland, 19 September 19 1956, Brian Defoe case record (1956).

46. Betty Markel case record (1962).

47. Arnie Goldman case record (1954).

48. Gallagher, "Rest and Restriction," *American Journal of Public Health* 46 (1956): 1425.

49. Pamela Cartwright case record (1957).

50. Ron Houston case record (1958).

51. Susie Barnard case record (1956).

52. Only about 6 percent of the cases examined from the 1950s were purely somatic illnesses. Most patients who were seen for organic diseases also had some sort of psychological problem that grew out of or was compounded by their physical illness. Although I was only able to sample private patient records for this book, a study by the Commonwealth Fund in 1954, which surveyed all of the patients seen at the Adolescent Unit during the period from 1951 to 1954, confirmed that at least two-thirds of all cases involved school problems, conflicts over adolescent behavior, and emotional problems of adolescence. See Charles O. Warren, "Harvard University Medical School. Program in Comprehensive Pediatric Medicine. Visit by Dr. Warren and Dr. Evans, December 15–17, 1954" (summary memorandum), December 23, 1954, Harvard Program in Comp. Med., CF Collection, Box 134, Folder 1225. This pattern persisted for at least the next twenty years. An interview with Dr. Masland, the chief of the Adolescent Unit at the time, conducted for *Parents' Magazine* in 1972 indicated the proportion of emotional

problems to physical diseases remained constant well into the early 1970s. According to Masland, "perhaps three patients out of ten have some organic disease . . . while the remaining seven complain of . . . symptoms that are warning signs of emotional distress." Linda Pembrook, "Adolescent Clinics: A Vital Step in Solving the Problems of Teenagers," *Parents' Magazine* 47/11 (November 1972): 113. This ratio was not unique to the Adolescent Unit at Boston Children's Hospital. An interview with Joseph Rauh at the Adolescent Clinic at Cincinnati Children's Hospital conducted for *Today's Health* in 1973 indicated that "at least 75 percent of all physical disorders diagnosed here [at the clinic] are accompanied by emotional factors." Englebardt, "Now: Health Care Teenagers Can Believe In," p. 19.

53. Out of a total of 191 cases from the 1950s, 103, or 54 percent, involved some kind of school-related problem, such as school failure or poor grades.

54. *Annual Reports of the Adolescent Unit,* 1952, 1953, 1954, 1957, Children's Hospital Archives; Nicolson, "The Adolescents Get a Doctor of Their Own," pp. 25–28.

55. Information on the course of treatment for learning disabilities at the Adolescent Unit comes largely from interviews I conducted with Robert P. Masland, 25 July 1990 and 19 February 1991; and with Ruth Mersereau, who was the secretary at the Adolescent Unit from 1952 to 1976, conducted 26 December 1991. Copies of the tape recordings of the interviews are deposited in the Children's Hospital Archives.

56. *Annual Reports of Adolescent Unit,* 1952, 1953, Children's Hospital Archives.

57. For example, see David O. Levine, *The American College and the Culture of Aspiration* (Ithaca: Cornell University Press, 1986); and David Tyack, *The One Best System: A History of American Urban Education* (Cambridge, Mass.: Harvard University Press, 1974).

58. For more on social science research demonstrating the link between education and income, see Gerald Coles, *The Learning Mystique: A Critical Look at "Learning Disabilities"* (New York: Pantheon Books, 1987), pp. 192–193.

59. Mills, *The Power Elite* (New York: Oxford University Press, 1956; Galaxy Books, 1959), pp. 64–65. See also Robert Hampel, *The Last Little Citadel: American High Schools since 1940* (Boston: Houghton Mifflin, 1986), pp. 32–34; and Peter W. Cookson, Jr., and Caroline Hodges Persell, *Preparing for Power: America's Elite Boarding Schools* (New York: Basic Books, 1985).

60. Thirty-two percent ($N = 61$) of the cases involved some kind of behavioral problem. Three of these patients were referred to the Adolescent Unit from juvenile court.

61. May, *Homeward Bound,* pp. 10–11.

62. Gilbert, *A Cycle of Outrage,* pp. 136–137, 153–154.

63. Harry Richardson case record (1957).

64. Tom Beimers case record (1954).

65. Out of a total of 103 school problem cases examined from the 1950s, 85 (83

percent) were male, and 18 (17 percent) were female. The total number of cases sampled from the 1950s was 191: of these, 136 (71 percent) were male, and 55 (29 percent) were female. Therefore, 63 percent ($N = 85$) of all male patients ($N = 135$) were referred for some kind of school-related problem.

66. Diane Reynolds case record (1959).

67. Hope Archer case record (1955).

68. Thirty-two percent ($N = 18$) of all female patients from the 1950s were referred for school problems. In contrast, a total of 19, or 35 percent, were brought to the clinic because of acne, weight problems, or other difficulties related to physical appearance.

69. Brumberg, *Fasting Girls;* idem, *The Body Project: An Intimate History of American Girls* (New York: Random House, 1997), pp. 59–94; Breines, *Young, White, and Miserable,* pp. 95–101.

70. Jean Berkman case record (1955).

71. According to Gallagher's grant application to the Commonwealth Fund in 1952, there was "no institution devoting a major portion of its effort" to a "program aimed at the care and study of the adolescent," although he does acknowledge that a few specialty clinics in endocrinology and dermatology around the city did see adolescents. However, adolescents were not the focus of these specialty clinics and consequently the numbers of teenagers they treated were quite small. Gallagher, "The Adolescent Unit at the Children's Medical Center," grant application dated 1952, Harvard Program in Comp. Med., CF Collection, Box 134, Folder 1222. I have not been able to find any evidence to the contrary at any of the hospitals in the greater Boston area.

72. Jones, *Taming the Troublesome Child.*

73. Joseph Veroff, Richard A. Kulka, and Elizabeth Douvan, *Mental Health in America: Patterns of Help-seeking from 1957 to 1976* (New York: Basic Books, 1981).

74. Gallagher, *Medical Care of the Adolescent,* p. 316.

75. J. Roswell Gallagher, interview by Heather Munro Prescott, 9 March 1991, Lexington, Mass., tape recording deposited in Children's Hospital Archives.

76. For more on Gallagher's concerns about the dangers of basing adolescent medical care on psychiatric diagnoses alone, see Gallagher, "A Clinic for Adolescents," pp. 167–169. For more on Gallagher's position on psychiatry in general, see Gallagher, *Medical Care of the Adolescent,* pp. 316–326; idem, "The Physician's Attitudes toward Adolescents' Everyday Emotional Problems," in *Modern Perspectives in Child Development,* ed. Albert J. Solnit and Sally A. Provence (New York: International Universities Press, 1963), pp. 442–457; and Gallagher and Harris, *Emotional Problems of Adolescents,* pp. 95–96.

77. Gallagher and Harris, *Emotional Problems of Adolescents,* pp. 95–96. For a similar case, see Gallagher, "A Clinic for Adolescents," pp. 169–170.

78. Gallagher, "A Clinic for Adolescents," p. 169.

79. Cindy Wilson case record (1958).

80. Mrs. Reinhardt to Masland, 2 August 1957, Richard Reinhardt case record (1957).

81. Gallagher, *Understanding Your Son's Adolescence* (Boston: Little, Brown, 1951), pp. 154, 156.

82. For more on how class relationships shaped theories about learning disabilities, see Coles, *The Learning Mystique;* James G. Carrier, *Learning Disability: Social Class and the Construction of Inequality in American Education* (New York: Greenwood Press, 1986); idem, "The Politics of Early Learning Disability Theory," in *Learning Disability: Dissenting Essays,* ed. Barry M. Franklin (London, New York, and Philadelphia: Falmer Press, 1987), pp. 47–66; Kenneth A. Kavale and Steven R. Forness, *The Science of Learning Disabilities* (San Diego: College-Hill, 1985); and Christine E. Sleeter, "Learning Disabilities: The Social Construction of a Special Education Category," *Exceptional Children* 53 (1986): 46–54.

83. Only 14 of the 103 school problem cases from the 1950s I examined involved patients who were diagnosed with learning disabilities.

84. Howard Baker case record (1956).

85. Janice Boyd case record (1958).

86. Jenny Parker case record (1960).

87. Tom Boucher case record (1958).

88. Lois Kent case record (1955).

89. Gallagher, *Medical Care of the Adolescent,* pp. 1, 13. Emphasis is in original text.

90. Ibid., p. 13.

91. Ibid., pp. 18, 21.

92. Masland to Frank J. Sladen, Headmaster, Harrisburg Academy, 22 July 1960, Masland Correspondence Files, Children's Hospital Archives.

93. Mike Barton case record (1956).

94. Patient testimony, Donald Edwards case record, (1960).

95. Derrick Benson case record (1960).

96. Joe Bramble case record (1957).

97. Lake, "What Teen-Age Medicine Can Do for You," p. 185.

98. Gallagher and Harris, *Emotional Problems of Adolescents,* p. 57.

99. Ibid., pp. 45–46.

100. Gallagher to Justice Frederick T. Iddings, 13 March 1958, Gallagher Correspondence Files, Children's Hospital Archives.

101. Session with father, Ted White case record (1958).

102. Mrs. Christine Darling to Masland, 16 March 1964, Amy Darling case record (1964).

103. Masland to Mr. and Mrs. Sands, 24 April 1959, Gary Sands case record (1958).

104. Clinical notes, Lloyd Bartley case record (1958).

105. Mrs. B. A. Justin to Masland, 18 August 1965; Deborah Henson to Masland, 18 October 1965, Deborah Henson case record (1965).

106. Gallagher, *Medical Care of the Adolescent*, pp. 66, 64.

107. Cindy Welter case record (1957).

108. Ron Horowitz case record (1964).

109. Gallagher, *Medical Care of the Adolescent*, pp. 66, 64.

110. Ibid., pp. 66–67.

111. May, *Homeward Bound*, pp. 10–11; Geoffrey S. Smith, "National Security and Personal Isolation: Sex, Gender, and Disease in the Cold-War United States," *International History Review* 14/2 (May 1992): 307–337.

112. May, *Homeward Bound*, pp. 100–101. Kinsey's studies were Kinsey, Wardell Pomeroy, and C. E. Martin, *Sexual Behavior in the Human Male* (Philadelphia: W. B. Saunders, 1948); and Kinsey et al., *Sexual Behavior in the Human Female* (Philadelphia: W. B. Saunders, 1953).

113. May, *Homeward Bound*, pp. 100–101.

114. Philip Wylie, *Generation of Vipers* (New York: Holt, Rinehart and Winston, 1942, rev. 1955); Edward A. Strecker, *Their Mother's Sons* (New York: J. B. Lippincott, 1946). For a historical analysis of the impact of "Momism" on postwar psychology, see May, *Homeward Bound*, pp. 74, 96; and Sonya Michel, "Danger on the Home Front: Motherhood, Sexuality, and Disabled Veterans in American Postwar Films," in *American Sexual Politics: Sex, Gender, and Race Since the Civil War*, ed. John C. Fout and Maura Shaw Tantillo (Chicago and London: University of Chicago Press, 1993), pp. 247–266.

115. Helene Deutsch, *The Psychology of Women*, vol. 2, *Motherhood* (New York: Grune & Stratton, 1944), p. 321.

116. Gallagher, "Dysmenorrhea and Menorrhagia in Adolescence," p. 470.

117. For more on this research project, see Commonwealth Fund Archives, Grant Series, Rockefeller Archive Center, North Tarrytown, N.Y. (hereafter referred to as CF Archives), Box 122, Folders 118–21; Felix P. Heald, Jr., Robert P. Masland, Jr., Somers H. Sturgis, and J. Roswell Gallagher, "Dysmenorrhea in Adolescence," *Pediatrics* 20 (1957): 121–127; Heald and Sturgis, "Adolescent Gynecology: A Five Year Study," *Pediatrics* 25 (1960): 669–677; Sturgis, *The Gynecologic Patient: A Psycho-Endocrine Study* (New York: Grune and Stratton, 1962); and Sturgis, "Management of Congenital Defects," in *Adolescent Gynecology*, ed. Felix P. Heald (Baltimore: Williams and Wilkins, 1966), pp. 58–68.

118. Lois Kent case record (1955).

119. Martha Humphrey case record (1955).

120. Gallagher and Harris, *Emotional Problems of Adolescents*, p. 31.

121. Josie McDonald case record (1960).

122. Gallagher, *Medical Care of the Adolescent*, p. 53.

123. Ibid., pp. 196–197.

124. Ibid., pp. 67–68. See also Gallagher, "Problems of the Adolescent," *Pediatric Clinics of North America* 5/3 (1958): 775–787.

125. Sturgis, "Management of Congenital Defects," pp. 66–67. Unfortunately I was unable to sample any Turner cases, because they were interfiled with adult case records from the Brigham and Women's Hospital.

126. Carolyn Douglas case record (1956).

127. June Goldwin case record (1957).

128. The results of this research are published in Sheldon and Eleanor Glueck, *Unraveling Juvenile Delinquency* (Cambridge, Mass.: Harvard University Press, 1950); Carl Seltzer and J. Roswell Gallagher, "Somatotypes of an Adolescent Group," *American Journal of Physical Anthropology* 4 (1946): 153–168; and idem, "Body Disproportions and Personality Ratings in a Group of Adolescent Males," *Growth* 23 (1959): 1–11. A follow-up study of the original delinquent subjects was conducted in the late 1970s and published in Emil M. Hartl, Edward P. Monnelly, and Roland D. Elderkin, *Physique and Delinquent Behavior* (New York: Academic Press, 1982).

129. Gallagher, *Medical Care of the Adolescent*, p. 16.

130. Gallagher and Harris, *Emotional Problems of Adolescents*, p. 34.

131. Ibid., pp. 41–42.

132. Steve Sussman case record (1956).

133. Untaped interview with Robert P. Masland by Heather Munro Prescott, 22 July 1994; "J. Roswell Gallagher, M.D.: Reminiscences," videotape interview with J. Roswell Gallagher, Robert P. Masland, Jr., Esterann Grace, and Jean Emans by Prescott and Joseph L. Rauh, 25 October 1993. Tape deposited in Children's Hospital Archives and available from JLR. Although the unit did not have any full-time female physicians on the staff until the early 1970s, there were a few female medical students, residents, and fellows who trained at the unit during the 1950s and 1960s.

134. Gallagher and Harris, *Emotional Problems of Adolescents*, p. 59.

135. Bob Russell case record (1956).

136. Gallagher and Harris, *Emotional Problems of Adolescents*, p. 38.

137. Gallagher, *Medical Care of the Adolescent*, p. 277.

138. Ronnie Feinstein case record (1957).

139. Gallagher and Harris, *Emotional Problems of Adolescents*, pp. 61–62.

4. Adolescent Medicine since the 1960s

1. For example, see Jim Miller, *Democracy Is in the Streets: From Port Huron to the Siege of Chicago* (New York: Simon and Schuster, 1987); David Caute, *The Year of the Barricades: A Journey through 1968* (New York: Harper and Row, 1988); David Farber, *Chicago '68* (Chicago: University of Chicago Press, 1988); Ronald Fraser et al., *1968: A Student Generation in Revolt* (New York: Pantheon Books, 1988);

George Katsiaficas, *The Imagination of the New Left: A Global Analysis of 1968* (Boston: South End Press, 1987); Hans Koning, *1968: A Personal Report* (New York: Norton, 1987); and Kim McQuaid, *The Anxious Years: America in the Vietnam-Watergate Era* (New York: Basic Books, 1989).

2. Dale C. Garell, "Adolescent Medicine: A Survey in the United States and Canada," *American Journal of the Diseases of Children* 109 (April 1965): 314–317.

3. Dale C. Garell, "Adolescent Medicine: Entering It's [sic] Own Adolescence?" *Adolescent Medicine: A Semi-Annual Letter in the Interest of Adolescent Medical Care* [hereafter referred to as *Adolescent Medicine*] 1/1 (February 1965): 1–2. *Adolescent Medicine* was a mimeographed newsletter for physicians interested in adolescent medical care that Garell began to compile and distribute among adolescent clinic directors in 1965.

4. Andrew Rigg and Rona C. Fisher, "Some Comments on Current Hospital Medical Services for Adolescents," *American Journal of Diseases of Children* 120/3 (1970): 193–196; Adele D. Hofmann, "Fellowships in Adolescent Medicine," *Journal of Pediatrics* 83/3 (1973): 512; Joseph L. Rauh, "Survey of Physician Fellows in Adolescent Medicine," *Journal of Adolescent Health Care* 1/1 (1980): 52; Joseph L. Rauh and Alice Passer, "Survey of Physicians in Adolescent Medicine, 1979–1984," *Journal of Adolescent Health Care* 7/1 (1986): 34; Victor Strasburger, "(W(h)ither Adolescent Medicine? A Mid-Life Crisis," *Journal of Adolescent Health Care* (1988): 449–451; and Elizabeth R. McAnarney, "Adolescent Medicine: Growth of a Discipline," *Pediatrics* 82/2 (August 1988): 270–272.

5. Gallagher, *Medical Care of the Adolescent* (New York: Appleton-Century Crofts, 1960).

6. Information on visits to the Adolescent Unit by other physicians and the development of the postgraduate course comes from the Annual Reports of the Adolescent Unit, Boston.

7. See meeting programs for the Society for Adolescent Medicine for content of meetings. I am grateful to Dr. Joseph Rauh of the Adolescent Unit at Cincinnati Children's Hospital Medical Center for preserving these programs and allowing me to consult them.

8. Halpern, *American Pediatrics: The Social Dynamics of Professionalism, 1880–1980* (Berkeley: University of California Press, 1988), p. 111.

9. Garell noted that by 1970, over half of population in the United States would be under age twenty-five, and the next five years would see the adolescent age population increase by 50 percent. Garell, "Adolescent Medicine," p. 314.

10. Interview with Thomas Shaffer by Heather Munro Prescott, 8 January 1994, Columbus, Ohio; and interview with Robert T. Brown by HMP, 6 January 1994, Columbus, Ohio; both tape recordings in Prescott's possession.

11. *Minutes of the Children's Heart Association,* Department of Pediatrics, Cincinnati General Hospital, Cincinnati, Ohio; *Cincinnati Adolescent Clinic, Division of*

Adolescent Medicine, 25th Anniversary, 1960–1985 (Cincinnati: Children's Hospital Medical Center, 1985).

12. Reports of Board of Directors, Board of Directors Files, Library, National Children's Hospital, Washington, D.C., hereafter referred to as Board of Directors Files, National Children's Hospital; interview with Dr. Robert Parrott by Heather Munro Prescott, 27 June 1994, Washington, D.C., tape recording in Prescott's possession.

13. Garell, "Adolescent Medicine," p. 315.

14. Ibid., p. 315.

15. Interview with Dr. Thomas E. Shaffer conducted by Heather Munro Prescott, Columbus, Ohio, 8 January 1994, tape recording in Prescott's possession. Shaffer was eventually coaxed back to Children's Hospital in 1964, after the adolescent unit received a grant from the Children's Bureau to fund staff salaries.

16. Interview with Dale Garell and Robert Blum conducted by Heather Munro Prescott, 19 March 1993, Chicago, Ill., tape recording in Prescott's possession.

17. Joseph P. Michelson, "The Jewish Hospital of Brooklyn Adolescent Clinic," *Adolescent Medicine* (November 1966): 15. An interview with Joseph L. Rauh at the Children's Hospital of Cincinnati indicates that he had some difficulties with other staff at the Hospital, although to a lesser degree than did Heald. Interview with Rauh by Heather Munro Prescott 9 April 9 1991, Cincinnati, Ohio, tape recording in Prescott's possession. See also interview with Garell and Blum.

18. Garell and Blum interview.

19. For more on the status of the Adolescent Unit in relationship to the rest of Children's Hospital Medical Center, see interview with Felix P. Heald by Heather Munro Prescott, 24 March 1990, Atlanta, Ga.; interview with Heald by HMP, 21 September 1990, Baltimore, Md.; interviews with Robert Masland by HMP, 27 December 1989, 25 July 1990, and 19 February 1991, Boston, Mass.; and interview with Thomas Cone by HMP, 9 November 1990, Cambridge, Mass. Tape recordings of all these interviews are deposited in the Children's Hospital Archives.

20. See Annual Reports of the Adolescent Unit, Boston, Children's Hospital Archives. My interview with Rauh indicates that he, as well as some of his colleagues, only spent a brief time at the Adolescent Unit in Boston before going on to found their own adolescent clinics.

21. Interview with Adele Hofmann by HMP 28 January 1991, conducted by telephone, tape recording in Prescott's possession.

22. Dale Garell, "Here We Go," *Adolescent Medicine,* (June 1968): 2; Charles Irwin, "Why Adolescent Medicine?" *Journal of Adolescent Health Care* 7/6S (November 1986, Supplement): 4S.

23. Garell, "Adolescent Medicine: Entering It's [sic] Own Adolescence," p. 1.

24. Gallagher, "The Origins, Development, and Goals of Adolescent Medicine," *Journal of Adolescent Health Care* 3 (1982): 60–61.

25. Joseph L. Rauh, "Felix Heald, M.D.: Scholar and Pioneer in Adolescent Medicine" (unpublished paper presented at Felix Heald Day, Baltimore, Md., September 22, 1990), p. 5; Felix Heald, "The History of Adolescent Medicine," in *Textbook of Adolescent Medicine,* ed. Elizabeth R. McAnarney, Richard E. Krelpe, Donald P. Orr, and George D. Comerci (Philadelphia: W. B. Saunders, 1992), p. 4.

26. "Topics of Discussion," *Adolescent Medicine* 1/2 (November 1965): 7.

27. Dale C. Garell, "Toward an Adolescent Medical Society," *Adolescent Medicine* 1/2 (November 1965): 2.

28. The expression "young turks" comes from Rauh's recollections of this period. See Rauh, "Felix Heald," p. 5; and interview with Rauh by HMP, 9 April 1991. The formation of the ad hoc committee is described in a "Special Announcement" published in *Adolescent Medicine* 3/2 (December 1967): 7.

29. Garell, "Here We Go," 1.

30. *Adolescent Medicine* 5/1 (June 1969): 4.

31. Garell, "Is the Adolescent Clinic a Specialty Clinic?" *Adolescent Medicine* 3/2 (December 1967): 1–4.

32. Quoted in Charles A. Janeway, "Pediatrics and the Adolescent: Presentation of the C. Anderson Aldrich Award to J. Roswell Gallagher," *Pediatrics* 51/3 (March 1973): 456.

33. "Topics of Discussion," *Adolescent Medicine* 1/2 (November 1965): 7.

34. "Excerpt from 'A Survey of Adolescent Medicine in the U.S. and Canada,'" *Adolescent Medicine* 1/1 (February 1965): 9.

35. "Topics of Discussion," *Adolescent Medicine* 1/2 (November 1965): 7.

36. Paul Starr, *The Social Transformation of American Medicine* (New York: Basic Books, 1982), p. 363.

37. Memorandum to members of attending staff from P. B. Swope, president of Board of Directors, September 3, 1959, Board of Directors Files, National Children's Hospital.

38. Board of Directors Reports, 1957–1960, Board of Directors Files, National Children's Hospital; Lawrence D'Angelo and Tomas J. Silber, "Adolescent Medicine at Children's Hospital National Medical Center," *Clinical Proceedings of the Children's Hospital National Medical Center* 40 (1984): 379–380.

39. Annual Report of the Adolescent Clinic, University of Cincinnati Medical Center, 1965.

40. Telephone conversation with Dale Garell, 16 November 1995.

41. Arthur Lesser, "The Origin and Development of Maternal and Child Health Programs in the United States," *American Journal of Public Health* 75/6 (June 1985): 593–594. For more on the early history of these Children's Bureau programs, see Kriste Lindenmeyer, *A Right to Childhood: The U.S. Children's Bureau and Child Welfare, 1912–1946* (Urbana: University of Illinois Press, 1997).

42. Programs funded by special project grants are listed in a letter from Dorothea Andrews to Alice Lake, October 21, 1966, Children's Bureau, Central Files, Box 101, Folder 4–5–12, National Archives, Washington, D.C., hereafter referred to as Children's Bureau, Central Files.

43. The files of the Children's Bureau contain numerous requests from adolescent unit directors for financial assistance, and regretful letters from bureau personnel informing them that the Title V appropriations were not sufficient to cover all the programs that needed financial assistance. For example, see Arthur J. Lesser to Dr. Samuel Karelitz, Chief of Pediatrics, Long Island Jewish Hospital, August 21, 1963, Children's Bureau, Central Files, Box 1003, Folder 4-9-4; Robert W. Deisher, Deputy Chief, Children's Bureau, to Harris D. Riley, Dept. of Pediatrics, University of Oklahoma, March 23, 1964, Children's Bureau, Central Files, Box 1003, Folder 4-9-4; Arthur Lesser to Dale Garell, Children's Hospital of Los Angeles, August 18, 1964, Children's Bureau, Central Files, Box 1003, Folder 4-9-4.

44. S. L. Hammar, "The University of Washington Adolescent Clinic," *Adolescent Medicine* 2/2 (November 1966): 21–24.

45. *Adolescent Medicine* 1/2 (November 1965): 3.

46. Arthur Lesser, "Report of Conference on Special Project Grants, June 27, 28, 1961," Children's Bureau, Central Files, Box 1059, Folder 12-0-4-8.

47. James T. Patterson, *America's Struggle against Poverty, 1900–1994* (Cambridge, Mass.: Harvard University Press, 1994).

48. Kennedy, "Special Message to Congress," *Papers of the Presidents: John F. Kennedy, 1963.* (Washington, D.C.: Government Printing Office, 1963), pp. 164–172.

49. Ibid., pp. 165–166, 171.

50. Michael Harrington, *The Other America* (New York, 1962); John Kenneth Galbraith, *The Affluent Society* (Boston, 1958).

51. Lesser, *Health of Children of School Age,* Children's Bureau Publication no. 427–1964 (Washington, D.C.: Children's Bureau, 1964). See also Clara Schiffer and Eleanor Hunt, *Illness among Children: Data on the United States National Health Survey* (Washington, D.C.: Children's Bureau, 1963).

52. For more on the history and shortcomings of the Medicaid program, see Karen Davis and Cathy Schoen, *Health and the War on Poverty: A Ten-Year Appraisal* (Washington, D.C.: Brookings Institution, 1978); Robert Stevens and Rosemary Stevens, *Welfare Medicine in America: A Case Study of Medicaid* (New York: Free Press, 1974); and Rashi Fein, *Medical Care, Medical Costs: The Search for a Health Insurance Policy* (Cambridge, Mass.: Harvard University Press, 1986).

53. Arthur J. Lesser, "The Origin and Development of Maternal and Child Health Programs in the United States," *American Journal of Public Health* 75/6 (June 1985): 596.

54. U.S. Dept. of Health, Education, and Welfare (HEW), *The Children and*

Youth Projects: Comprehensive Health Care in Low Income Areas (Washington, D.C.: Government Printing Office, 1972), p. 5.

55. Quoted in Lesser, "The Origin and Development of Maternal and Child Health Programs," p. 596.

56. For a summary of these amendments, see U.S. Congress, House, Committee on Ways and Means, *Summary of Major Provisions of Public Law 89–97, the Social Security Amendments of 1965* (Washington, D.C.: Government Printing Office, 1965), pp. 8–9.

57. Lesser, "The Origin and Development of Maternal and Child Health," pp. 595–596; Davis and Schoen, *Health and the War on Poverty*, pp. 131–134.

58. U.S. Dept. of HEW, *The Children and Youth Projects*, pp. 7, 16–18. It is difficult to say with precision how many of the C & Y programs had a "special emphasis" on adolescents. The HEW report only mentions Alabama and Roosevelt specifically, and notes that "a number of other C & Ys have or are planning special adolescent health programs."

59. Davis and Schoen, *Health and the War on Poverty*, p. 124.

60. Lesser, "The Origin and Development of Maternal and Child Health," p. 595.

61. Davis and Schoen, *Health and the War on Poverty*, p. 139.

62. Constance Nathanson, *Dangerous Passage: The Social Control of Sexuality in Women's Adolescence* (Philadelphia: Temple University Press, 1991), p. 42.

63. Ibid., pp. 43–44.

64. Hilary Millar, *Approaches to Adolescent Health Care in the 1970s* (Rockville, Md.: U.S. Dept. of Health, Education, and Welfare, 1975), p. 30. There were legal complications barring fuller adolescent participation in these programs, which are described in further detail below.

65. Davis and Schoen, *Health and the War on Poverty*, p. 163. The phrase "maximum feasible participation" was coined by Richard Boone, aide to Jack Conway, one of Sargent Shriver's aides in the OEO. Patterson, *America's Struggle against Poverty*, p. 145.

66. U.S. Department of Health, Education, and Welfare, Office of the Secretary (Planning and Evaluation), *Delivery of Health Services for the Poor* (Washington, D.C.: Government Printing Office, 1967), pp. 5a, 52.

67. Schoen and Davis, *Health and the War on Poverty*, p. 170. This fell far short of the OEO's goal to expand the program to include 1,000 centers, serving 25 million low-income people.

68. Lee B. Macht, Donald J. Scherl, William J. Bicknell, and Joseph T. English, "The Job Corps as a Community Health Challenge," *American Journal of Orthopsychiatry* 39/3 (April 1969): 504–511; William J. Bicknell, Lee B. Macht, Donald J. Scherl, and Joseph T. English, "Evolution of a Health Program: The Job Corps Experience," *American Journal of Public Health* 60/5 (May 1970): 829–837; Lee

Macht and Donald J. Scherl, "Adjustment Phases and Mental Health Interventions among Job Corps Trainees," *Psychiatry* 37 (August 1974): 229–239; Jon E. Fielding and Scott H. Nelson, "Health Care for the Economically Disadvantaged Adolescent," *Pediatric Clinics of North America* 20/4 (November 1973): 975–988; Jon E. Fielding, ed., *Problems in Comprehensive Ambulatory Health Care for High Risk Adolescents* (Washington, D.C.: Dept. of Labor, 1973); and Charles R. Hayman and Arthur Frank, "The Job Corps Experience with Health Problems Among Disadvantaged Youth," *Public Health Reports* 94/5 (September-October 1976): 407–414. The Office for Health for Health Affairs also supervised health programs for other OEO programs, including VISTA and the Community Action Programs.

69. Dale Garell, "Adolescent Medicine and the Poverty Programs," *Adolescent Medicine* 2/1 (June 1966): 2–3.

70. Board of Directors Report, February 1969, Board of Directors Files, National Children's Hospital.

71. *Adolescent Medicine* 3/1 (June 1967): 6–9; *Adolescent Medicine* 3/2 (December 1967): 10, 13; *Adolescent Medicine* 4/1 (June 1968): 5–7.

72. *Adolescent Medicine* 3/1 (June 1967): 7–9; *Adolescent Medicine* 3/2 (December 1967): 11–13; *Adolescent Medicine* 4/1 (June 1968): 5–7; *Adolescent Medicine* 4/2 (December 1968): 17–18.

73. Electronic mail message from William Daniel to Heather Munro Prescott, 2 December 1995; U.S. Dept. of HEW, *The Children and Youth Projects*, pp. 16–17. Interest in the adolescent medicine program waned after Daniel's retirement, and there is currently no adolescent service at the University of Alabama.

74. *Adolescent Medicine* 3/1 (June 1967): 5; *Annual Reports of the Adolescents' Unit*, Boston Children's Hospital, 1966–67, 1967–68.

75. Los Angeles, for example, worked with Neighborhood Health Centers in Watts and East Los Angeles as well as those in South Central. *Adolescent Medicine* 3/1 (June 1967): 9–10; *Adolescent Medicine* 3/2 (December 1967): 10, 15; *Adolescent Medicine* 4/1 (June 1968): 7, 12; *Adolescent Medicine* 4/2 (December 1968): 14, 24.

76. Masland, Annual Report of the Adolescent Unit, Boston, 1967–68, Children's Hospital Archives.

77. Joseph M. Conforti, "Attitudes toward Health and Health Care Facilities among Low Income Youth," *Social Science Quarterly* 50 (1969): 689–694.

78. An article published in 1973 described youthful alienation as "the phenomenon of a youth group, members ranging from mid-adolescence to young adulthood, which rejects the traditional status system based on educational and occupational achievement through competition. Instead, they embrace a value system that emphasizes the search for a simple stress-free way of life which they hope will provide emotional satisfaction and the preservation of self-esteem." Donald C. Ross, Sr., and Donald C. Ross, Jr., "Youthful Alienation and Social Mobility," *Clinical Pediatrics* 12/1 (January 1973): 22.

79. David E. Smith, "Runaways and Their Health Problems in Haight-Ashbury during the Summer of 1967," *American Journal of Public Health* 59/11 (November 1969): 2046–2047.

80. For more on the history of the Haight-Ashbury clinic, see David E. Smith, *Love Needs Care: A History of San Francisco's Haight-Ashbury Free Medical Clinic* (Boston: Little, Brown, 1971); and Richard B. Seymour and David E. Smith, *The Haight-Ashbury Free Medical Clinics: Still Free after All These Years, 1967–1987* (San Francisco: Partisan Press, 1987).

81. D. Marsh, "New Program Reaches Out to Street Youth," *Massachusetts General Hospital News* 30 (1970): 5.

82. For more on the Cambridgeport Medical Clinic, see Joseph Brenner, "A Free Clinic for Medical Care," *New York Times Magazine* (October 1970): 30–31, 107–117; and interview with Dr. Joseph Brenner conducted by Heather Munro Prescott, 19 February 1991, tape recording in Prescott's possession.

83. For more on Guthrie's work with the Bridge and the mobile medical unit, see Marsh, "New Program"; Andrew D. Guthrie, Jr., and Mary C. Howell, "Mobile Medical Care for Alienated Youth," *Journal of Pediatrics* 81/5 (November 1972): 1025–1033; Guthrie, "For the Street Scene: Mobile Medical Care," *Journal of Social Issues* 30/1 (1974): 173–180; Millar, *Approaches to Adolescent Health Care*, pp. 34–35; and interview with Guthrie conducted by Heather Munro Prescott, 13 February 1991, tape recording deposited in Children's Hospital Archives.

84. Irene R. Turner, "Free Health Centers: A New Concept?" *American Journal of Public Health* 62/10 (October 1972): 1348.

85. Seymour and Smith, *The Haight-Ashbury Free Medical Clinics*, pp. 125–152.

86. Herbert J. Freudenberger and Arlene P. Freudenberger, *1973—The Free Clinic Picture Today—A Survey* (New York: American Psychological Association, 1974), p. 6.

87. The term "new breed" comes from Turner, "Free Health Centers," p. 1351. The comment on the liberal political views of clinic personnel comes from Freudenberger and Freudenberger, *1973—The Free Clinic Picture Today*, pp. 11–12.

88. Seymour and Smith, *The Haight-Ashbury Free Clinics*, pp. 27–28.

89. Promotional materials on The Door: A Center of Alternatives; Millar, *Approaches to Adolescent Health Care*, pp. 34–35; Sidney Lecker, Loraine Henricks, and James Turanski, "New Dimensions in Adolescent Psychotherapy: A Therapeutic System Approach," *Pediatric Clinics of North America* 20/4 (November 1973): 883–900; Loraine Henricks, "The Door—A Center of Alternatives: Developmental Features of an Innovative Multiservice Center and Health Care Facility," from Conference Packet, "Youth, Health, and Social Systems," Breckenridge, Colo., October 28–November 1, 1973, pp. 1–17.

90. Seymour and Smith, *The Haight-Ashbury Free Medical Clinics*.

91. Marsh, "New Program," p. 5, mentions that medical students and residents

from the Children's Hospital were among the many physicians who volunteered their services to the medical van.

92. Henricks, "The Door—A Center of Alternatives," pp. 1–2.

93. For example, see Alice Lake's health advice columns in *Seventeen* magazine, including "What Teenage Medicine Can Do for You," *Seventeen* 29 (June 1970): 132–133, 185–187; and idem, "What Happens behind the Doctor's Door," *Seventeen* 26 (December 1967): 102–103, 137. See also Betty Klarnet, "One of Their Own," *Family Health* 1/2 (November 1969): 26–30; Linda Pembrook, "Adolescent Clinics: A Vital Step in Solving Problems of Teenagers," *Parents' Magazine* 47 (November 1972): 68–70, 113; and Stanley Englebardt, "Now: Health Care Teenagers Can Believe In," *Today's Health* 51 (June 1973): 16–19, 60–62.

94. Garell, Report on Current Activities of Division of Adolescent Medicine at Children's Hospital of Los Angeles, *Adolescent Medicine* 4/1 (June 1968): 12; Millar, *Approaches to Adolescent Health Care*, p. 34; interview with Dale Garell and Robert Blum by Heather Munro Prescott, 19 March 1993, Society for Adolescent Medicine meeting, Chicago, Ill., tape recording in Prescott's possession.

95. Millar, *Approaches to Adolescent Health Care*, pp. 29–30; Katherine A. Zsoldos, "Montefiore's Experiment in Adolescent Medicine," *Medical Dimensions* (April 1972): 54–56.

96. *Adolescent Medicine* 2/2 (November 1966): 8.

97. Masland, Annual Report of the Adolescent Unit, Boston, 1967–68, Children's Hospital Archives.

98. Information on the Breckenridge Conference comes from "Problems of Health Programming Related to Minority Youth," Conference Program, Youth, Health, and Social Systems, Breckenridge, Colo., October 29–November 1, 1973; and Millar, *Approaches to Adolescent Health Care*, pp. 38–39.

99. Conference Program, Youth, Health, and Social Systems.

100. Ibid.

101. Somers H. Sturgis, "Introduction," in Felix P. Heald, ed., *Adolescent Gynecology* (Baltimore, Md.: Williams and Wilkins, 1966), pp. 5, 7.

102. Somers H. Sturgis et al., *The Gynecologic Patient: A Psycho-Endocrine Study* (New York: Grune and Stratton, 1962), p. 67.

103. Nathanson, *Dangerous Passage;* Rickie Solinger, *Wake Up Little Susie: Single Pregnancy and Race before Roe v. Wade* (New York and London: Routledge, 1992)

104. Solinger, *Wake Up Little Susie*, p. 42.

105. Nathanson, *Dangerous Passage*, p. 245n14.

106. E. Goodman and E. Gerber, "She Won't Be Back," *American Education* 3/9 (1967): 6–8; Marion Howard, *The Webster School: A District of Columbia Program for Pregnant Girls* (Washington, D.C.: U.S. Dept. of Health, Education, and Welfare, Children's Bureau, 1968); Howard J. Osofsky, *The Pregnant Teenager: A Medical, Educational, and Social Analysis* (Springfield, Ill.: Charles C. Thomas, 1968); Lor-

raine V. Klerman and James F. Jekel, *School-Age Mothers: Problems, Programs, and Policy* (Hamden, Conn.: Linnet Books, 1973); and Frank R. Furstenberg, *Unplanned Parenthood: The Social Consequences of Teenage Childbearing* (New York: Free Press, 1976), cited in Nathanson, *Dangerous Passage*, p. 245n14.

107. Solinger, *Wake Up Little Susie*, pp. 214–215.

108. Some historians have argued that the sexual revolution of the 1960s actually began at least a decade earlier. See Rosalind Pollack Petchesky, *Abortion and Woman's Choice* (Boston: Northeastern University Press, 1990), pp. 205–238; Nathanson, *Dangerous Passage*; Solinger, *Wake Up Little Susie*; Kristin Luker, *Dubious Conceptions: The Politics of Teenage Pregnancy* (Cambridge, Mass.: Harvard University Press, 1996); and Beth Bailey, "Sexual Revolution(s)" in *The Sixties: From Memory to History*, ed. David Farber (Chapel Hill: University of North Carolina Press, 1994), pp. 235–262.

109. Kinsey, *Sexual Behavior in the Human Female* (Philadelphia: Saunders, 1953).

110. Jerome S. Menaker, "Teenage Obstetrics," *Pediatrics Clinics of North America* (February 1958): 141–142.

111. Rauh, Annual Report of the Adolescent Clinic, Children's Hospital Medical Center, Cincinnati, October 2, 1961, Rauh History Files, Children's Hospital Medical Center, Cincinnati, Ohio.

112. Southam, "Metropathia Hemorrhagica and Nonpsychogenic Amenorrhea," in *Adolescent Gynecology*, ed. Heald, p. 51.

113. Data on gender ratios in adolescent medicine come from Garell, "Adolescent Medicine," p. 316; and Joseph L. Rauh and Alice Passer, "Survey of Physician Fellows in Adolescent Medicine, 1979–1984," *Journal of Adolescent Health Care* 7 (1986). 36

114. Jean Emans and Donald Peter Goldstein, *Pediatric and Adolescent Gynecology* (Boston: Little, Brown, 1982), p. 10. Goldstein was gynecological consultant to the Adolescent Unit at Boston Children's Hospital during the 1970s and 1980s. Emans has been on the staff of the Adolescent Unit for the past two decades, and replaced Masland as director of the Adolescent Unit in 1992.

115. Joan Jacobs Brumberg, *The Body Project: An Intimate History of American Girls* (New York: Random House, 1997), pp. 171–192.

116. Fielding and Nelson, "Health Care for the Economically Disadvantaged Adolescent," pp. 975–988; Millar, *Approaches to Adolescent Health Care*, pp. 38–39.

117. Sally Irving to Masland, undated circa December, 1969, Masland correspondence files, Children's Hospital Archives. As with the patient case records, Sally's name has been changed.

118. For more on the laws and court decisions governing minors' access to medical care during this time, see Harriet F. Pilpel, "Minors' Rights to Medical Care," *Albany Law Review* 36 (1972): 462–487; and Lawrence Wilkins, "Children's

Rights: Removing the Parental Consent Barrier to Medical Treatment of Minors," *Arizona State Law Journal* (1975): 31–92.

119. Masland to Jerome T.Y. Shen, 28 July 1971, Masland Correspondence Files, Children's Hospital Archives.

120. Telephone interview with Adele Hofmann by Heather Munro Prescott, 28 January 1991, tape recording in Prescott's possession. See also Hofmann and I. Ronald Shenker, "Medical Care of Adolescents and the Law," *New York State Journal of Medicine* 70 (October 15, 1970): 2603–2611; Hofmann and Harriet Pilpel, "The Legal Rights of Minors," *Pediatric Clinics of North America* 20/4 (November 1973): 989–1004; and Hofmann, "Consent, Confidentiality, the Law, and Adolescents," *Delaware Medical Journal* 45 (February 1973): 35–39.

121. Smith, *Love Needs Care.*

122. Pilpel, "Minors' Rights to Medical Care," p. 466.

123. *In re Gault,* 387 U.S. 1 (1967); *Tinker v. Des Moines Independent School District,* 393 U.S. 503 (1969). For more on the movement to expand the legal rights of minors during this period, see Joseph M. Hawes, *The Children's Rights Movement* (Boston: Twayne Publishers, 1991), pp. 80–95.

124. Garell, "Due Process," *Adolescent Medicine* 3/1 (June 1967): 2–4.

125. D. E. Greydarus, "Abortion in Adolescence," in *Premature Adolescent Pregnancy and Parenthood,* in E. R. McAnarney (New York: Grune and Stratton, 1983), p. 355.

126. Gallagher, *Medical Care of the Adolescent,* p. 13.

127. Greydarus, "Abortion in Adolescence," p. 355. See also Nathanson, *Dangerous Passage;* Solinger, *Wake Up Little Susie.*

128. Millar, *Approaches to Adolescent Health Care,* pp. 30–31; Davis and Schoen, *Health and the War on Poverty,* pp. 159–160.

129. Davis and Schoen, *Health and the War on Poverty,* pp. 170–173.

130. Garell, "On Being Relevant," *Adolescent Medicine* 5/1 (June 1969): 2–3.

131. For more on the history of the American Academy of Pediatrics, see Halpern, *American Pediatrics,* pp. 80, 94–95, 102–103.

132. Minutes of Executive Board, November 1970, Society for Adolescent Medicine Archives, Pediatric History Center, Bakwin Library, American Academy of Pediatrics, Chicago, Ill., hereafter referred to as SAM Archives.

133. Hofmann, "Fellowships in Adolescent Medicine," *Adolescent Medicine* 8/1 (Summer 1972): 2–31.

134. "Retreat/Planning Session, October 12, 1972," *Adolescent Medicine* 9/1 (Spring 1973): 6.

135. "Minutes of the Executive Council–Committee Chairman Retreat, October 17, 1974," *Adolescent Medicine* 11/1 (Spring 1975): 14–15; "Executive Council Meeting Minutes, October 19, 1978," *Adolescent Medicine* 15/1 (Spring 1979): 3.

136. Michael I. Cohen, "Importance, Implementation, and Impact of the Ado-

lescent Medicine Components of the Report of the Task Force on Pediatric Education," *Journal of Adolescent Health Care* 1/1 (1980): 2.

137. Task Force on Pediatric Education, *The Future of Pediatric Education* (Evanston, Ill.: American Academy of Pediatrics, 1978).

138. Cohen, "Importance, Implementation, and Impact," p. 2.

139. Minutes of Executive Council Retreat, October 1976, SAM Archives.

140. "Executive Council Retreat, October, 1976," *Adolescent Medicine* 13/1 (Spring 1977): 4.

141. Adele D. Hofmann, "Society for Adolescent Medicine Statement of Purpose," manuscript, 1977, SAM Archives.

142. For more on the distinction between the American Academy of Pediatrics, the American Pediatric Society, and the Society for Pediatric Research, see Halpern, *American Pediatrics,* pp. 118–119.

143. Heald, "History of Adolescent Medicine," p. 15.

144. Heald, "Special Communication: History of the Society for Adolescent Medicine," *Adolescent Medicine* 15/1 (Spring 1979): 28–29.

145. "Retreat. Washington, D.C., January 25, 1979," *Adolescent Medicine* 15/1 (Spring 1979): 6.

146. Letter from John Edlin to Heather Munro Prescott 15 January 1996.

147. "Retreat. Washington, D.C., January 25, 1979," *Adolescent Medicine* 15/1 (Spring 1979): 6.

148. Ibid.

149. "Retreat/Planning Session, October 12, 1972," *Adolescent Medicine* 9/1 (Spring 1973): 6.

150. Rosemary Stevens, *American Medicine and the Public Interest* (New Haven: Yale University Press, 1971), p. 325. According to Sydney Halpern, most medical segments that attempted to gain autonomous boards after World War II encountered the same kinds of problems. Since 1950 the ABMS has awarded only four primary boards: family practice, nuclear medicine, allergy and immunology, and emergency medicine. Halpern, *American Pediatrics,* pp. 110–111. For a timeline of medical specialties and subspecialties, see Dorothy Susan Indyk, "The Emergence of Perinatal Medicine: A Paradigm for the Study of the Process of Differentiation and Integration in Medicine" (Ph.D. diss., Columbia University, 1987), p. 51.

151. "Minutes of the Executive Council Meeting, October 18, 1975," *Adolescent Medicine* 12/1 (Spring 1976): 7–8.

152. See results of survey in "Committee on Education: Where From and Where To? Report to Executive Council, May 12, 1976," *Adolescent Medicine* 12/2 (Fall 1976): 27–28.

153. For example, see Bob Latta's testimony, "Minutes of the General Business Meeting, October 18, 1975," *Adolescent Medicine* 12/1 (Spring 1976): 11.

154. See testimony of Adele Hofmann, "Minutes of Executive Council Meeting,

October 18, 1975," p. 8; and testimony of Dr. Oberst, "Minutes of the General Business Meeting, October 18, 1975," p. 11, SAM Archives.

155. See testimony of Dr. Piel and Dr. Shenker, "Minutes of Executive Council Meeting, October 18, 1975," p. 8, SAM Archives.

156. "Committee on Education: Where From and Where To?" p. 28.

157. Gallagher's views on adolescent patient care come from interviews conducted by Heather Munro Prescott on 28 December 1989 and 9 February 1991, Lexington, Mass., tape recordings in Children's Hospital Archives; and from Gallagher's numerous articles on adolescent medicine. For example, see Gallagher, "A Clinic for Adolescents," *Children* 1 (1954): 167; and Gallagher and Heald, "Adolescence: Summary of Round Table Discussion," *Pediatrics* 18 (1956): 1019.

158. See interviews with Masland.

159. Letter to Society for Adolescent Medicine from Board of Trustees of the American Medical Association—Subject: Actions of AMA Board of Trustees re: New Specialties, December 8, 1977, quoted in Tomas Silber, "Adolescent Medicine: A Sociological Perspective," *Adolescent Medicine* 14/2 (Fall 1978): 15.

160. Silber, "Adolescent Medicine," p. 15.

161. Executive Council Meeting Minutes, November 4, 1977, SAM Archives.

162. Executive Council Meeting Minutes, October 19, 1978, in *Adolescent Medicine* 15/1 (Spring 1979): 3. For more on the history of the use of "fellow" status to distinguish members of medical societies with special expertise, see Stevens, *American Medicine and the Public Interest*, p. 94.

163. Richard G. MacKenzie, "President's Message," *Society for Adolescent Medicine Mini-Newsletter* (formerly *Adolescent Medicine*), 1/1 (Spring 1980): 2.

164. Richard G. MacKenzie, "Editorial: The First Issue," *Journal of Adolescent Health Care* 1 (1980): 63.

165. For discussions of the Fellow status in SAM, see Executive Council Minutes for October 28, 1981; May 10, 1982; October 20, 1982; and May 2, 1983; and the Minutes of the Annual Business Meeting for the membership at large, October 22, 1982, and October 21, 1983, SAM Archives.

166. Strasburger, "W(h)ither Adolescent Medicine."

167. After reaching a peak of 44 training programs in 1984, the number declined to 36 in 1985 and to 35 in 1986. Data from listing of Specialty Training Programs in the *Journal of Pediatrics*, compiled by Indyk, "The Emergence of Perinatal Medicine," p. 87. The number of teenagers in the U.S. shrank from a high of 70 million in 1970 to 63 million in 1980. Bruce Chadwick and Tim B. Heaton, *Statistical Handbook on Adolescents in America* (Phoenix, Ariz.: Orynx Press, 1996), p. 3.

168. Strasburger, "Looking for an Academic Job in Adolescent Medicine: A Personal Odyssey," *Journal of Adolescent Health Care* 10 (1989): 578–581.

169. G. Commerci, "Report of Ad-Hoc Committee on Pediatric Residency

Training," read before the SAM Annual Meeting, Denver, 1985, quoted in Irwin, "Why Adolescent Medicine," p. 5S.

170. Gail B. Slap, "Adolescent Medicine: Attitudes and Skills of Pediatric and Medical Residents," *Pediatrics* 74 (1984): 191–197; Michael D. Resnick, "Use of Age Cut-Off Policies for Adolescents in Pediatric Practice: Report from the Upper Midwest Regional Physician Survey," *Pediatrics* 73 (1983): 420–427; and L. S. Neinstein and J. R. Shapiro, "Pediatricians' Self-Evaluation of Adolescent Health Care Training, Skills and Interest," *Journal of Adolescent Health Care* 7 (1986): 18–21.

171. Strasburger, "W(h)ither Adolescent Medicine," p. 450.

172. This chronology comes from Charles Irwin's presentation at a Panel Discussion on Board Certification held at the Society for Adolescent Medicine Business Meeting, Atlanta, Ga., March 24, 1990, SAM Archives.

173. Ibid.

174. Minutes of Panel Discussion on Board Certification, Society for Adolescent Medicine Business Meeting, Atlanta, Georgia, March 24, 1990, SAM Archives.

175. Charles E. Irwin, "Interim Report Regarding the Subspecialty Boards in Adolescent Medicine," *Society for Adolescent Medicine Newsletter,* n.s. 2/2 (Fall 1991): 1.

176. Interview with Charles E. Irwin conducted by Heather Munro Prescott, 20 March 1993, Chicago, Ill., tape recording in Prescott's possession.

177. Interview with Victor Strasburger, 13 November 1993, Albuquerque, N.M., tape recording in Prescott's possession.

178. "Retreat of the Society for Adolescent Medicine, Dallas, Texas, February 10, 1984," SAM Archives.

Conclusion

1. For an overview of these studies, see U.S. Congress, Office of Technology Assessment (OTA), *Adolescent Health—Volume I: Summary and Policy Options, OTA-H-468* (Washington, D.C.: Government Printing Office, April 1991), pp. I-26–I-27.

2. U.S. Congress, OTA, *Adolescent Health;* Janet E. Gans, *America's Adolescents: How Healthy Are They?* (Chicago: American Medical Association, 1990).

3. Christopher Lasch, *Haven in a Heartless World: The Family Besieged* (New York: Basic Books, 1977).

4. Linda Gordon makes a similar point about the interference of social workers in domestic violence cases. Gordon argues that while social welfare agencies did undermine the authority of the abusers—usually fathers—in their client-families, the victims of abuse often asked for, and often even benefited from, social workers' intrusion into family affairs. Gordon, *Heroes of Their Own Lives: The Politics and History of Family Violence, Boston, 1880–1960.* (New York: Viking Press, 1988), pp. 294–295.

5. "Access to Health Care for Adolescents: Position Paper of the Society for Adolescent Medicine," *Journal of Adolescent Health* 13 (1992): 162–170.

6. Sydney Lewis, *"A Totally Alien Life-Form": Teenagers* (New York: New Press, 1996), p. 83.

7. The most concise statement on the resurgence of politically conservative views regarding the American family is Arlene Skolnick, *Embattled Paradise: The American Family in an Age of Uncertainty* (New York: Basic Books, 1991).

8. Allan M. Brandt, "Behavior, Disease, and Health in Twentieth Century America: The Moral Valence of Individual Risk," in *Morality and Health*, ed. Allan Brandt and Paul Rozin (New York and London: Routledge, 1997).

9. Catherine Stevens-Simon, "Letter to the Editor: Working with the 'Personal Fable,'" *Journal of Adolescent Health* 14 (1993): 349; Victor Strasburger, *Getting Your Kids to Say 'No' in the '90s When You Said 'Yes' in the '60s: Survival Notes for Baby Boom Parents* (New York: Simon and Schuster, 1993), pp. 29–30.

10. The term "super predator" was coined by the juvenile justice expert John Diiulio and popularized in William Bennett, *Body Count: Moral Poverty and How to Win America's War against Crime and Drugs* (New York: Simon and Schuster, 1996). For more on how race influences juvenile justice decisions, see Madeline Wordes, "Locking Up Youth: The Impact of Race on Detention Decisions," *Journal of Research in Crime and Delinquency* 31 (1994): 149–165.

11. Stuart L. Kaplan, "A Note on Racial Bias in the Admission of Children and Adolescents to State Mental Health Facilities versus Correctional Facilities in New York," *American Journal of Psychiatry* 149 (1992): 768–772.

12. Constance A. Nathanson, *Dangerous Passage: The Social Control of Sexuality in Women's Adolescence* (Philadelphia: Temple University Press, 1991).

13. J. Kahn and K. Smith, *Familial Communication and Adolescent Sexual Behavior* (Cambridge, Mass.: American Institutes for Research, 1989).

14. L. H. Bearinger and E. R. McAnarney, "Integrated Community Health Delivery Programs for Youth: Study Group Report," quoted in U.S. Congress, OTA, *Adolescent Health*, p. I-45.

15. According to the most recent survey of pediatric diplomates by the American Board of Pediatrics, approximately 30 percent of pediatric residents choose to pursue subspecialty training. Approximately 0.7 percent of the pediatric residents surveyed chose to pursue fellowship training in adolescent medicine. By comparison, the most popular subspecialty, neonatal/perinatal medicine, attracted 6.3 percent of all pediatric residents. See Thomas R. Oliver et al., "Pediatric Workforce: Data from the American Board of Pediatrics," *Pediatrics* 99 (1997): 241–244.

16. The work of Mike Males is particularly compelling on this point. See Males, *The Scapegoat Generation: America's War on Adolescents* (Monroe, Maine: Common Courage Press, 1996).

17. Strasburger, *Getting Your Kids to Say 'No.'*

18. For more on adolescents' compliance with medical advice, see Ira M. Fried-

man and Iris F. Litt, "Adolescents' Compliance with Therapeutic Regimens," *Journal of Adolescent Health Care* 8 (1987): 52–67.

19. David Elkind, *The Hurried Child: Growing Up Too Fast Too Soon* (Reading, Mass.: Addison-Wesley, 1981); idem, *Ties That Stress: The New Family Imbalance* (Cambridge, Mass.: Harvard University Press, 1994).

20. Barbara A. Mitchell and Ellen M. Gee, "'Boomerang Kids' and Midlife Parental Marital Satisfaction," *Family Coordinator* 45/4 (October 1996): 442.

21. "A Position Statement of the Society for Adolescent Medicine," *Journal of Adolescent Health* 16/5 (May 1995): 413. For more on the debate about the proper age classification for adolescence, see Richard R. Brookman, "The Age of 'Adolescence,'" *Journal of Adolescent Health* 16/5 (May 1995): 339–340.

22. U.S. Congress, OTA, *Adolescent Health*, p. I-31; Oliver et al., "Pediatric Workforce."

23. Tomas J. Silber, "Adolescent Medicine: Origins, Segmenting, Synthesis," *Journal of Adolescent Health Care* 4 (1983): 136.

24. Information on the percentage of medical schools with adolescent divisions comes from the Society for Adolescent Medicine central office in Independence, Mo.

25. U.S. Congress, OTA, *Adolescent Health*, p. I-108.

26. Robert H. Durant, "Adolescent Health Research as We Proceed into the Twenty-first Century," *Journal of Adolescent Health* 17 (1995): 201.

27. Ibid.

Index

ALSO BY ADAM THIRLWELL

Politics
The Delighted States

THE ESCAPE

THE ESCAPE

A NOVEL

ADAM
THIRLWELL

FARRAR, STRAUS AND GIROUX

NEW YORK

Farrar, Straus and Giroux
18 West 18th Street, New York 10011

Copyright © 2009 by Adam Thirlwell
All rights reserved
Printed in the United States of America
Originally published in 2009 by Jonathan Cape, Great Britain
Published in the United States by Farrar, Straus and Giroux
First American edition, 2010

Library of Congress Cataloging-in-Publication Data
Thirlwell, Adam, 1978–
    The escape : a novel / Adam Thirlwell. — 1st American ed.
      p. cm.
    ISBN: 978-0-374-14878-2 (ha : alk. paper)
     1. Older men—Sexual behavior—Fiction.   2. Adultery—Fiction.
  3. Inheritance and succession—Fiction.   4. Alps Region—Fiction. I. Title.

PR6120.H575E83 2010
823'.92—dc22   2009042321

www.fsgbooks.com

10 9 8 7 6 5 4 3 2 1

TO ALISON,
FOR MY FAMILY

Contents

PART ONE

Haffner Unbound

1

And so the century ended: with Haffner watching a man caress a woman's breasts.

It was an imbroglio. He would admit that much. But at least it was an imbroglio of Haffner's making.

He might have been seventy-eight, but in Haffner's opinion he counted as young. He counted, in the words of the young, as hip. Or as close to hip as anyone else. Only Haffner, after all, would have been found in this position.

What position?

Concealed in a wardrobe, the doors darkly ajar, watching a woman be nakedly playful to her boyfriend.

This was why I admired him. Haffner Unbound! But there were other Haffners too – Haffner Pensive, Haffner Abandoned. He tended to see himself like this; as in a dream, in poses. Like the panels of a classical frieze.

A tzigani pop album – disco drumbeats, accordions, sporadic trumpets – was being broadcast by a compact-disc player above the minibar. This weakened his squinting concentration. He disliked the modern zest for sex with music. It was better, thought Haffner, for bodies to undress themselves in the quiet of the everyday background hum.

In Naples once, in what, he had to say, could only be described as a dive, in the liberated city, the lights went suddenly out, and so the piano stopped, and in the ensuing silent twilight Haffner watched a woman undress so slowly, so awkwardly, so peacefully – accompanied only by the accidental chime of wine glasses, the brief struck fizz of matches – that she had, until this moment, more than fifty years later, remained his ideal of beauty.

Now, however, Haffner was unsure of his ideals.

He continued looking at Zinka. It wasn't a difficult task. Her hair was dark; her nipples were long, and almost black, with stained pools of areolae; her stomach curved gently towards her hips, where the bone then steeply rose; her legs were slender. Her breasts and nose were cute. If Haffner had a type, then this was it: the feminine unfeminine. The word for her, in his heyday, would have been *gamine*. She was a *garçonne*. If those words were, he mused, at the end of his century, still used for girls at all.

They were not.

A suckling noise emerged from Niko, who was now tugging at Zinka's nipples with the pursed O of his mouth.

Haffner was lustful, selfish, vain – an entirely commonplace man. It was the unavoidable conclusion. He had to admit it. In London and New York he had practised as a banker. His life had been unremarkable. It was the twentieth century's idea of the bourgeois: the grey Atlantic Ocean. The horizontal fretting waves of the grey Atlantic Ocean. With Liberty at one extreme, and the Bank of England at the other. But Haffner wasn't straddling the Atlantic any more. A hotel in a spa town was now Haffner's temporary home. He was landlocked – adrift in the centre of Europe, aloft in the Alps.

And now he was hidden in a wardrobe.

He was not, however, the usual voyeur. It was true that Niko was unaware of his presence. But Zinka – Zinka knew all about this spectral form in the wardrobe. Somehow, in a way which had

4

seemed natural at the time, Zinka and Haffner had developed this idea of Haffner's unnatural pleasure. The causes were obscure, occasioned by some random confluence of Haffner's charm and the odd mixture Zinka felt of tenderness for Haffner and mischief towards her boyfriend. But however obscure its causes, the conclusion was obvious.

So, ladies and gentlemen, maybe Haffner was grand, in a way. Maybe Haffner was an epic hero. And if Haffner was a hero, then his wallet, with its creased photographs, was his mute mausoleum. Take a look! Haffner in Rome, wonkily crowned by the curve of the Colosseum, a medusan mess of spaghetti in front of him; Haffner and Livia at a garden party in Buckingham Palace, trying to smile while hoping that Livia's hat – a plate on which lay a pile of flowers – would not erupt and blow away; Haffner's grandson, Benjamin, aged four, in a Yankees baseball cap, pissing with cherubic abandon – a live Renaissance fountain – in the gardens of a country house.

All photo albums are unhappy, in the words of the old master, in their own particular way.

2

And me? I was born sixty years after Haffner. I was just a friend.

I went to see him, in a hospital on the outskirts of London. His finale in the centre of Europe had been a decade ago. Now, Haffner was dying. But then Haffner had been dying for so long.

—The thing is, he said, I just need to plan for the next forty-eight hours. We just need to organise the next few days of the new era.

And when I asked him what new era he meant, he replied that this was exactly what we had to find out.

Everything was ending. On the television, a panel was discussing the crisis. The money was disappearing. The banks were disappearing. The end, as usual, was continuing. I wasn't sorry for the money, however. I was sorry for Haffner. There was a miniature rose in bud on the table. Haffner was trying to explain. Something, he said, had gone very very wrong. Perhaps, he said, we just needed to get this closed – pointing to a bedside cabinet, whose lock was gone.

He was lower than the dust, he told me. Lower than the dust. After an hour, he wanted to go to the bathroom. He started trying to undress himself, there in his armchair. And so I called a nurse and then I left him, as he was ushered into the women's bathroom, because that bathroom was closer to the room in which Haffner was busily dying.

Standing in the hospital's elliptical concrete drive, as the electric doors opened and closed behind me, I waited for the taxi to take me to the trains – back to the city. Across the silver fields the mauve fir trees kept themselves to themselves. It was neither the country nor the city. It was nowhere.

And as I listened to the boring sirens, I rehearsed my memories of Haffner.

With my vision of Haffner – his trousers round his ankles, his hands nervous at his cream underwear – I began my project for his resurrection. Like that historian looking down at the ruins of Rome, in the twilight – with the tourists sketching their souvenirs, and the bells beginning, and the pestering guides, and the watersellers, and the sun above them shrinking: the endless and mortal sun.

3

His career had been the usual success story. After the war Haffner had joined Warburg's. He had distinguished himself with the money he made in the exchange crisis. But his true moment had arrived some years later, when it was Haffner who had realised, as the fifties wore on, the American crisis with dollars. Only Haffner had quite understood the obviousness of it all. The obtuseness of Regulation Q! Naturally, more and more dollars would leave, stranded as they were in the vaults of the United States, and come to Europe – to enrich themselves. This was what he had explained to an executive in Bankers Trust, who was over in London to encourage men like Haffner to move to New York. In 1963, therefore, Haffner left Warburg's for America, where he stayed as a general manager for eleven years. He was the expert in currency exchange: doyen of the international. Then, in 1974, he returned as Chief General Manager in the London office of Chase Manhattan. Just in time for the birth of his grandson – who had promised so much, thought Haffner, as another version of Haffner, and yet delivered so little. Then, finally, there came Haffner's final promotion to the board of directors. His banishment, joked Haffner.

Haffner, I have to admit, didn't practise the usual art of being a grandfather. Cowardice, obscenity, charm, moral turpitude: these were the qualities Haffner preferred. He had bravado. And so it was that, a decade ago, in the spa town, when everything seemed happier, he had avoided the letters from his daughter, the telephone calls from his grandson, the metaphysical lamentation from his exasperated family. Instead, he continued staring at Zinka's breasts, as Niko clumsily caressed them.

Since Zinka was the other hero of Haffner's finale, it may be useful to understand her history.

To some people, Zinka said she was from Bukovina. This was where she had been born, at the eastern edge of Europe – on a night, her mother said, when everything had frozen, even the sweat on her forehead. Her mother, as Zinka knew, was given to hyperbole. To other people, Zinka said she was from Bucharest; and this was true too. It was where she had grown up, in an apartment block out to the north of the city: near the park. But to Haffner, she had simply said she was from Zagreb. In Zagreb, she had trained in the corps de ballet. Until History, that arrogant personification, decided

7

to interrupt. So now she worked here, in this hotel in a spa town, in the unfashionable unfrequented Alps, north of the Italian border – as a health assistant to the European rich.

This was where Haffner had discovered her – in the second week of his escape. Sipping a coffee, he had seen her – the cute yoga teacher – squatting and shimmying her shoulders behind her knees, while the hotel guests comically mimicked her. She was in a grey T-shirt and grey tracksuit trousers: a T-shirt and trousers which could not conceal the twin small swelling of her breasts, borrowed from an even younger girl, and their reflection, the twin swelling of her buttocks, borrowed from an even younger boy. Then she clasped her hands inside out above her back, in a pose which Haffner could only imagine implied such infinite dexterity that his body began to throb, and he felt the old illness return. The familiar, peristaltic illness of the women.

Concealed in a bedroom wardrobe, he looked up at what he could see of the ceiling: where the electric bulb's white light was converted by a dusty trapezoid lampshade into a peachy, emollient glow.

He really didn't want anything else. The women were the only means of Haffner's triumph – his ageing body still a pincushion for the multicoloured plastic arrows of the victorious kid-god: Cupid.

4

Reproductions of these arrows could now be found disporting on Niko's forearms, directing the observer's gaze up to his biceps, where two colourful dragons were eating their own tails – dragons which, if he could have seen them in detail, would have reminded Haffner of the lurid mythical beasts tattooed on the arms of his CO in the war. But Haffner could not see these dragons in detail. Gold bracelets tightly gilded Niko's wrist. Another more abstract tattoo spread over the indented muscles of his stomach – a background, now, to his erect penis, to which Zinka – dressed only in the smallest turquoise panties – was attending.

Situations like these were Haffner's habitat – he lived for the women, ever since he had taken out his first ever girl, to the Ionic Picture Theatre on the Finchley Road. Her name was Hazel. She let him touch her hand all through the feature. The erotic determined him. The film they had seen had been chosen by Hazel: a romance involving fairies, and the spirits of the wood. None of the effects – the billowing cloths, the wind machines, the fuzzy light at the edges of each frame, the doleful music – convinced sarcastic Haffner of their reality. Afterwards, he had bought her two slices of chocolate cake in a Lyons Tea House, and they looked at each other, tenderly – while, in a pattern which would menace Haffner all his life, he began to wonder when he might acceptably, politely, try to kiss her.

He was mediocre; he was unoriginal. He admitted this freely. With only one thing had Haffner been blessed – with the looks. There was no denying, Haffner used to say, mock-ruefully, that Haffner was old – especially if you took a look at him. In the words of his favourite comedian. But Haffner knew this wasn't true. He was unoriginal – but the looks were something else. It was not just his friends who said this; his colleagues acknowledged it too. Now, at seventy-eight, Haffner possessed more hair than was his natural right. This hair was blond. His eyes were blue; his cheeks were sculpted. Beneath the silk weave of his polo necks, his stomach described the gentlest of inclinations.

Now, however, Haffner's colleagues would have been surprised.

Haffner was dressed in waterproof sky-blue tracksuit trousers, a sky-blue T-shirt, and a pistachio sweatshirt. These clothes did not express his inner man. This much, he hoped, was obvious. His inner man was *soigné*, elegant. His mother had praised him for this. In the time when his mother praised him at all.

—Darling, she used to say to him, you are your mother's man. You make her proud. Let nobody forget this.

She dressed him in white sailor suits, with navy stripes curtailing each cuff. At the children's parties, Haffner acted unconcerned. As soon as he could, however, he preferred the look of the gangster: the Bowery cool, the Whitechapel raciness. Elegance gone to seed. His first trilby was bought at James Lock, off Pall Mall; his umbrellas came from James Smith & Sons, at the edge of Covent Garden. The royal patent could seduce him. He had a thing for glamour, for the mysteries of lineage. He could talk to you for a long time about his lineage.

The problem was that now, at the end of the twentieth century, his suitcase had gone missing. It had vanished, two weeks ago, on his arrival at the airport in Trieste. It had still not been returned. It was imminent, the airline promised him. Absolutely. His eyesight, therefore, had been forced to rely on itself – without his spectacles. And he had been corralled into odd collages of clothes, bought from the outdoor-clothes shops in this town. He walked round the square, around the lake, up small lanes, and wondered where anyone bought their indoor clothes. Was the indoors so beyond them? Was everyone always outdoors?

He was a long way from the bright lights of the West End.

Zinka leaned back, grinned up at Niko, who pushed strands of her hair away from her forehead: an idyll. He began to kiss her, softly. He talked to her in a language which Haffner did not know. But Haffner knew what they were saying. They were saying they loved each other.

It was midsummer. He was in the centre of Europe, as high as Haffner could go. As far away as Haffner could get. Through the slats on the window he could see the blurred and Alpine mountains, the vague sky and its clouds, backlit by the setting sun. The view was pricked by conifers.

And Haffner, as he watched, was sad.

He lived for the women. He would learn nothing. He would learn nothing and leave everyone. That was what his daughter had said of him, when she patiently shouted at him and explained his lack of moral courage, his pitiful inadequacy as a husband, as a father, as a man. He would remain inexperienced. It seemed an accurate description.

But as Zinka performed for her invisible audience, Haffner still felt sad. He thought he would feel exultant, but he did not. And the only explanation he could think of was that, once again, Haffner was in love. But this time there was a difference. This, thought Haffner, was the real thing. As he had always thought before, and then had always convinced himself that he was wrong.

5

The pain of it perturbed him. To this pain, he had to acknowledge, there was added the more obvious pain in his legs. He had now been standing for nearly an hour. The difficulty of this had been increased by the tension of avoiding the stray coat hangers Haffner had not removed. It was ridiculous, he thought. He was starting to panic. So calm yourself, thought Haffner. He tried to concentrate on the naked facts – like the smallness of Zinka's breasts, but their smallness simply increased his panic, since they only added to the erotic charge with which Haffner was now pulsing. They were so little to do with function, so much to do with form – as they hung there, unsupported. The nipple completed them; the nipple exhausted them. They were dark with areolae. Their proportions all tended to the sexual, away from the neatly maternal.

Haffner wasn't into sex, after all, for the family. The children were the mistake. He was in it for all the exorbitant extras.

No, not for Haffner – the normal curves, the pedestrian features. His desire was seduced by an imperfectly shaved armpit, or a tanning forearm with its swatch of sweat. That was the principle of Haffner's mythology. Haffner, an admirer of the classics. So what if this now made him laughable, or ridiculous, or – in the newly moralistic vocabulary of Benji, his Orthodox and religious grandson – sleazy? As if there should be closure on dirtiness. As if there should ever be, thought Haffner, any shame in one's lust. Or any more shame than anyone else's. If he could have extended the epic of Haffner's lust for another lifetime, then he would have done it.

In this, he would confess, he differed from Goldfaden. Goldfaden would have preferred a happy ending. He was into the One, not the Many. In New York once, in a place below Houston, Goldfaden had told him that some woman – Haffner couldn't remember her name, some secretary he'd been dealing with in Princeton, or Cambridge – was the kind of woman you'd take by force when the world fell apart. Not like his wife, said Goldfaden: nothing like Cynthia. Then he had downed his single malt and ordered another. At the time, helpful Haffner's contribution to the list of such ultimate women was Evelyn Laye, the star of stage and screen. The most beautiful woman he had ever laid eyes on, when she accompanied her husband to his training camp in Hampshire, in 1939. They arrived in a silver Wolseley 14/16. Goldfaden, however, had contradicted Haffner's choice of Evelyn Laye. As he contradicted so many of Haffner's opinions. She was passable, Goldfaden argued, but it wasn't what he had in mind. And Haffner wondered – as now, so many years later, he watched while Niko stretched Zinka's slim legs apart, displaying the indented hollows inside her thighs, the tatooed mermaid's head protruding from her panties – whether Goldfaden would have agreed that in Zinka he had finally found this kind of woman: the unattainable, the one who would be worth any kind of immorality. If Goldfaden was still alive. He didn't know. He didn't, to be honest, really care. Why, after all, would you want anyone when the world fell apart? It was typical of Goldfaden: this macho exaggeration.

But Haffner no longer had Goldfaden. Which was a story in itself. He no longer had anyone to use as his silent audience.

This solitude made Haffner melancholy.

The ethos of Raphael Haffner – as businessman, raconteur, wit, jazzman, reader – was simple: no experience could be more pleasurable than its telling. The description was always to be preferred to the reality. Yet here it was: his finale – and there was no one there to listen. In the absence of this audience, in Haffner's history, anything had been known to take its place; anything could be spoken to in Haffner's intimate yell: himself, his ghosts, his absent mentors, even – why not? – the more neutral and natural spectators, like the roses in his garden, or the bright impassive sun.

He looked at Zinka, who suddenly crouched in front of Niko, with her back to Haffner, and allowed her hand to be elaborate on Niko's penis.

As defeats went, thought Haffner, it was pretty comprehensive. Even Papa never got himself as messed up as this.

Was it too late for him to change? To undergo one final metamorphosis? I am not what I am! That was Haffner's constant wish, his mantra. He was a man replete with mantras. He would not act his age, or his Age. He would not be what others made of him.

And yet; and yet.

The thing was, said a friend of Livia's once, thirty years ago, in the green room of a theatre on St Martin's Lane, making smoke rings dissolve in the smoky air – a habit which always reminded Livia of her father. The thing was, he was always saying that he wanted to disappear.

She was an actress. He wanted this actress, very much. Once, in their bedroom with Livia before a party, he had seen her undress; and although asked to turn away had still fleetingly seen the lavish shapeless bush between her legs. With such memories was Haffner continually oppressed. It wasn't new. With such memories did

Haffner distress himself. But he couldn't prevent the thought that if she'd undressed in front of him like that, then it was unlikely that she looked on him with any erotic interest – only a calm and uninterested friendliness.

Yes, she continued, he was always saying how he'd prefer to live his life unnoticed, free from the demands of other people.

—But let me tell you something, Raphael, said Livia's friend. You don't need to disappear.

Then she paused; blew out a final smoke ring; scribbled her cigarette out in an ashtray celebrating the natural beauty of Normandy; looked at Livia.

—Because no one, she said, is ever looking for you.

How Haffner had tried to smile, as if he didn't care about her jibe! How Haffner continued to try to smile, whenever this conversation returned to him.

Maybe, he thought, she was right: maybe that was the story of his life, of his century.

And now it was ending – Haffner's twentieth century. What had Haffner done with the twentieth century? He enjoyed measuring himself like this, against the grand categories. But that depended, perhaps, on another question. What had the twentieth century done with him?

6

The era in which Haffner's last story took place was an interregnum: a pause. The British empire was over. The Hapsburg empire was over. Over, too, was the Communist empire. All the ideologies were over. But it was not yet the time of full aromatherapy, the era of celebrity: of chakras, and pressure points. It was after the era of the spa as a path to health, and before the era of the spa as a path to beauty. It was not an era at all.

Everything was almost over. And maybe that was how it should be. The more over things were, the better. You no longer needed to be troubled by the constant conjuring with tenses.

In this hiatus, in the final year of the twentieth century, entered Raphael Haffner.

The hotel where Haffner was staying defined itself as a mountain escape. It had the normal look. It was all white – with a roof that rose in waves of red tile and green louvred shutters on all three floors, each storey narrower than the one below. The top storey resembled a little summerhouse with a tiny structure made of iron shutters on the roof, like an observation post or a weather station with instruments inside and barometers outside. On top of it all, at the very peak, a red weathercock turned in the wind. Every window on every floor had a balcony entered through a set of French doors. Behind the hotel rose the traces of conifered paths, ascending to a distant summit; in front of it, pooled the lake, with its reflections. Beside this lake, on the edge of the town, there was a park, with gravel diagonals, and a view of a distant factory.

Once, the town had been the main location for the holidays of the Central European rich. This was where Livia's family had spent their summers, out of Trieste. They had gone so far, in 1936, as to purchase a villa, with hot and cold water, on the outskirts of the town. In this town, said Livia's father, he felt happy. It had style. The restaurants were replete with waiters – replete, in their turn, with eyebrow. Then, in the summer of 1939, when she was seventeen, Livia and her younger brother, Cesare, had not come to the mountains, but instead had made their way to London. And they had never come back. Seven years later, in a hotel dining room in Honfleur, where Haffner had taken her for the honeymoon which the war had prevented, she described to Haffner, entranced by the glamour, the dining rooms of her past. Crisp mitres of napkins sat in state on the tables. The guests were served not spa food but the classics of their heritage: schnitzel Holstein, and minestrone. The

Béarnaise sauce was served in a silver boat, its lip warped into a moue. There was the clearest chicken soup with the lightest dumplings.

And now, when this place belonged to another country, here was Haffner, her husband: alone – to claim the villa, to claim an inheritance which was not his.

The hotel still served the food of Livia's memory. This place was timeless: it was the end of history. The customer could still order steak Diane, beef Wellington – arranged on vast circles of china, with a thin gold ring inscribing its circumference. Even Haffner knew this wasn't chic, but he wasn't after the chic. He just wanted an escape. An escape from what, however, Haffner could not say.

No, Haffner could never disappear.

In 1974, in the last year of his New York life, when Barbra – who was twenty-nine, worked in the Wall Street office as his secretary and smoked Dunhills which she kept in a cigarette holder, triple facts which made her desirable to Haffner as he passed middle age – asked him why it was he still went faithfully back every night to his wife, he could not answer. It didn't have to be like that, she said. With irritation, as he looked at Barbra, the steep curve between her breasts, he remembered his snooker table in the annexe at home, its blue baize built over by Livia's castles of unread books. He knew that the next morning he would be there, at home: with his breakfast of Corn Chex, morosely reading the *Peanuts* cartoons. He knew this, and did not want to know it. So often, he wanted to give up, and elope from his history. The problem was in finding the right elopee. He only had Haffner. And Haffner wasn't enough.

Zinka turned in the direction of the wardrobe. Usually, she wore her hair sternly in a pony tail. But now she let it drift out, on to her shoulders. And Haffner looked away. Because, he thought, he loved her. He looked back again. Because, he thought, he loved her.

No, there was no escape. And because this is true, then maybe in my turn I should not always allow Haffner the luxury of language.

He was burdened by what he thought was love. But therefore he did not express it in this way. No, trapped by his temptations, Haffner simply sighed.

—Ouf, he exhaled, in his wardrobe. Ouf: ouf.

7

In this vacant hotel room to which Zinka had lured Niko, Zinka had arranged things so that she was facing the mirror which hung above the bed. Behind her, stood Haffner – in the wardrobe. Before her, sat Niko, his legs and his testicles dangling over the edge of the bed. His foot protruded close to Haffner's lair. One of his toenails, Haffner noted, was blackened – the badge of Niko's fitness, of the dogged distances he jogged every day.

But Haffner felt no grievance at the disparity between their bodies. He had perspective. This was one reason to love him. He had the sense of humour I admired. It wasn't just that it was possible to imagine that what was higher could derive always and only from what was lower – in the words of another old master. No, one could go further. And so it was also possible to imagine that – given the polarity and, more importantly, the ludicrousness of the world – everything derived from its opposite. day from night, frailty from strength, deformity from beauty, fortune from misfortune. Victory was made up exclusively of beatings.

This defeat, therefore, could be a victory too. It seemed unlikely, perhaps, but Haffner rarely wanted to be burdened with the problems of probability. Haffner found perks everywhere.

Niko's face was now smothered by the dark nipples of his girlfriend. He was blinded by her body. He therefore couldn't see that, in the mirror, she was looking at the wardrobe, where Haffner was looking at her. Her lips were parted. She was smiling at him: at the invisible Haffner she knew was lurking there, having first splashed a tangle of coat hangers hurriedly into a drawer. Haffner happily smiled back. Then he stopped himself. It felt obscurely comical for a man to be smiling when concealed in a wardrobe. So, shyly, Haffner looked away. He gazed at her thin back instead, gently imprinted with vertebrae.

A thought arrived to Haffner. Was this it? he considered. Was this love?

When he was seventeen – so Haffner once told me, when we were both drunk on vodka cokes, at a golden-wedding party themed for no obvious reason to gangster films of the American 1970s – Haffner had gone to sleep each night imagining the girl he would meet, who would be his perfect girl. This was very important, he said. She would be a woman of the world, attractive, with a hint of something more, if I knew what he meant. I knew what he meant: he wanted the urban, he wanted a vision of cool. And, he told me, he continued to do this – even after the advent of his wife (and his girlfriends, his collection of lovers). Even there, in this spa town, at seventy-eight, he still calmed himself to sleep imagining this girl who would be so infinitely charmed by him. But now, something had changed.

As of now, this girl was simply Zinka.

This was not, of course, what Haffner was meant to be thinking. But then Haffner had a talent for not thinking the orthodox thoughts.

It wasn't enough that Haffner was failing to accomplish the bureaucratic task, which was why he was here, in this spa town: to oversee the legal restoration to his family of the villa – appropriated first by the Nazis, then by the Communists, and finally by nationalist capitalists – which now, in the absence of any other surviving relative, belonged theoretically to Haffner and his descendants. No, even here, in the centre of Europe, he had managed to complicate matters even more mythologically. In addition he had already managed to concoct this unusual story with Zinka. Not content with this, he had also managed to concoct another more ordinary story: an affair with a married woman, staying at the hotel. Her name was Frau Tummel. She said that she adored him; and one aspect of Frau Tummel's soul was its sincerity.

Haffner, however, at this moment, didn't care about Frau Tummel's soul. He knew that he was meant to have been with her – regarding a sad sunset. But Zinka's sudden plan had possessed an overwhelming power of persuasion.

He was not a good man. He didn't need to be told. The jury wasn't out on Haffner's ethics. The case was closed. As a businessman, he had tended to the risky; as a husband, to the unfaithful. He hadn't really cared about his duties as a father or a grandfather. He cared about himself.

How fluently Haffner could self-lacerate! Then again: how easily Haffner could be distracted from his tribunal.

Niko began to whimper, gently. Why, thought Haffner, in his cupboard, did Haffner have to be old? It was devastating; it was Sophoclean. How could this love for Zinka have arrived so late in his life? Yes, Haffner was lyrical. He understood the language of inspiration. Here it was. Yes, here it was. He was inflated: a Silenus raised from his stupor, made buoyant by a force which was beyond him, as he stood there, neatly framed by a hotel wardrobe.

8

I should pause on that adjective Sophoclean, that noun Silenus.

Haffner was an admirer of the classics.

He had always watched the television dons; he had listened to the radio intellectuals. And now, at this late stage, in his retirement, Haffner had embarked on a programme of enlightenment – a succession of evening classes. Even if he would learn nothing about himself, he still wanted to know everything about anything else. So there they were: the old and unemployed, the desperate to learn. Into this group came Haffner. In these classes, Haffner read history. That was his idea of the classic. Occasionally, after he had returned to London, until Haffner's dying took over, I came with him. We grappled, in the introductions to the classics, with the concept of philosophic history. History which was ironic, clever, unimpressed.

The course on the *Lives of the Caesars* was Haffner's late education. He listened to a man berate the Caesars for their immorality. What a lesson it was, said Errol – sitting behind a desk which was too small for him, being made for a lissom teenager, not a distended middle-aged man – what a lesson in vanity, in the way power corrupted. To which the group, all seated at miniature desks, solemnly assented. A poster on the wall displayed a range of fluorescent vegetables and their appropriate names in German. Then Haffner asked if he could say something. He understood that they had all been very moved by the book which was the subject of this course. And he would like to say that he had been the most moved of them all. He had been converted, he said: and now he fully understood the grandeur of the Romans. He hadn't cared for them before, but now, said Haffner, reading about the glorious crimes of the emperors, he saw how truly great they really were.

At this point, Haffner paused for the expected laugh. It did not come.

Blissfully, Haffner had roamed along the shelves of the hotel library, parsing its eccentric selection of the classics. Beside his bed, there was now an abridged edition of Edward Gibbon, underneath his copy of the *Lives of the Caesars*. By his lounger at the side of the pool, with its view of the snow-shrouded mountains, was a novel by Thomas Mann. He liked to stretch himself. Only after a week here had Haffner realised he was the only one who read. Everyone else favoured sleep; they favoured chatter. But Haffner respected those things over which he had no authority. Those things made him want to accrue their authority too. His will was all vicarious.

Haffner hadn't been to university. His daughter had been, and his grandson, but not Haffner. He had been to war instead. But

Haffner felt no insecurity. He had his own triumphs. It was Haffner, for instance, who had persuaded the Chancellor of the Exchequer, the Governor of the Bank of England and the Emeritus Professor of Economic Theory at the LSE – Goldfaden, hero of the Brains Trust, doyen of the radio lecture – to be gathered in one unheard-of trio at the annual dinner of the City branch of the Institute of Bankers, in 1982. He wasn't nobody.

And now he was a student of philosophic history. With this knowledge, he weighed up his biography: he studied the story of Livia, his wife; and Goldfaden, Haffner's friend and counsellor. Goldfaden: the celebrity economist, famed on both sides of the Atlantic.

Goldfaden was a capitalist; but a capitalist who liked to tease. Where, Goldfaden would ask his baffled listeners, was the greatest monument to international esprit? Who had inherited the mantle of Isaac Leib Peretz, the Jewish cosmopolitan? The man who had once argued, at the beginning of the century, that it was a unique culture rather than its patrolled borders that guaranteed a nation its independent existence. True, maybe. But you couldn't beat patrolled borders to help you sleep at night, thought Haffner. Couldn't beat them. While Goldfaden carried on his party trick. They couldn't guess? They couldn't say which was the most cosmopolitan country on earth? The Soviet Union, of course! The greatest federation of nations this world had seen since the Roman empire. Communism! The highest stage of imperialism. What Jew wouldn't love an empire? An empire, continued Goldfaden, was the greatest political system on earth – a confederation of states, blithe to the problems of ethnicity. The zenith of liberalism. But its era was now over; and Goldfaden mourned it. Or so he said, thought Haffner.

But Haffner was still not ready to consider the problem of Goldfaden.

One time, having finished the classic novel I had told him to read, Haffner told me that it had prompted certain thoughts. Think about it: the novel of education was lost on the young. It was the old who were the true protagonists. It was the old, thought Haffner, who deserved the love stories. Return, Monsieur Stendhal! Let yourself go, Mr Dickens! Feast on Haffner! Write a sentimental education for the very old, the absolute advanced.

But no one would.

It was a pity, because Haffner was a folk hero. These were the stories I grew up with – about Haffner. He was a man of legend: his anecdotes were endless. Like this, his final story.

Because there it was, once more, the lust – extravagant: like a sprinkler in the rose garden of Haffner's suburban home, automatically turning itself on to soak the lawn already soaked with rain.

9

Niko was now spread on the bed, his legs twitching. His eyes were shut. Zinka was poised, leaning over his face. His mouth was blindly searching – a kitten – for her breasts.

Then Haffner swayed and chimed against the hangers.

Niko was stilled. Haffner was stilled, his heart an amplification. Only Zinka continued as if nothing had happened. She tended to Niko; she asked him to carry on. And Haffner stood and listened to his heart as if he were only an outsider – as if he were the minicab driver waiting outside a nightclub, in the dawn, in the East End of London, or the Meatpacking District of New York, listening to the deep bass rhythm through the guarded doors while swapping two Marlboros for two much stronger and harsher cigarettes illegally imported from Iran.

To Haffner's slow relief, he noticed that slowly Niko was slowly distracted, slowly.

He really should have been somewhere else, thought Haffner. He should have been with Frau Tummel. Or, even more morally, he should have been in his own room, in his own bed, asleep, with his head slipping off the bolster's irritating cylinder – before returning

22

once again, the next morning, to the Town Hall and its endless offices, where the subcommittees sat, the subcommittees which included the Committee on Spatial Planning. The Committee over which Haffner was here to exercise his charm. Yes, he should have been performing his role as a family man. But Haffner, somehow, still preferred this wardrobe with a view.

Livia's own erotic style, he remembered, watching Zinka, had been subtler. She would meet him in the foyer of the municipal pool in Golders Green, having just performed a synchronised swimming routine, and Haffner would say to her, laughing, that she was his emissary in the world of women. He would beg her to tell him what she saw, in the changing rooms. Livia sat him down. She touched him with the tips of her fingers absently resting on his penis through the button fly of his trousers, for this was how gentlemen dressed, and she told him about the girls in their changing room, the ones who shaved the hair between their legs into neater triangles, the ones who stood there, naked, pretending nobody could see, a festival of women. And Haffner would ask her not to stop, not to stop, and Livia would say that she wasn't stopping, dear heart: she wasn't stopping.

Then Zinka and Niko came to their own conclusion.

Haffner relaxed, relieved. He was beginning, he realised, to be too preoccupied by the practical difficulties of this display. Now that it was over, he began to long for his own bed. But Niko, to Haffner's irritation, seemed to be in a languid state of abandon. He wanted to lie there; he wanted Zinka to rest in his arms.

This was not, thought Haffner, at all what he had been led to expect.

And Haffner waited, in a wardrobe, while a couple held each other: amorous.

Oh Haffner had stamina! So often, in the bedroom, Haffner surpassed everyone's expectation. So many people thought they knew him! As if anyone could really know him. But Haffner would often argue that in this matter of Haffner's monstrosity one could draw some distinctions. He wasn't, for example, a monster like Caligula. The incest didn't move Haffner. Whereas Caligula used to commit incest with each of his three sisters in turn. And very possibly his mother. And his brothers. His mother and his brothers and his aunts.

Haffner was the generalissimo of hyperbole. Unlike a real generalissimo, however, he had to perform the hyperbole himself.

My poor Haffner: his own shill.

No one else, for instance, was so sure that the obvious comparison to Haffner was Caligula. It wasn't so much Haffner's monstrosity which troubled his family, but his absolute mundanity. Whenever his daughter, Esther, brought up the issue of his adultery, his bed tricks, she said he was banal. She would stand there, in her business suits, with their badly cut trousers; her silk blouse; the sleek blonde bob which Haffner regretted, taming as it did the cuteness of her curls. This belittling idea of hers had always unnerved Haffner. He felt a distant sense of pique. Surely, he would reason, unconvincingly, afterwards – to an unconvinced Haffner, or an unconvinced anonymous drinker, or the indignant husband of his daughter – the infidelity had contained infinite riches, if only you knew how to look? From one perspective, pure vanity: yes maybe. But from another – what gorgeous vistas! What passes, what valleys, what pastoral hillocks!

Was there really anything so wrong, thought Haffner, in a crescendo of impatience, as he waited for Niko and Zinka to leave, as Zinka paused in the doorway, looking back to the innocent wardrobe – was there really anything so wrong, thought Haffner, as he finally emerged, with being a man of feeling?

The classics were full of it. The loves of the gods were various. The loves of Jupiter, for instance, were a festival of costume change, of metamorphosis. He mated with Aegina as a flame, Asteria as an eagle, Persephone as a snake; with Leda he took the form of a swan, with Olympias a snake. To Semele he appeared as a blazing fire, to Io as a fog, to Danae as a shower of gold. When he first slept with Juno, his wife, he became a cuckoo. Alcmena and Callisto were won by his impersonations of humans. Yes, the loves of Jupiter were famous. They had heft.

With these stories Haffner sought consolation.

But, I have to add, in the many stories of Haffner, he was always only himself.

Haffner Amorous

1

Returning to his room, Haffner rounded a corner and passed a coiled roulade of fire hose pinned to the wall, as he happily imagined his bed and its crisp sheets, a single circle of chocolate laid out on one diagonal fold. And then he discovered the weeping monumental form of Frau Tummel.

For what was up was also down, and what seemed a victory, after all, was really a defeat: so Haffner's happiness must always be subject to swift reversals.

Frau Tummel was in a cotton nightgown, with ruched lace at the breasts, and a cotton bathrobe stitched with pink tight roses. There, in front of his door, Haffner confronted her – outlandish in his sky-blue and pistachio ensemble. He looked around, to see if anyone else might be there. He felt burdened with concern: for Frau Tummel, and for himself. He didn't want to explain why it was that he had returned to his room this late, in such exhaustion.

Frau Tummel raised her face, displaying the ravages of her mascara: a harlequin.

—What are you doing here? said Haffner, brightly.

—We had a rendezvous, she said.

—Come now, said Haffner, less brightly.

Maybe it was over, she said, sadly.

—Over? said a Haffner transformed into the sign for a smile: a single reclining parenthesis.

Yes, continued Frau Tummel. It would end with him leaving her. She knew this. And it was right. For sure. It was understandable.

He tried to reassure her. Of course he wasn't going to leave! The idea of it! And Frau Tummel said that yes, she knew this. She knew he thought this was true. But how could he know this? There were so many complications. She really thought they needed to discuss this.

The sign for Haffner was no longer a supine parenthesis.

He knew what he was meant to say. He didn't want to say it. He wanted to be alone; to go to sleep. But Haffner had his code of honour. This was one aspect of his undoing. He was an admirer of the classics, and no man with a classical education could deny the wills of women. The classics taught one, he had decided, to trust in the pagan gods. Trust Cupid. Trust him in all his other guises, as cherubs, or as Eros. The men must always allow themselves to be led by the women. So he said what he was meant to say. He wondered if she would like to come into his room.

Frau Tummel raised her ravaged face: a joyful harlequin.

So ended, in one swift exchange, the swift moment of Haffner's happiness.

2

The imbroglios seemed so fluently to come to Haffner.

He was here to claim his wife's inheritance – therefore, naturally, he became involved with other women. This seemed to be the logic of his life.

They had met two weeks ago, on the second day of his stay, at the swimming-pool complex in the hotel's basement. There were three pools – three adjacent water lilies, each attached to the other by a miniature set of steps. The smallest was a Jacuzzi – for the indolent, or the fat. In it could therefore be found Haffner, who was indolent, and Frau Tummel, who was fat.

The voice of Frau Tummel, he soon discovered, was husky, it was rasping. She had class. She wrapped herself in a towel to go and lie on a lounger outside, to smoke three rapid cigarettes, pinched in the contraption of her extravagant cigarette holder – which unfolded and then unfolded one more time, just when you thought it could not be extended further. Then she relapsed into the boiling Jacuzzi, to Haffner's charmed curiosity.

He wasn't normally so devoted to swimming pools. He preferred the gyms – the exercise machines which prolonged to such a surprisingly toned extent the overlong life of Haffner. The gym was another place where we had fleetingly made conversation. Occasionally, I would happen on Haffner in the changing room: and, delighted, he maintained a naked conversation – our penises dolefully looking away – while I stood there on the bobbled tiles wishing I were not faced by the superior nature of Haffner's so much older muscles. Although the gym was really a place of yearning for Haffner. It was, quite frankly, most often a place of rest. In the gym, a slothful primate, he could let his arms droop over the bars on the chest press. Below the slope of his T-shirt, his arms were white and darkly speckled, like a photocopy. From here, he could observe the varieties of breast movement – some solid in sports bras, others fragile, unsupported, tenderly visible. He developed a stare for this purpose, an alibi – heavy-lidded with exhaustion, hypnotically unfocused, unable to look away.

Frau Tummel worked in the perfume industry. She was here in this spa hotel with her husband – whose nerves, she told Haffner, were gone, whose blood pressure was abnormal. He spent his days on the veranda, looking at the silent mountains: sipping peppermint tea. It was, thought Haffner, the old old story: the loyal wife who was bored of her loyalty – the century's normal story of a spa.

When Frau Tummel had gone, Haffner leaned back in the Jacuzzi, letting the movement of the bubbles absorb his concentration with their frantic foam – and then he padded off, leaving dark echoes of his feet on the floor's lukewarm tiling. In one room, he discovered a table with flowers: gentian, violets. In another room there was a sauna, where a woman was lying, motionless, on the pine slats of the highest step. Haffner paused, considered not. And then he pushed open another door, and discovered Frau Tummel again, in the process of being massaged. She was lying on her front, on a towel monogrammed in stitched gold thread with the hotel's invented crest. And in her shock she leaned up, so exposing to Haffner's gaze the moles on her breasts, the beginnings of her pink areolae, cobbled with cold.

He apologised, and went outside. Twenty minutes later he apologised to her again, in the rest room, illuminated by low lighting, and inventively perfumed candles – tuberose, lily, pomegranate. They decided to go for a walk. They made for the peak of the mountain. Light shimmered on her hair. She was uninterested in Haffner's ability to name the varieties of Alpine star, the daisies and the grasses – names he had culled from a colour-coded children's botany book, the white flowers in one section, the pink in another, bought in a fit of nostalgia for Haffner's earnest youth when buying chocolate in a tabac. She wanted to talk about love. She wanted to talk about her marriage, which entailed discussion of Haffner's marriage. It involved so many sacrifices, did he not think? The conversation so absorbed them that soon she was back in the hotel with Haffner, sitting on his bed. This did not surprise Haffner. Nor was it surprising that, as she lit a final cigarette, then stubbed it out, Haffner discovered that, without realising, as he kissed her, he had gone too far. He had overstepped, or overreached.

Yes, because nothing in this world occurs without a backstory: and what is higher always derives from what is lower and every victory contains its own defeat.

That day, Frau Tummel's feelings had been a little depleted. She had been demoralised by a fractious meeting with her husband's doctor in the morning; and then by an unhappy phone call from her mother at lunchtime. The massage had been suggested by her husband – it would, he said, cheer her up. The casual flirting with Haffner was an improvised addition of her own. But nothing, thought Frau Tummel now, as she stubbed out her final cigarette, was improvised. Nothing was casual. Everything was fate.

Like Haffner, she saw signs everywhere.

She turned round, and Haffner kissed her. And Frau Tummel kissed him back – for he was the magical combination of clever and kind. He understood her. But at this point, her body overtook her.

Frau Tummel was fifty-five. Her periods, as she used to tell her girlfriends, in a spirit of European openness, were becoming more and more erratic. Her cycle was unpredictable. The night before, after an absence of three months, a period had begun. And so she did not want to have sex with Haffner. She did not even want to undress. He must not touch her. Gently, Frau Tummel tried to explain her feelings to Haffner.

She didn't want to say, she said. He should not make her say.

And Haffner did not mind, he told her, gently. For he knew why – the constant coyness of unfaithful wives. So Haffner continued to kiss her. Through his trousers, hesitantly she touched the nub of his penis, blunted by his briefs.

Born with a different kind of soul to Haffner, Frau Tummel's husband was repelled by her periods. Quickly they had developed an unspoken rule that they would never have sex at these times; nor would he even touch her. Frau Tummel was therefore amazed when Haffner was so undisgusted. Such elegance!

Such delicacy! It even tempted her, for a moment, to relinquish her scruples. But no, she thought, gathering herself, she really shouldn't.

Perhaps if she had slept with Haffner, she might not have been so moved. But she did not. So Frau Tummel could nurture her feelings, invulnerable to complication. On returning to her husband, she could wonder why it was she was so impatient with desire.

Haffner didn't know how seriously Frau Tummel took her moment with Haffner. He thought this was what she did. He thought she had done this before. She would go so far, and then back off.

Frau Tummel, however, had never been unfaithful. She was not trained at it. The guilt of it confused and overtook her, the next morning, as she woke up beside her husband, cutely rumpled in a mess of pillow and pyjama.

The guilt of it confused and overtook her – Frau Tummel! who was fifty-five! but at fifty-five you can still, after all, be inexperienced – that this feeling she felt for Haffner must be love.

3

She didn't know that love was always the beginning of Haffner's downfall. She didn't know that this was what Haffner was gloomily concluding, as he observed Frau Tummel's weeping form, sipping a gin and tonic he had invented from the minibar.

Mainly, the love belonged to other people. Once, it had been Haffner's.

When he was courting her, in the summer of 1939, Haffner used to take Livia dancing in metroland, the green and pleasant suburbs of north London. Since Haffner was a little perturbed by this girl who had the glamour of a foreign accent, Italianate, a flutter, he tried to impress her with the gorgeousness of his dancing, for at that time Haffner – so Haffner said – had the finest pair of feet in north London. And in Highgate once they sat down after a dance, and looked at each other, while Haffner worried about the visibility of his erection, mummified in his underwear. They had been dancing a foxtrot. He crossed his legs, making sure that Livia could not see or know about it. But she knew. And it intrigued her. She sat there, and she wondered if Haffner would do anything so bold as try to kiss her. They had been courting for some time now. She had just turned eighteen. And she wondered if she would be interested if Haffner did indeed do something. Yes, she thought, she would. But it needed Haffner first. While Haffner, who was shy despite his fleet feet, his slick blond hair, decided that he could do nothing without her visible approval. And so Haffner and Livia sat together and neither touched nor talked.

Two weeks later, at a dance hall in Hendon, they argued about this.

She was sorry, concluded Livia, but it didn't happen and if it didn't happen then it couldn't happen. Haffner asked if this had to be true. Yes, said Livia, it did. And she left Haffner outside, and went back in on the arm of another man. There was a small wart on the right-hand side of his neck, like a piece of gravel. So Haffner had nowhere to go. He walked away from home, towards the river, for an hour, into the dismal city. He reached the Gray's Inn Road, then High Holborn, where the family law firm was, the family law firm which he was destined never to enter, and then wandered back, finding himself in Clerkenwell. This, he discovered, was a mistake. All the Italian shops made him even more nostalgic for his Livia. He passed Chiappa & Sons, the organ makers on Eyre Street Hill; the working men's club – the Mazzini Garibaldi – where her brother, Cesare, would later sit and play morra: teased for his elegant accent, his neat small hands. In the cab shelter opposite Hatton Garden, by the Italian church, Haffner sat at a table beside an initial pool of gravy which he mopped up with the folded triangle of a napkin. He looked out the window. Up on Leather Lane, a jumper was caught in a tree. It settled, sodden, between a collection of branches. And as he gazed at this wrecked jumper, improbably in the branches of this silver birch, Haffner realised that it wasn't a kiss he wanted: it wasn't even the body of Livia. He wanted her for ever. He wanted to marry her. And so he concocted an imaginary conversation between an imaginary Haffner and an imaginary Livia, as he looked at the way the foggy rain made the occasional lamp outside a sieved and shimmering haze, a delicate gold.

These thoughts returned to Haffner, sentimental, in the Alpine rain, observing the different gold of a Central European desk light.

4

He knew this was all very wrong, said Frau Tummel.

—Oh I don't know, said Haffner, airily.

She had decided that she really must cheer up. She must not be so down. She must not show him this face of hers.

What he did to her, what he made her feel: was wrong, said Frau Tummel. He was a bad man, she said – tapping him on the nose: a disgruntled, startled puppy. He was a bad man.

She may have been delicious, thought Haffner, sadly – with her joyful breasts, her trembling thighs – but her concerns were not his concerns. It was undeniable. The flirting surely could have possessed slightly more élan. But Frau Tummel didn't want sophistication. Frau Tummel's thing was love. She went for the serious. And Haffner was not in the mood for love; or the serious. Or maybe I should say: he didn't go for love now, with her. With Frau Tummel he would have liked, instead, to be delirious with appetite.

The love was all for Zinka.

—Yes, yes, said Haffner. You told me that.

And maybe this was not fair. Maybe this wasn't accurate to the difficulty Frau Tummel was feeling.

Did he know, she asked him, how lucky they were?

—How lucky? queried Haffner.

Yes, how lucky they were, repeated Frau Tummel.

He looked at her. She stepped forward, let the belt of her bathrobe undo itself, pushed it off her shoulders, on to the floor. Then she unbuttoned her nightgown to her breasts, and pulled it down over her shoulders. Now, therefore, she was naked – except, to Haffner's surprise, for her bra. The bra saddened him; it added to her pathos. Like the bathrobe, it was dotted with stitched pink roses.

In this bra, Haffner confronted the problem of love.

Haffner was not all barbarian, not all the time. He was helpful. He tried to please. Weakly, not wanting to sadden her, he wondered if they should order some champagne.

Stricken, he watched Frau Tummel smile.

—Oh, said Frau Tummel, it is a good life, is it not?

Haffner's deepest wish was to possess the total independence of a mad imperator; a classical god. But the stern line of Haffner's cruelty was always complicated by the kink of his kindness.

Frau Tummel leaned across the bed, on to her stomach, and picked up the phone. She talked to reception as she lay there, her legs kicking in the air. It was such a girlish gesture, this kicking in the air.

While somewhere else – but where? Dubrovnik? La Rochelle? – a younger Livia opened the wardrobe in their hotel room so that the mirror reflected the bed on which she flung herself, face down, thus able to be ravaged from behind by her marauder, the angel Raphael, while simultaneously watching her angel rear devastatingly above her.

But where? Dover, in 1949!

Haffner leaned forward, and spread Frau Tummel's legs apart:

revealing their symmetrical Rorschach stain – like a picture of a butterfly once solemnly presented to him by his grandson, Benjamin, constructed by pressing one half of the paper over the other – already stained with Benji's idea of a butterfly's smudged if multicoloured pattern. Haffner began to lick her, gently, as she tried to finish the call. And as he licked her, as he parted her, she started to invent more and more food. They would have champagne, she said, yes – and also caviar. And blini. And a Russian salad. And pickled cucumbers. And oh, she said. No, oh, she said. She was fine. She was very well. If they could bring everything in, if they could just come up and put everything in her room. If they could bring it up. If they could bring it up. And put it in. Then she put the phone down, and revelled in the pleasure of Haffner's flesh.

If he was touching her like this, then of course it was love. No one except her husband had ever touched her in this way. Not even her husband had touched her in this way.

Too soon, the room service arrived. She gathered herself back into the bathrobe. Haffner, in his dishevelled tracksuit, tipped the waiter, wondering if he could induce him to stay, deciding that he couldn't.

—You aren't angry with me? she asked.

But why, asked Haffner, would he be angry?

But it was so complicated. She was sorry. She was sorry for being so complicated. But he had to understand. She had a husband.

Haffner understood.

He must think it was like Romeo and Juliet, she said.

Haffner did not reply: he had no idea how he could reply.

—You know, she said, I am not. This is not me. But it is difficult to hide the secrets of the heart.

—Hide what? said Haffner, appalled.

—Raphael! said Frau Tummel. You are too much.

And Haffner considered the extraordinary way in which a life repeated itself. For Livia had used this phrase for him. Just once. Or a phrase resembling this phrase. Maybe he was too much for her, she said. Maybe in the end he was too much even for her. And when he had tried to tell Livia, this was in 1982, the night of his triumphant dinner for the Institute of Bankers, that all he wanted was her, she turned away. They were sitting in the kitchen. She was in a nightgown which Haffner had never liked – being made of a blue towelling, which tended to make her look, he argued, unattractive: he never wanted the cosy, the comfortable, only the erotic. That was one form, he now considered, of his immaturity. So maybe everyone had him right. He could understand it. He was too much for himself.

He put his fingers to Frau Tummel's lips. She began to kiss them. Each finger she curled into her mouth.

What could really go wrong, thought Haffner, in a hotel, in a spa town? It seemed safe enough.

But then he had to correct himself. He allowed his will to follow the wills of women. That was his classical principle. But he knew that this had its problems too. He freely admitted this. When the women were in love with him, then Haffner was no longer safe. This was one aspect of his education. It had happened with Barbra. It had happened before Barbra. And now, he worried, it was happening again.

This was one aspect of his education. But Haffner would never learn.

5

Haffner acceptingly approached the women who approached him as if they were portents. They were Haffner's irresistible fate.

He didn't, he once said – in a conversation which was now legendary in Haffner's family, when confronted by Esther after

Livia's death with accusations of his truly infantile excesses – he didn't want to regret anything. No, he didn't see why he should be left with any regret. He said this without really thinking, as he said so many things. Or so argued Haffner afterwards – after it had become his definition. As if a man's marriage, said Esther, triumphantly, with the absolute agreement of her family, should ever make him regret anything. Esther's husband, Esmond, did not continue the conversation. And although it had passed into the annals of his family as the epitome of Haffner's selfishness, as recounted to me once by Benjamin, I was not so convinced. Awkward he may have been, but Haffner was not malicious. And Benjamin, with his new-found devotion to his religion, his new-found devotion to the family, was not, I thought, a reliable moral guide: he had lost his imagination.

Nor, I tried to say to Benjamin, had Livia ever been public with her disapproval. If she really disapproved. So maybe this should make us pause as well.

One can be so rarely sure, Haffner once said to me, that what one has done is right. So maybe it was possible that in his self-defence Haffner was being truthful, rather than self-deceiving. He was simply being faithful to his refusal of self-denial; his absolute distrust of the philosophy on which it was based, the puritanical certainty.

Which was one reason, surely, why Livia might love him. For Haffner's absolute sense of humour.

6

Oh the comic pathos of dictators! Haffner's sense of humour!

Maybe they were never really given their moral due. More and more, as Haffner lay beside the swimming pool, or sat on a bench in front of an Alpine view, he approved of the scandalous emperors. He couldn't understand the world's astonishment.

Like Augustus, who had absolute faith, so wrote his historian, in certain premonitory signs. Once, when a palm tree pushed its way between the paving stones in front of his home he had it transplanted to the inner court beside his household gods, and lavished care on it. Just as Haffner found it difficult to reject the women who entered his sphere of orbit. Who could have the hubris to reject the artistry of chance? If Augustus didn't, then why should Haffner? Even if it was unclear how much his meetings with women were to do with chance, rather than the machinations of Haffner's will. But then again, Augustus could be a mentor here as well, since it was Augustus who justified his adulterous affairs as the necessary burden of an emperor – charged with knowing the secrets of his subjects, his closest advisers. Of course an emperor had to sleep with his counsellors' wives! How else would he know what they were thinking? There was nothing in it for Augustus: his sexual life was all in service to the state.

And in fact this was not a new discovery of Haffner's. Perhaps he had forgotten, but the emperors had entered his moral universe before. Years ago, Livia had been reading about these Roman dictators. They were all in Dubrovnik, in the wilds of Europe, during one of Esther's summer holidays. They lay underneath a parasol, moving their position in relation to it as the day wore on, a live performance of a sundial – and, to the shuffle of the sea, Livia read aloud to Haffner from the book which her brother had given her. A new translation. Haffner was slowly sunburning. And she had mischievously read out to Haffner the story of Tiberius – the man who had built a private sporting-house, where sexual extravagances were performed for his secret pleasure. Hundreds of girls and young men, whom he had collected from all over the empire as adepts in unnatural practices, and known as *spintriae* – but what did *spintriae* mean? wondered Haffner: it must have been dirty; it must have been good, or the man would have translated it: no, said Livia, there was no footnote, nothing – would perform before Tiberius in groups of three, to excite his waning passion. Some aspects of his criminal obscenity were almost too vile to discuss, much less believe, read Livia. Imagine training little boys, whom he called his minnows, to chase him while he went swimming and get between his legs to lick and nibble him! Or letting babies not yet weaned from their mother's breast suck at him – such a filthy old man he had become! So wrote his historian. But neither Livia nor Haffner was so prone to judgement.

Filthy old man or not, they seemed to get Tiberius. The experimenter with pleasure: a pioneer of power – always minuscule before the infinite.

A few years later, at the time of the Brazilian coup, they had been in São Paulo – some deal with a bank which didn't work out. The deal, and the bank. With their host, who impressed Haffner with the beauty of his wife, and the cultural beauty of his life, they were sitting in a theatre, watching a classic of contemporary theatre. And even Haffner was amused when the police burst in, and called up everyone involved on stage. They took a programme and began to intone the names: the actors, the stage manager, the lighting designer. Dutifully, the arrested provocateurs lined up on stage. And finally, stated the policemen, confident in their authority, they demanded that the arch instigator, the impresario of this whole production should present himself to the police as well: a man with the unlikely Brazilian name of Bertolt Brecht. Everyone looked concernedly around. Mr Brecht appeared, they thought, to have disappeared.

And what Haffner now remembered was how that night, in their hotel room, Livia had confessed that however much she found it funny, however much she had laughed with their hosts, with the audience, with the entire tropical night – deep in her worried thoughts was a regret. She still felt sorry for the deluded dictatorial policemen.

The poor dictators! Even the dictators, after all, were the dupes of accident and defeat.

7

At this moment, for instance, Frau Tummel was trying, in the words of the comics, to offer Haffner pleasure. Perhaps this might not obviously seem like a defeat. But look closer, dear reader – look closer. Enter Haffner's soul. Haffner was beginning to feel melancholy. Soft in Frau Tummel's mouth, his penis had no point to it.

If the ghost of Livia were looking down, at this moment, perhaps she would have found this funny, thought Haffner. And so could he. It was just another instance of the accidental.

He touched Frau Tummel, gently, on her grey and golden hair – on the combed grey roots. Could he ask her, politely, he said, to stop doing what she was doing?

Frau Tummel looked up, the head of his slumped penis slumped on the slump of her lower lip. A thin trail of saliva, unnoticed, connected the two. Haffner tried to be romantic: he tried to maintain the tone. She still loved her husband, he told her. She was being silly. But no, said Frau Tummel. It was over a long time ago. And she bent down, continuing to show her affection to Haffner. While Haffner despaired. His soft penis was not moving. It hung there: obeisant to the law of gravity.

It wasn't, obviously, the first time this kind of event had occurred. The despair was local. It had placed Haffner in a difficult social situation. On the one hand, it meant that he could not experience the pleasures he had previously experienced with Frau Tummel. But, on the other hand, he could not ask her to leave. His pride would not allow it. So he was trapped into a conversation – where Frau Tummel had the power. She pitied him; she pored over him; she looked after him. She stated the permanence of their love.

His impotence had trapped Haffner in a conversation he wanted to be over. This sadness was creating so much more intimacy than he ever wanted. He tried to concentrate on images of the erotic: he tried to think about Zinka's breasts. But Zinka eluded him. He remembered the way Livia had touched him, the first time, at the ponds on Hampstead Heath – her hand dipping under his briefs, under the curve of his tense strained penis, a hand which he delightedly and immediately made wet with his semen. Neither of them had spoken. She simply withdrew her hand, took out a handkerchief, wiped it gently – a gesture which for Haffner still seemed fraught with tenderness.

And maybe that had been the moment when he decided to marry Livia: when he knew that he was in love. Just because it had happened so fast. All his triumphs, he began to think now, were just defeats reconfigured. Like the time he batted for five hours in Jerusalem, in 1946, thus securing an improbable draw on a pitch destroyed by three days of tropical rain.

He looked at Frau Tummel. Frau Tummel was looking with tenderness at him: an absolute maternal tenderness. A tenderness which made Haffner afraid with its intimacy. And she bent down, kissed his penis, at its tip.

—Whatever you want, she said. Whatever you want, I will do.

He looked down at his drooping penis – once faithful in all his infidelities. Its defeat now should not, he reflected, have surprised him.

—You can have me, said Frau Tummel, anywhere. If that will help. You can have me where my husband has not had me.

Frau Tummel believed in the reality of their love. She believed that this love was truth. Frau Tummel was not a libertine: for her, the erotic was an aspect of love. She was a Christian woman. She had been brought up to trust and worship the instincts of her soul.

Or was now not the right time for her little lamb? she wondered. Perhaps not, replied her little lamb. Perhaps not.

—We must, said Frau Tummel, talk to my husband. It is the only right thing.

She said this with no enjoyment, no glory. She had come here with her ill husband. She was a model wife. And she would leave with her life destroyed, she thought. She could not live without her husband, and now she could not leave without Haffner. To Haffner, however, it seemed so unnecessary. He talked about the need to take their time. He talked about the need not to injure the blossom of their love.

The dawn was just beginning, in the window. There was a light sparse rain.

But maybe it was possible, she added, for Haffner to forget. If he would only let another woman into his life – to care for him, to be his companion.

8

Frau Tummel's will was just another way in which the twentieth century was conspiring to entrap Haffner. Once more, he had entered *Mitteleuropa*. It was a place which had always amazed him. Its endless capacity for seriousness! The intellectual fervour! Whenever he thought about the Europeans, he became hysterical with exclamations. Ever since he discovered, through Cesare, that the Russians wrote to each other with exclamation marks, Haffner had liked this theatrical way of talking. The European vocative – addressing absent abstractions. Love! Death! Fame! Bohemia! Wherever Bohemia was. It was how he always thought about Cesare. Whom Haffner had loved. Of whom Haffner despaired.

Cesare used to come up with Livia from Charlton, in south London, where they were boarding, at the home of a paint salesman from Trieste. Haffner used to sit with him on Wimbledon Common.

He was about twenty; Cesare was about eighteen. Cesare delighted in deckchairs. And patiently Haffner explained the rules of cricket. Cesare was slightly deaf in one ear – after an accident when he was a child. He didn't mind, however, because in Cesare's opinion it added lustre to him. His deafness was distinguished. He listened to Haffner with one hand cocked, like the flower of an ear trumpet. A hollyhock, thought Haffner. Patiently, he convinced Cesare that just because the two batsmen were at opposite ends of the wicket, this didn't mean that they were on different sides. Cesare could not understand this. He tried, but he could not.

Haffner loved him, but had never quite got him. Never, in his entire life, did Cesare lose his comical Italian accent. His hair was white by the time he was twenty; but his eyebrows for ever were black. And Haffner never asked him if this was due to nature or nurture. Yes, Cesare would sit there, reading *War and Peace*, while Haffner watched the cricket. This must have been 1940, thought Haffner. When the BBC was supporting the Russian cause with its radio version of Tolstoy's novel. Haffner must have been on leave, or about to ship out. He would test Cesare on the characters' names from the bookmark on which was printed each family, and a guide to pronunciation.

And then, as always, they discussed the politics of Europe. To Cesare, this was natural. So natural that from that point on it had marked his life, thought Haffner, these discussions of European politics: the endless problems Cesare found with any kind of state. Problems to which Haffner was oblivious. He had the arguments with anarchists, with Socialists, with social democrats and liberal democrats. He had talked them through with Fascists and with Communists. Cesare himself had preferred a modified form of Communism. Haffner, the Englishman, had demurred. He wouldn't be swayed by Cesare's assertion that Haffner, like Cesare, was a Jew, not an Englishman; that as a Jew he really should be more mindful of the rights of minority peoples.

Cesare was European; and Haffner was not.

Haffner did care about the rights of minorities. His way of displaying this was simply less exhibitionist than others – or so Haffner told himself. In 1938, for instance, at the Scarborough Cricket Festival, a week or so before Chamberlain set off for Munich, he had remonstrated with his father, who had offered the opinion that a Nazi Britain might have its advantages – less obsessed with money, less nouveau riche – unconvinced as he was that Hitler really meant to do away with every Jew. First, Raphael had reminded him, Hitler really did want to do away with every Jew; and secondly – he continued – what was so wrong with the plutocrats? Who had a problem with the City of London? He wasn't bothered by the vulgar, Haffner. He didn't see why Papa should so look down on people.

But then, sanity had never been Papa's hallmark. In the Great War, he had joined up in the Rangers. He served in the Dorsetshire Regiment, a machine-gunner. He served throughout the battle of Passchendaele, until he was wounded.

—Anything is better than war, said Papa. Anything.

And although Haffner thought he was the opposite of Papa, I am not so sure. No, like Papa, Haffner never took the Europeans seriously. Like Papa, he never quite understood their rages.

—My theory of course is that Cohen is not a real Jew, Haffner once said to me, talking about Goldfaden's friend, a Canadian Marxist Jewish academic: the son of immigrant pioneers. He's too Jewish to be true. My theory is, continued Haffner, that at a certain point in, say, the 1950s, he realised that his career could flourish if he were Jewish – not true now, of course, not true now – and that he there-fore took on the persona of a Marxist Jewish intellectual.

—In reality, he concluded, his ancestry is Polish. Working-class anti-Semitic Polish. He denies this, of course. But then, finished Haffner, pouring himself another drink, smiling at me, ignoring my empty proffered glass, he would.

Haffner was silent. He kissed Frau Tummel, gently, on the cheek.

—I have an idea, said Frau Tummel. We will swim. Yes? We will have *eine kleine* dip. You have a wife. I have a husband. We must forget them both. For an hour.

But Haffner, he was realising, could forget nothing. Haffner was still ancient. He was wondering if Trajan had come here. Was this the land of Dacia, or Dalmatia? Pannonia? The Romans had conquered everywhere; their triumph was total. So presumably the legionaries had ended up in these mountains too – blistered, their groins chafed, their cracked nipples greased with duck fat to protect them against the coarse fabric of their shirts – and then afterwards, on their return to Rome, they had set up that column with its curving wrap-around frieze, like a stick of candy – or like the light-house on Cape Hatteras in the Outer Banks, where Haffner had spent a weekend with Livia, where they had seen the dolphins shimmying after each other, their sheen dappled and mottled in the water. Yes, that column which I Haffner had seen when he was twenty-four and remembered nothing about the Romans except the fact that an orator called Cicero made many speeches – speeches, Livia told him, which had been delivered in that sad and empty brick building on the edge of the Forum. It hadn't moved Haffner then. It seemed to move Haffner now.

He had understood Livia, and Livia had understood him. She had borne with fractious grace the obvious signs of infidelity; the crazy signs of infidelity – like the moment when she saw a woman driving down the high street in Hendon, in Haffner's car. A car, he told her that evening, he had donated to the garage because it was out of order. How could he control what the garage had done with it next (folding his napkin, finding his pipe, leaving the room, aggrieved)? Yes, she understood the dictators. Livia – the most nat-urally elegant woman he ever knew: who once played tennis naked, he suddenly remembered, in the rain, after two gimlets and three martinis, at some friend's house in the Cotswolds. Oh he was stricken!

—Raphael! said Frau Tummel. Are you listening?

And yes yes, said Haffner, in another world entirely – where a rejuvenated version of Haffner issued giggling directions from the passenger seat, as Livia drove them back to London, tipsy and still naked except for a towel across her waist, the seat belt tight between her freezing breasts.

Haffner Amphibious

1

The lake in this town was not the kind which Haffner admired: it had no follies – no ruined grottos, no temples to Venus. Its spirit was civic, not aristocratic. Politics possessed it, not pleasure. It lay in front of the hotel, on the edge of the park. In the distance, made fuzzy to Haffner – bereft, as ever, of his glasses – were the twin peaks of the mountains, and their thinner silhouettes, the twin peaks of the factory chimneys. And all the cement apartment blocks: the random codes of their illuminated windows like the punched cardboard sheets for street organs.

Beside this lake, as the dawn freshened, Frau Tummel began to undress. Haffner looked around, nervously. They were sheltered, here, by two clustering beech trees. They did not reassure him very much. He looked at Frau Tummel, who was bending over, folding her nightgown. The tuft of hair between her legs was visible then invisible as she leaned further forward, arranging her bathrobe on top of the nightgown: a neat arrangement of squares.

An echo in Haffner's mind, Zinka bent over to extract her stocking from the bed's scalloped valance.

Reluctantly, Haffner undressed. He displayed his slighter breasts to the gathered winds: the voyeuristic zephyrs. They made for his pink nipples, the droop of his ghostly pectorals. He let his shirt drop where it wanted: it tumbled to the ground, a dying swan.

Just as after yet another late night of working he would undress in his dressing room, or on the landing, leaving puddles of clothes behind his tiptoeing footsteps – and then enter the bedroom, feeling the carpet on his bare feet, the densely corrugated metal strip at the door where the carpet ended, and then be suddenly surprised by Livia turning on an enquiring lamp, so that he paused there, a satyr, stalled in the pursuit of an invisible prey.

2

At the jetty, Haffner paused. The wood was greasy. Frau Tummel was already in – treading water, only her head visible. Her face had transformed itself into a smile.

—It is delicious, she said. You must come in.

Haffner was not amphibious, not normally. But nothing, at the moment, seemed normal. Their affair had been marked by water. Water was its motif. First the swimming pool, the Jacuzzi: and now this. It was unusual in the life of Haffner. In general, he avoided water. Although it was true that there had been that night in the baths at Rome – the day after they had liberated the city. The opened city.

Silk reflections from the water had unfolded on the ceiling. The building was Haffner's most exalted idea of the grand. It was monumental. It was imperial. The largest bronze eagle he had ever seen was spread, like a mounted butterfly, against a wall.

There had been other moments in Jacuzzis, whirlpool baths. There had been, also, Livia's love of swimming competitions, with her hair invisible in its sleek white cap. But, in these scenes, the water was an accessory. It was almost furniture.

He put a foot in, holding on to the jetty's post: paused. He retracted his foot.

—It is very cold, he said, gravely.

He looked around. The wind was breathing through the trees. But Haffner didn't want the nymphs, the naiads and dryads: the sylvan pastoral.

It wasn't that Haffner was immune to nature. Haffner was a member of the Royal Horticultural Society. Its journal would arrive, a precise oblong, in its plastic wrapper. It was the only society to which he felt allegiance: a community which shared his love of the cultivated, the meekly tended – the romance of the rose.

Haffner was an expert in breeding roses. He loved the extraordinary lottery of each new specimen. All the textbooks talked of the evolution of a species in temporal terms; for them, everything proceeded in a logical order. The first was always the most important. But breeding, Haffner decided, proved this could not be true. It was a pure fluke, if a new variety of rose was formed, and therefore propagated, before another one. Its place in the species had nothing to do with time. It was much more like a jigsaw puzzle. In nature, Haffner found the self-sufficiency of art. But he didn't describe it like this; which is how I might have described it. For Haffner, this insight had other vocabulary. That things could happen according to a logic which one could not understand was no argument against that logic's existence. But perhaps this was not right, either; perhaps Haffner didn't use words to describe the pain it caused him, the lush pain as he looked at the photographs of gardens in exotic places, full of grace, these places in another hemisphere – Persia, Pakistan, Afghanistan.

You have no idea how therapeutic it can be – he would tell bored Benji, bovine – to take the secateurs and go out into the garden, after a hard day's work. Everyone, he would add, must have a hobby; and Benjamin, who at this point, when he was fifteen, wanted no hobbies, no bourgeois attributes, absently nodded.

Now, however, Haffner was oblivious to the pastoral: he wanted to be anywhere but here. He wanted sirens, emergencies, the asphalt and the smoke. The asphalt jungle and the big smoke. He wanted the transparent lethal purity of carbon monoxide.

So Haffner looked away, into the landscape, and there discovered to his dismay a shape which was walking with a staccato lilt, and which therefore would soon resolve itself into the more solid flesh of Zinka. Presumably, thought hampered Haffner, she was on her way back to work at the hotel. He looked down: at his slight breasts, his bright nipples, the hair around his belly button: his penis dwindling in the cold. An acorn, it blended in with the arboreal theme. There seemed no obvious hiding place, thought Haffner, rapidly assessing the bleak and empty parkland – and in any case it was too late. Zinka had seen him. Shame possessed Haffner – a shame that she was seeing him like this, so unclothed; and a greater shame of seeing her so soon after the escapade of the night before. He was not quite sure how one was to behave, when one has just concealed oneself inside a wardrobe in a vacated hotel room, to watch a woman nakedly converse with her boyfriend. But most of all, he felt embarrassed of her seeing him with Frau Tummel: in this illusion of intimacy. Because love was his downfall. And with Zinka, he was concerned that the love this time belonged to Haffner.

If only he could have explained how little Frau Tummel meant to him! Then, perhaps, he would have been glad to see Zinka. But he could not. So, in an ecstasy of embarrassment and shame – the only forms of ecstasy which seemed still available to Haffner – he jumped in.

3

As he sank, the everlasting problems of Haffner's life concentrated themselves into more particular problems of the body. He felt sheathed in cold; enveloped. It seemed unlikely that he would ever feel warm again. The water was dark, slubbed with weeds.

At first, Haffner thought that he was only sinking. But this was premature. Gradually, he felt his body ascend: gifted with buoyancy.

Finally, he reached the surface, where Frau Tummel joyfully greeted him. He tried to tread water. It seemed harder than he remembered. His heart was gripped by cold. He felt it slow, then slow some more. This scared him. His breathing became more difficult. He looked around for safety. No safety seemed visible.

—It is wonderful, no? said Frau Tummel.

Carefully, trying to swim suavely, Haffner made as if to disport himself, a porpoise, in the water. He tried to move towards the jetty, where he could cling to a step, or a pole.

—And how are you? asked Zinka: above him.

—Oh we are very well! said Frau Tummel. Is it not wonderful?

Zinka smiled at Haffner: a bubble of intimacy. Haffner, his hair slick over his forehead, a bedraggled pony, tried to smile winningly back.

Then he felt the weather begin. It started to rain on Haffner, and his mistress, gently, in the lake.

He clung to the jetty, and found no solace. He was out of his depth, thought Haffner. In all the possible senses.

They seemed to be having fun together, said Zinka. They weren't together, said Haffner. They thought it would be charming, said Frau Tummel. That wasn't right, Haffner tried to say.

The rain became stronger. In response, Haffner maintained a casual grin. Glancing with mock-helplessness at the heavens, Zinka said that she really had to be getting to work. Was it really necessary? asked Haffner. Frau Tummel glared at him. Yes, said Zinka, she felt so – after all, they didn't want her there, did they, interrupting them? Oh, said Haffner. He was sure that wasn't true. Was it? he asked Frau Tummel.

She didn't want to make Zinka late, said Frau Tummel.

It wasn't special to Haffner, the desperation he felt as reality crowded in. Haffner was special only in his hyperbole: his unusually stubborn refusal to accept the order of the facts. And because he was determined in his refusal of reality, hyperbolic with effort, Haffner said to Frau Tummel that of course Zinka wouldn't be late. It really wouldn't happen. In any case, if there were any trouble, he would take care of the matter. Indignantly Frau Tummel splashed away. Haffner looked at her. Zinka looked at her. Then, before Haffner could turn back to Zinka, Zinka had looked away.

—I should be going, said Zinka.

Surely, thought Haffner, he could think of something to say? Surely at this point he could come up with the sentence which would charm Zinka, and make her stay?

No, said Zinka. She really had to go. Frau Tummel splashed noisily in the calm water. Momentarily, Zinka was distracted. But she would see them later, no – perhaps for the aerobics? She smiled at Frau Tummel; then at Haffner. It would be at twelve. And she turned around, while Haffner gazed after her: her retreat in the grey towelling of her tracksuit.

Well, that went well, he thought, brightly. One should build on that. They weren't far off, he decided, mordantly, from reaching an understanding.

And this was how I could have depicted Haffner as an allegory, if I had wanted to make Haffner an allegory – with a woman walking away from him and a woman swimming away from him, while he clung to a jetty, frantically thinking, failing, possibly dying.

4

Now, announced Frau Tummel, they must swim. She offered Haffner the prospect of catching her, and then set off, with swift strong choppy strokes – the fat shaking beneath the curves of her biceps – towards what might, to Haffner's straining eyes, have been an island: or might have been just debris, floating in the lake.

Around him, the horizons gathered, and their attendant mountains.

He set off. Mistakenly, he swallowed some cold and soiled water. Very soon he wallowed back. If he could only move his arms, thought Haffner, then he might survive. The prospect seemed unlikely. It seemed improbable that Haffner's body would ever work again.

He was not, it was true, famous for the accuracy of his self-diagnosis. The day he thought he had cancer, he asked Livia if he could show her his testicles. She had just come out of the shower – in a perfume of synthetic citrus fruits. Her hair was flattened against her face, which emphasised the way her face with its perfect cheek-bones looked old, looked mournfully mature. He proffered her a testicle, asked her to feel it. She declined. Over breakfast, he pointed out that he should probably go to see Ordynski. Livia tightened the lid on the marmalade and agreed that he probably should. If it was absolutely necessary, then of course he should. And so it was that Haffner went to his doctor, who told him that no, there was nothing to worry about: there was no evidence of any tumour.

Haffner corrected Ordynski.

—Not yet, he sadly said.

He was the recorder on the grandest scale of all the ways in which life was unjust to him. These ways were mainly physical. And maybe Haffner was right: maybe this was one way of living healthily – minutely to record a list of all the unfair weaknesses he endured: a heart murmur, an attack of asthma, exploratory tests on his kidneys and aorta in an effort to discover the causes of Haffner's exorbitant blood pressure. Then the possible cancers, the lingering viruses. If this made him a hypochondriac, so be it. So what if he was still alive? It didn't prove the irrelevance of his symptoms. It didn't prove that one day they wouldn't unfurl themselves into truths.

What no one seemed to understand, he used to tell his daughter, as they watched Benjamin play cricket, on some sports ground in the bucolic environs of London – before Benjamin developed his intellectual difficulties with the idea of sport – was how the imagination of disaster was such a burden. He wouldn't wish it on anyone. It was no joke, living with illness in the way that Haffner lived with it. It was debilitating. Churchill, in Marrakech, got through his pneumonia on pills. He knew that. But that was Churchill. And Esther had simply got up, silently, straightened the creases in her slacks, and gone to buy herself a tea.

And as he mournfully watched the distant image of his grandson perform the neat parallelogram of a forward defensive stroke, Haffner considered the sad truth that his fears were never believed. Haffner was always alert to the way a life became a system of signs. It didn't seem unreasonable to Haffner. Greater men than Haffner, he reminded the now imaginary Esther, had been caught in the trap of a justified paranoia. Wasn't it well known, thought Haffner, that an emperor, of all people, was the most miserable of men – since only his actual assassination could convince the people that the manifold conspiracies against his life were real? This was one resemblance of Haffner to the emperors. Only Haffner's death would convince his family that he had been right all along.

In the mercurial water, this death seemed finally imminent. Frau Tummel had swum back. Such a kitten he was, to dislike the joys of water! And angrily Haffner had gestured at Frau Tummel – a gesture which was meant to signify absolute irritation, but because this gesture meant that he let go of the jetty, he suddenly found himself underwater, then hoisted by Frau Tummel in an ungainly manner back towards a pole which he grabbed at, gratefully, spouting water like a respiring whale.

Frau Tummel asked after him, but Haffner could not speak. Breathing heavily, he looked across the lawns. On the edge of the park, there was what to Haffner seemed another park. This one was an area of tarmac, for children's games. Yearningly – because Haffner adored all games – he imagined the roundabout, the swings, the rocking horses with their bellies pierced by springs. The springs beneath one swaying horse were creaking in the wind: as if, thought Haffner, the horse were neighing.

This playground seemed a refuge to Haffner.

Frau Tummel had plunged underwater, to tug at his legs, pulling him away from the safety of the jetty, into the abysmal open water. There was sun as well, true, but the sun was no help to him now. The rain was coming down, thought Haffner, really quite hard.

Behind the hills arc'd a fuzzy rainbow.

—You are so Englishman! said Frau Tummel. Enjoy yourself, my love. Express your feelings!

He couldn't help thinking that Frau Tummel was angry with him. No other explanation seemed plausible for her oppressive joyfulness. Swimming wasn't how Haffner expressed himself. When he wanted to express himself, he turned to his clarinet.

He wouldn't do it, he told Frau Tummel. He wouldn't swim. He was finished. And he raised himself gradually out of the water, the sheen streaming off him in the pale beginning sunlight.

5

And as he stands there, rubbing at his body with a towel which seemed of an unnaturally limited size, gathering his clothes about him, I feel a little sad that Haffner's moments of self-expression should be so absolutely historical. Let Haffner be allowed his chapter of jazz!

For he played his clarinet with abandon, in the suburbs of north London. Dutifully, he studied Benny Goodman's exercises for the modern player: the complex intervals of his jazz arpeggios. The greatest melody of all time, thought Haffner, was 'Begin the Beguine', as rendered by the genius Artie Shaw. For its outlandish, unhummable length. Its reckless shape which defied all normal ideas of the proper lifespan of a melody. That was self-expression. But self-expression, so often, was banned for Haffner. Gently, Livia would beg him to think of the neighbours. And Haffner would reply that he was thinking about the neighbours: it was a generous gift, this performance by Haffner of 'Begin the Beguine'.

Some saw in his love of jazz songs an irrevocable flippancy. He had no respect, Goldfaden used to say, for authority. It was quite extraordinary. But Haffner wasn't so sure that this was true. His authorities were simply different from those of other people. Esmond tried to find authority in his wife; his grandson found it in his rabbi. Other people depended on their manager, their marriage-guidance counsellors. Haffner found it in jazz. He took what he could. How strange was it anyway to listen to Cole Porter? Had anyone else come up with better descriptions of the heart's affections? Not Shakespeare, as his daughter argued; not the writer of the Psalms, as Benjamin now argued.

Every time we say goodbye, I die a little. That was all it took for Haffner to shiver with emotion.

There was a stringent division in the record collection which Haffner shared with Livia. Haffner owned the jazz. Livia admired her opera singers, her great conductors. She was the one who owned the cumbersome box sets – the collected symphonies, the complete quartets. As an encouraging birthday present, she had given Haffner Mozart's *Haffner Symphony*. He had tried to listen, but he had to confess that he saw no interest in it. Not even with such a title. No, if Haffner tried to improve himself, he preferred to read. That was his chosen domain of education. Whereas when it came to music, he preferred the songwriters: Arlen, Gershwin, Mercer. The songs from the era when Haffner was young: the songs from before the era when Haffner was young.

According to the liner notes on the record Haffner loved most – of Ella Fitzgerald singing Cole Porter – the qualities which made Porter great were Knowledge, Spunk, Individuality, Originality, Realism, Restraint, Rascality. Haffner had no problem with this list. Its last term, however, was a problem for Haffner's idea of the aesthetic. The last quality on the liner notes was Maturity. And Haffner could do without maturity. As if that was an ideal. The greatest education possible, thought Haffner, would not lead its citizens into an age of responsibility, but instead would escalate them to the rarefied heights of dazzling, starlit, spangled immaturity.

6

He was saying goodbye, said Haffner to Frau Tummel: and then he turned away.

—Raphael, said Frau Tummel.

Haffner turned back.

But Frau Tummel did not say anything. She smiled at him, in a way which she hoped was happy. And Haffner, once more, turned away.

He had finally become his father. The man who drifted away. It had never been his aim. He had done his best to avoid becoming Papa. At least, for instance, it had only been the one wife for Haffner. He had that over him. But still, all the motifs were there.

His father had been the quietest man he ever knew. One finger was missing, due to an accident in the Great War, for which Papa never offered an explanation. A photograph survived somewhere – in a box in some attic, acrid with asbestos – of Solomon Haffner, smiling as he held a grenade in his muddy hand: like the proud cultivator of a prize marrow at a provincial gardening show. But Solomon never talked. So Haffner had been forced to imagine the reasons for his missing finger: chewed off in hunger, blown away by a bullet, poisoned to the root by acid. The word for his father, said his mother, was *destroyed*. Some of Papa had been destroyed. Raphael had to understand this. She said this to Haffner when yet another cook was sitting in the hall, waiting to be interviewed, since her predecessor, along with several others, had condescended to treat Solomon Haffner in ways which went beyond the normal domestic duties of domestics. She only hoped (oh Mama!) that Raphael would not behave in this way when he was a man.

And as if the powers governing Haffner wished to demonstrate how comprehensively he could be entrapped, Haffner's phone went – stowed in his tracksuit pocket. The voice of his grandson asked him if things were fixed yet. Had he managed to get any further?

Really, thought Haffner, Mama had been correct all along. It wasn't right, for Haffner to be adult. The duties were beyond him.

At the moment, the twenty-three-year-old Benjamin was in Israel, somewhere near Tel Aviv. He was at a summer school in a rabbinical seminary, where he was educating himself about the history of his people. His people and their invented traditions. As Haffner argued. In Tel Aviv, in his self-imposed isolation, Benjamin had taken on – for reasons which were obscure to his grandfather – the burden of his family's disappointment in Haffner. Every day, he had called Haffner: wondering when the matter would be fixed. Because no one understood, said Benjamin, why it was taking so long. He couldn't understand it himself. He really thought, he said, that Haffner should at least be explaining what was going on.

—Your mother put you up to this? said Haffner.

Benjamin assured him that this wasn't true. He was only, he was only trying to understand what was going on.

Everyone was tired of the grandfathers. Everyone was bored with the everlasting males. This seemed fair.

Was it possible that Haffner wasn't the father of his child? He envied his brother-in-law, Cesare, who had lived his life only for himself, unencumbered. Cesare's lone state had always worried Livia. It had never worried Haffner. Or there were those other men, the cuckolds, with their blissful state of non-paternity. He could see the point of that as well. Oh Haffner so wanted to desert! It was just, he never had a clear idea of what he would desert for: no, he was not a natural elopee. Haffner had never joined the truant train of Bacchus – Bacchus, with his gang of heartbreakers, his absconding crew. Always, the final disappearance had been beyond him.

7

The first time he had heard the music of Artie Shaw was in his training camp in Hampshire, listening to the wireless with Evelyn Laye. She had expressed admiration. So, quickly, Haffner became a connoisseur; he developed a taste for the lyrics of Johnny Mercer, the music of Hoagy Carmichael. Haffner loved the USA – that land of opportunity, of the Ritz, and razzmatazz. One night, waiting to find out what to do next at Anzio, when the options seemed decidedly limited, Haffner chatted to a black man in a US cavalry unit. His name was Morton. He was Haffner's double; his twin. They spent the night amusing themselves by coming up with the names of the great women songwriters: Kay Swift, of course; and Alice Wrubel. The geniuses for the standards.

But Morton was now dead too. Like everyone else whom Haffner loved, including Haffner's wife.

Haffner walked home, to the hotel. In the distant landscape, there were concrete buildings. These were the buildings of the Socialist renaissance. Their facades were stained concrete and patched glass. There was no ornament. A small sports complex, with its dank swimming pool and dark sauna. A home for the mentally ill. And out on the absolute edge of the town, where the motorway began, were the beginnings of the capitalist renaissance: the warehouses and their associates: the strip club, the pool hall, the strangely Chinese restaurant.

It was hard to see the attraction of this spa town. It was melancholy: chlorinated, salty, sulphuric. It wasn't the spa town which Haffner had imagined. It wasn't for Haffner. He wished he were anywhere else but here. He'd rather, quite frankly, be in a provincial town in Britain, standing at a bar where coked-up girls drank Malibu through fluorescent plastic straws. Haffner's image of the sanatorium had been a lustful, tubercular hothouse. That was surely what it had been like, in the era of the Great War – before Haffner had even been born. The stories Livia had reported! Of docile and female patients, their legs akimbo in stirrups. The women would invent symptoms, just so they could be treated by the stern philandering doctors, there, on the examination table. They would lay themselves out, tense specimens to be relaxed and galvanised by massage. Or even, wondered Haffner, they would begin to enjoy the tenderness of the speculum. Because it was very possible, Haffner had once been told, by a girl whom he believed was flirting with him, that one could climax through these examinations: it had once been very embarrassing for her, but the nurse assured her it was entirely normal. A fact which, when relayed idly to Livia, received only an abrupt refutation.

On Livia, Haffner paused.

She used to refute him, often. She was Haffner's educator. This seemed like Haffner's ideal of marriage. Without her, he was adrift. But adrift as he was, now that she was absent, he could still admit that not even in Haffner's moral philosophy was it possible to argue that his attempt to secure her inheritance should have transformed itself into this Haffnerian farce: the bored affair with a married woman; the excited affair with a girl who was half a century younger than him. In neither of which, thought Haffner, did Haffner seem to be in control. No, it rather seemed to be Haffner on the massage table, supine: Haffner himself in stirrups.

A cold remorse flowed through him. Today, he thought, would be the day he finished this business of Livia's villa. Let his grandson be proud of Haffner! He would go back to that committee room, he would try once more. No one would vanquish Raphael Haffner.

And so he strode in his damp sportswear through the hotel's uniform gardens. The electric doors of the entrance hissed open, and Haffner hurried in, only to be called back by the receptionist. He hadn't, presumably, forgotten about his early massage?

Mr Haffner, thought Haffner – who? Him? That schmuck could forget anything.

But Haffner was in a new era of maturity. He asked if the massage could wait. The receptionist thought that it could. So Haffner strode on, and returned to his room.

He stood there, looking in the mirror – contemplative at the sketchy portrait of Haffner. The diminutive slope of his belly seemed suddenly sad to him now: the fat, the mark of the human. His penis hung there, in its brief tuft of hair, so oblivious, thought Haffner sadly, to the history of its glories and disasters The veins on his chest were turquoise behind his skin. Bruises, like passport stamps, lay on his shins and arms.

It seemed unlikely, he admitted, that Zinka could love him.

But Haffner was not downcast. He was unmockable when it came to his body. And in this, truly, he was greater than Julius Caesar, who was so disturbed by his lack of hair that he combed the thin strands forward over his head. Which was one reason, and perhaps the most important, why Caesar, it was said, so coveted the laurel wreath.

Haffner was not vain. He dismissed the love Frau Tummel felt for him; he dismissed the love he might feel for Zinka. He was an emperor, a dictator.

Now, he had to deal with his inheritance.

PART TWO

Haffner Enraged

1

Haffner walked into town. At first, he proceeded through a suburban and universal neatness – past the front gardens embroidered with roses; the garbage cans topped with sedge hats; the open garages displaying workbenches and shelves of car accessories: the serried oblongs of oil cans – like the retrospective Manhattan skyline as one stands on the ferry, and the sun is everywhere, and everyone is in love. Haffner's Saab 900 returned to him, isolated in the car show of his memory: the avant-garde slope of its trunk, the sky blue of its paintwork, the luminous orange quiver of its speedometer. A car which Livia had driven into their garden wall. Which Haffner had driven into the new glass frontage of an evangelical church. Thus continuing a grand family tradition, begun in 1922 when Papa crashed the new Mercedes, blaming first the wind conditions, then the road conditions, and finally an assortment of malevolent historical enemies, the most powerful of whom were the Bolsheviks.

Two men walked past him, carrying a wardrobe, one of whose doors had fallen open, so exposing to the outside world a mirror which was now reflecting the unimpressed landscape, behind which disported the tremulous picturesque mountains.

A variety of apartment blocks arranged themselves around an absent centre. Then a road adorned with nothing: no building, no monument, not even slick patches of well-kept grass. Just dust and the sky and a view of a factory. This landscape then softened into more apartment blocks. By the side of the road was a cement mixer and its accompanying builder – in T-shirt, socks and jeans – who was slapping the soles of his trainers together to dislodge the dry mud, his arms flapping up and then down.

He really did have no idea why the family so insisted on reclaiming a villa in this benighted country. He hardly envisaged the family holidays, the relaxing weekend breaks. But then Haffner, having reached this obvious conclusion, could see the force of an obvious question. If this was the case, then why was Haffner here?

Haffner was disinclined, at this point, to undertake the self-examination. Already, too many people seemed to want to understand his motives. It didn't need Haffner to enquire into them as well.

Instead, Haffner entered into the old town. Just off the main square, in the courtyard of a church, there was a kiosk topped with a cross, with lit candles for the dead. The air was weeping above the flames. A woman lit a small stub then changed her mind. She plucked then dabbed its wick, then selected the tallest, most powerful candle. Beside the church, set back in its railed-off enclosure, stood the Writers' Club. It advertised coffee. Haffner wandered in. The Writers' Club was also marked by candles, which lit the dining room, pointlessly illuminating the coffered dark ceiling, the mahogany sideboards. In the foyer were gilt candelabra, gripped in their mouths by silenced lions. At each corner of the room, there was a mirror; caryatids in the eaves of the roof, which displayed a peeling fresco of a fleshy muse, airborne in a toga. On the terrace, an emblematic writer was scribbling at a table, throwing away crumpled carnations of paper. On the table beside him, two slices of melon rind had been laid crossways over each other by an artistic vanished diner: an impromptu four-pointed crown.

Yes, here Haffner was: in what he only knew as Bohemia. It wasn't Bohemia, of course. But Haffner's idea of geography, like his idea of history, was eclectic. It had been taught to him by his Uncle Ernie. Uncle Ernie! – who ran a brewery business and whose hatred of women developed intricate disguises, so that once, from Nice, he sent a postcard to the young Haffner describing how Mrs Jay had once more collared him for a dance, but thank good ness this time she didn't have her monkey with her. Haffner always wondered if this monkey were real, or allegorical. Uncle Ernie's theory of Europe was simple: there was England, there was France, and then began Bohemia – a land which stretched from Gdansk to Vienna, from Strasbourg to Odessa. A minute version of Haffner tried to query this, but was rebuffed. So although Bohemia had disappeared in 1918, before the era of Haffner, it was now Haffner's central country: wherever Haffner was in Europe, that place became Bohemia.

He couldn't really say that the architecture of this town was truly modern. It was, he thought, as he left the club, a place which seemed unobtrusively to have opted for excess. What might have been a palace or at least the grandest of condos rose proudly in the sunlight. Over the porch curved a glass shell, with strutted ribs, a petal of glass: on either side of it were twin balconies, made of iron: these balconies were furious with detail. Curlicues of foliage melted into each other, in black mazes, twisted into dripping florets and stems – like the rose bushes Haffner had so coveted, in Pfeffer's garden. Pfeffer, Haffner's schoolfriend, was a lawyer in the City. His rose bushes were all tended by a gardener – and yet it was Pfeffer whose picture was found in the horticultural journals, Pfeffer who wrote in with exquisite botanical notes describing impossible species; Pfeffer who sentimentally named each of his new breeds with the name of one of his grandchildren. Above these railings, the brickwork was scrolled and crenellated. The facades had terracotta highlights, small statues which carried flaming torches in an upstretched hand, dead goddesses, proud heroes. The entire classical corpus. And the walls of the Town Hall's foyer bore bas-reliefs, mosaics. *Industry Leading the Spirit of the People. The Triumph of the Working Man. The Fecundity of the New Woman.*

No, nothing here was modern. But then, Haffner's twin domains – the islands of Manhattan and the City of London – weren't modern either. Everywhere was decorated in the junk of the Hapsburg nineteenth century. The junk was inescapable.

2

On his arrival, Haffner had come to the Town Hall, and been given a variety of forms to be filled out. These confused him, but Haffner persevered. Yes, Haffner had tried to do the dutiful, the proper thing. He had never planned on his private imbroglio. He had just thought that the legal process would be a formality: his last duty to the dead, which he could be done with in one day. For it had been Haffner who had placated his rivals at J.P. Morgan with artfully capped and collared contracts; Haffner who had perfected the art of the butterfly spread. These residential forms, he thought, could therefore not be beyond him. They simply involved him proving that he was who he was; and that Livia had been who she had been; and the house was what it was. With these forms neatly completed, he came back, to be told that the only person in the building who could translate for him was away. She was having a hernia operation. Two days later, by this time embroiled with Frau Tummel, and touched by Zinka, he had returned once more, greeted his oddly healthy translator, handed in the forms, and been told that the process was still in its initial stages.

Now, then, for the fourth time, he ascended the stairs, slowly, and entered the building. A security guard, sitting inside a plastic box, with a dog asleep at his feet, acknowledged him with a movement of one eyebrow. Haffner waved at this man, cheerily. For one should always be good to the staff. You never knew when they might become useful. He had been taught this by his first ever superior at Warburg's, in the Long Bar at Slaters in the welcome spring of 1947: and Haffner had never forgotten. The bellboy, the receptionist, the driver: Haffner knew them all by name. Even if, so often, he reflected, Haffner got it wrong: the temping busboy, the relief lift attendant . . .

Haffner's goal was the Committee on Spatial Planning. The room which contained the secretaries to the Committee on Spatial Planning was adorned by no painting, no mirror, no poster. Its walls were bare, except for a cork noticeboard, pinned with reminders of rota systems, memos about departmental protocol. A handwritten invitation to a party from two months ago was beginning to curl at the bottom: a stalled wave.

The single window seemed to offer a view of nothing: a back garden, a washing line. Just as on the tenement roofs below Grand Street the washing used to hang there like the urban signal for surrender. Haffner would look out over the shining city: at the World Trade Center, and its ancestor, the Chrysler, all his beloved monuments. The feats of prowess! The tricks of engineering! He looked out and basked in that new capital of speed.

But was the villa worth it? This was the question which Haffner still pursued. After all, the villa didn't belong to them: not any more. Long before the death of Livia's father and mother, in Buchenwald, in 1944, it had been transferred to the Nazi authorities. A German family had lived there for two years, until the Soviets arrived, and instituted their Communist utopia. The villa was then occupied by a functionary in the department of education. His soul was bucolic. He had relandscaped the gardens. Then, following the events of perestroika, and all its unintended consequences, the new democratic regime had auctioned it, and it was bought by a Czech microchip company – who used it as a vacation cottage for their favoured, bonus-earning employees. And now, following the policy of reappropriation, the villa was legally to be returned to Livia's family.

None of this, thought Haffner, explained why the villa was worth his protracted effort. The history of this century, in Haffner's opinion, was rarely an adequate explanation. Instead, the private history of his century seemed more relevant. Haffner knew the concealed grievances of his family. He didn't believe that Esther really wanted this villa: not for herself. No, it wasn't about the villa. Haffner was here as a symbol. His daughter's constant theme was that Haffner should pay for his mistakes: the carelessness of his parenting; the flippancy in his friendships; the breakdown of his marriage. Just once, as Esther put it, he would act unselfishly.

Yes, thought Haffner sadly: it was always about Haffner. And the judgement on Haffner was simple: Haffner had failed.

3

Livia had not shared this mournful disappointment in Haffner. Her moments of reproach occurred more unexpectedly, there where Haffner felt most safe. Like the time when she rebuked both Haffner and her brother – in the seclusion of a booth in Sheekey's, watched over by a black-and-white scene from a drawing-room farce – after a night out in theatreland. She was unconvinced by Haffner's lack of commitment to an omnipotent God. No, she said, as Cesare tried to talk, let her finish. This was not because she was an Orthodox believer. She was simply unconvinced by Raphael's refusal to believe that this world could not be the only world. But then, Cesare defended him, he thought that Raphael was very right to be unconvinced by their inherited God – that bearded legal system. Here, he accidentally dropped a piece of bread under the table. Together, both Haffner and Cesare motioned to pick it up. They bent; they paused: they left it to its fate. No, continued Cesare, he had always preferred a certain Jewish renegade, Spinoza (—Who?

said Haffner; Spinoza, repeated Cesare, refusing all explication), who had observed that humans were mistaken if they thought that God was a superman, an elongated version of your average Joe. Absolutely! agreed Haffner. He couldn't agree more – rebending down to recover the bread, avoiding Livia's unimpressed gaze – thus hearing from between the stockinged calves of Livia, the trousered calves of Cesare, how there was no more reason to believe in such a myth, in Cesare's opinion, than there was to believe that God's form was that of a benign and bearded anteater, or a trident-wielding koala.

4

With this koala still perched on a branch of his mind, chewing on a eucalyptus leaf and resembling uncannily the koala which the young Benjamin had adored until its polyester fur lost all its shine and volume, Haffner went to a guichet. He loped over in a now stilted imitation of the walk which had marked the heyday of Haffner: suave, indolent, assured. Or all the other adjectives to which Haffner had aspired. He was told that he needed a ticket, with a number. Haffner questioned this. He pointed out that he was the only customer in the room. He asserted that no one had minded before. But no, said the woman: he still needed a ticket. He went to the red plastic box on the wall, which was sticking its tongue out, and extracted a ticket; sat down, and waited. He waited for ten minutes. No one else came in. Finally, his number was called. He returned to the guichet. At this point, he was told that if he had to speak in English, then they must wait for the interpreter. And so Haffner sat down again.

Such vacancy of waiting rooms! When Haffner wanted something done, it had been done. The fluency of the West – this was Haffner's expectation. He came from a world of anxious secretaries, divine stenographers. Not for him the sullen service, the dejected functionaries. The office as a place of pleasure – this was Haffner's norm. He sighed. He tried to read the notices. The notices gave nothing away.

With a heartbeat of flickering anticipation, Haffner saw a man come in: he was tall, and he looked tired. His air was Slavic. Perhaps, thought Haffner, this was his interpreter. The man began to talk in an incomprehensible language, then switched to Italian, then switched, to Haffner's relief, into English. His name was Pawel, he said. He was not an interpreter. Like Haffner, he was here as an applicant. He was here because his wife had – he was here to manage his wife's estate. Haffner nodded. In a way which he hoped indicated a funereal solidarity.

Together, they sat in silence.

Finally, Haffner's interpreter entered the room. Her name was Isabella. She was blonde. Her legs were long. Perhaps not the longest that Haffner had ever seen – in the matter of women only, he was not given to hyperbole – but they were extensive. She looked at Haffner, looked at the woman framed in the guichet like the image of the most venerated saint, and then nodded. Haffner moved over to the window. A relay involving sentences by Haffner and Isabella tried to reach the infinitely receding finish line of the woman in the guichet. Haffner was told that if he wished to discover information on the stages of the Committee's deliberation, he was at the wrong guichet. The room he needed was two doors down, across the corridor.

Haffner smiled encouragingly to Isabella.

They entered the new office. An anglepoise lamp, without a bulb, was folded in on itself. A woman was filing her nails with slow long strokes. Another woman was staring at what looked like absent space, but which was really the image of her daughter, playing trombone, who did not practise enough, and who therefore was unlikely to succeed in the brass competition in four days' time.

The lassitude of the ages spread its stain through Haffner's soul. He went up to the woman who was staring into space. As he spoke, she began to categorise papers into nine piles on her desk.

He began with what he considered to be a minuscule request.

Haffner wondered if at least it might be possible for a visit to be arranged inside the villa, even if the process were not yet fully complete. He had only, as it happened, seen photographs.

The woman then spoke in what seemed to Haffner to be a paragraph. A long, eventful, dense paragraph. He looked inquisitively, hopefully, at his translator.

—No, said the interpreter.

Haffner sighed.

There followed a much shorter sentence from the woman inside the guichet.

—Perhaps we could do this without a bribe, but maybe you don't need the stress, said the interpreter, interpreting.

There was a pause. They looked at Haffner. In this pause, the trio considered how corrupt this Haffner might be

5

Haffner's moral code belonged to the previous century – to the tsarist world of his great-grandfathers. His ideal was his great-great-grandfather: the emigrant – off the boat in the north of England, at a seaport no destitute Lithuanian cared or knew about. A miracle of survival, of charming strategy. Which was to be found also, he had to admit, in the history of Goldfaden and his family – unintentionally escaped from Warsaw in May 1940, their only possessions being two trunks of holiday clothes. For Goldfaden had only avoided the terror of the Ghetto because he had been in London with his family, to celebrate his sister's marriage. Strategic corruption, then, was Haffner's ideal: not the guarded lavishness of Haffner's parents, or the slick luxury of his contemporaries.

No, Haffner had no problem with the bribes. It was all a matter of survival. But in this case, he doubted if a bribe was worth the effort. He doubted if this woman really did possess the power she tried to flaunt.

And so, as often happened in Haffner's life, he accepted the facts and tried to re-create them according to Haffner's version of reality: he tried to discover an ally. He had never been hampered by the British ethos of the queue – its hopeful stance, its doleful allegiance to the scarcity, the want. He very much doubted, he used to say, if there was anyone who couldn't be corrupted. He went for friends: the deep connection. In Isabella he saw this possible ally in his route to justice. He offered to buy her a coffee. She looked at him. Resolutely, he did not look at her legs. And she said yes. Why not?

—Just five minutes, said Haffner, to the woman inside the guichet.

There had been many stories of Haffner. According to Haffner, this was because events conspired to ruin him. His innocence was always unimpeachable. But perhaps this was not so true. Was Haffner not to blame for the series of amatory notes sent to the rabbi's wife, which culminated in her flight to his house and the much talked about scene with Livia, who talked her through the crisis, and sent her home? Was it not Haffner who had spontaneously suggested an orgy in the London office after a retirement party – before swiftly and unobtrusively absenting himself? He couldn't deny it. All the facts of his legend were true.

6

She was so sorry, said Isabella. This was her country! So what could they do? He was Jewish, yes? And his wife as well. Such terrible suffering the Jews had faced. She felt very close to the Jews. She understood. She felt, she said, very close to every people that had suffered. For so many others had suffered too. This Haffner had to understand. Her people had also suffered so very terribly.

Once more, the horrified angel of history had come to roost on Haffner's shoulder: its wings gently flapping.

No, she said, it was true. Her grandmother was put into a cattle truck and taken to Siberia. Did Haffner know of this? Her grandmother saw a woman give birth to a child and then throw it over the side of the truck. These were horrors. Was he going to deny this?

Haffner was not going to deny it.

Her grandmother, she continued, had started smoking to make herself less hungry. She was hungry every day, in this Russian state. As if her country ever had anything to do with Russia! How she hated the idea of Eastern Europe – an invention of the West. This was the kind of tragedy her people had suffered. And no one cared.

—Well let's be precise here, said Haffner.

Like everyone else, she wanted to burden him with a past which was not his.

So, wearily, Haffner sat down to talk. But Haffner had not understood. He thought she wanted to deny the Jews their suffering. He thought she wanted to subject it to some diminuendo. All his life, he had tried to give this up – the talk of Jews and those who hated them. It belonged to a place which Haffner did not want to visit. It belonged to the conversations of his relatives. But now here he was, trapped: in the former Hapsburg empire, the former Soviet empire: high in the Alps, deep in the problem of grievances: and Haffner, if he had to, would fight.

—I don't know why, said Haffner, we need to be talking about the Jews.

—But I am not, said Isabella.

—Yes, said Haffner. You are. I know this is what you are saying.

—But I am not, said Isabella.

And she was right.

7

I should say this now, in this chapter on Haffner's inheritance: Haffner was not Jewish in the way that other people were Jewish. He was a minor sect of one. He always said that he never really cared about his religion at all. If Haffner had been an intellectual, if Haffner had been Goldfaden, the ever so fucking verbal Goldfaden, then perhaps he would have tried to explain his sympathy for the half-Jews, the non-Jewish Jews. Haffner could even see the worth of the self-hating Jew. It didn't seem reprehensible to Haffner. It had a rationale: the refusal to be burdened by the past of other people. But he wasn't an intellectual. This wasn't his way. He just knew that he only found amusing the attempts by the Orthodox communities of London to re-create a shtetl. When it was decided, late in Haffner's life, to re-create an eruv in the suburbs of north London, Haffner found this deeply comical – with Esther, as they walked to the car, having lunched at some new and disappointing Chinese eatery, Haffner sarcastically pointed out the string hung from lamp posts, a dejected line which sagged like the bunting at the saddest village fête, in the rain, in the centre of England, in the absent summer. He was bored by his friends who kept kosher, by the women who married and then developed a religious side, by the friends who wanted to visit historic synagogues, or remnants of ghettos, on their otherwise bourgeois summer holidays. Schmaltz! All of it! They weren't for him, the Jewish museums – with their nineteenth-century oil paintings of Torah scribes; the postcards thrown from moving trains, with the saddest phrases (*We must always think of the good things in life*) underlined. He wouldn't let it sadden him. It was not, he thought, his heritage: this European disaster.

Haffner had no sympathy for the manias of the twentieth century. The grand era of decolonisation; the century of splinter groups. All the crazed ethnicity. Was this such a triumph for the human spirit? It seemed to Haffner that it was a distinct defeat. All Haffner wanted was the conservative; the inherited; the right.

But the twentieth century was all he had.

And at this point I must describe a final loop in this aspect of Haffner's character. He disliked the burden of a tragic heritage.

He wished to live in a world free of this kind of inherited loyalty. But if anyone else, who was not Jewish, tried to agree with Haffner, he rebelled. No one else, he thought, had the right to criticise.

This was one of the marks of Haffner. Disloyal among his friends; and loyal among his enemies.

And so once more, in his exile, against his instincts, Haffner was becoming more Jewish than he wanted to be. Hyper-English among the Jews, this was Haffner – the blond and blue-eyed boy. But Jewish with everyone else.

8

As he prepared to defend his people, to argue the case of his embattled race, in a trance of passionate and unnecessary boredom, Haffner's phone rang. Hopefully, he looked at it, wishing for a respite from the history of Europe. For a brief moment, before remembering that this was impossible, he imagined it might be Zinka. But it was Europe all over again.

Once more, he heard the voice of Benjamin: the disappointment of Haffner's old age: as Haffner was the disappointment of Benjamin's youth.

—Poppa, said a voice which emanated from a payphone in some Tel Aviv hall of residence.

The recent mystery of Benjamin still confused Haffner. Each time Benji called, he said he wouldn't call again. And then he called again. And maybe if Haffner had only paused to consider this, then he might have seen the mute obviousness of Benjamin's behaviour: the slapstick of his reticence. He might have seen that Benjamin was in a crisis of his own. But Haffner was rarely good at that kind of thinking. He tended to believe that everyone said what they wanted. Just as, he maintained, he always said what he wanted. So it did not occur to him to wonder whether Benjamin might have more personal reasons for calling Haffner, the family's legendary immoralist. No, he did not imagine, for instance, ensconced as he was in his own romantic crisis, that Benjamin could be in a romantic crisis as well. Since Haffner never chose to believe in his own mysteries, why should he be forced to believe in the mysteries of others?

—Call me back, said Haffner, swiftly. I'm busy.

The voice of Benjamin swooned into silence.

And Haffner, in the unexpected glory of his triumph in so peremptorily dismissing Benjamin, returned to Isabella. He couldn't understand it. Yes, let him change the conversation for just one moment. He had now been to this office four, perhaps five times. And no one seemed interested. Did they realise they had a legal duty? Had they no respect for the law?

Isabella replied that there was no reason to raise his voice.

He demanded that they stop this conversation, he said to Isabella, and that they go back in. She would smoke one final cigarette, said Isabella. And Haffner loped away: to fume.

This pause lasted for as long as Haffner could contain himself, while staring at Isabella, angrily, with Isabella staring back. The pause, therefore, was short. He walked over to her again.

Why, he enquired, did she have to care so much about the past? It wasn't difficult, after all – remembering the past. It hardly needed to be an obligation.

You didn't need to remind Haffner about remembrance. He couldn't help it. So many of the atrocities were his. But why then should Haffner remember them? What use was the guilt? Since when, he asked Isabella, was suffering the criterion of a life? Why not the charm? Why not the fun?

—This country! sighed Isabella.

The smoke on her cigarette, noted Haffner, listlessly, was being redundantly echoed by its imperfect twin, the smoke from a distant chimney.

What kind of civilisation was it, she asked Haffner – who had no answer, just as he so rarely had answers to the absolute questions – where a girl was scared to go to church? Where a girl was told never to tell her friends that her family went to church? Because if they heard about it, they would send her family away. What kind of civilisation? This was reality, she said. This was real.

Could he have a cigarette? he asked. Moodily, Isabella extracted one. She lit it behind Haffner's hand. He inhaled: and felt sick.

It was the first cigarette he had smoked for twenty years. That seemed right. Smiling, therefore, in this moment of complicity, Haffner tried to create a truce.

Isabella pressed her cigarette out against the wall with her thumb: the butt bent. They went back into the cool of the building, and its humidified air.

9

This time, Haffner received a new answer.

There was, they had ascertained, a problem which no one had quite anticipated. He had not given them all the information required. Haffner paused them here. He could assure them, he said, that all the necessary information had been supplied, on more than one occasion. Perhaps, they said. But they needed to be sure. And Haffner was then asked where his wife had been born. He replied that he had given them this information already. Nevertheless, they said. Nevertheless what? said Haffner to Isabella, who declined to reply or to translate. If he gave this information again, thought Haffner, he gave it only to show how generous he could be. He wasn't one to bear grudges.

It turned out that, as they had feared, they could not help him at all.

His wife, you see, said Isabella, his late wife was a citizen not of this country but of Italy. He understood? So it was very difficult. They understood. But it was very difficult.

He had come, he pointed out, a very long way. They appreciated this, said Isabella, but their hands were tied. It was a problem of citizenship.

Were they serious? said Haffner. Isabella replied that absolutely. She was very sorry, she added. These were the ways of the world.

But did they understand, Haffner wondered, that the question of ownership was completely separate from whatever problem of citizenship they wanted to invent?

Isabella asked him to slow down. Could he please repeat himself?

Haffner, in his fury, awkwardly leaned into the guichet: an avenging, unsteady god.

He had no intention, he announced, of repeating himself to these people. He had had enough.

—Everyone is very sorry, said Isabella.

—It's not happening today? Haffner asked her.

—Today, no. I do not think so, she said.

—I just wanted to know, said Haffner, coldly.

As the gambler who plays cards, knowing they are rigged – the deal-box with its top-sight-tell, the coffee mill, the loaded dice – yet still believing in the efficacy of his luck, so Haffner confronted the miniature conflicts which the century placed in his path. That one had lost before the game had started was no reason not to play. And after all: surely he was still owed one great win: one absolute and effervescent triumph? He believed in it as other people believed in the more likely cascade of the slot machines: a parallel line of green apples, with jaunty stems.

—I am so sorry, said Isabella: melancholy for all the exiled and dispossessed.

Haffner only wanted a triumph. This was true. In the full panoply of his Jewishness, he had now experienced a moment of conversion. He wasn't doing this for Esther. Now, he was going to recover this villa in a gesture of piety. Yes, Haffner's triumph now consisted in his vision of the villa. And he knew his record when it came to obtaining triumphs. They proved, so often, beyond Haffner's talent. But Haffner, thought Haffner, was ready for the fight.

No wonder, thought Haffner, the emperors all went manic. He sympathised; he understood their frustration at reality's recalcitrance. No wonder they amused themselves with killing sprees.

10

In the *Lives of the Caesars*, the only ones who interested him were the monsters: Caligula, Tiberius, Nero. He liked the overreachers. How could you choose between them? If pressed, however, maybe Haffner would have gone for the god Caligula – who was happy to do it with anyone, male or female, active or passive. Caligula, continued Haffner, talking to himself, was famous for the comprehensiveness of his taste. He would give dinners to which he invited all the noble couples: the couples of the blood. This story in particular commanded Haffner's respect. It displayed a grand disregard for the niceties of public opinion. The wives would have to process up and down, passing a couch on which lay – untroubled by its stains, its cheap upholstery – the emperor Caligula. If one of them tried to avoid his gaze, he lifted up her chin. Like an animal. When the moment seemed right, he would send for one of them, and then the happy couple would retire. On their return, he would talk about her performance; mentioning a flaw here, a perfection there. He listed the movements for which she had no talent.

That, concluded Haffner, was the moment when Caligula rightly deserved his deification.

Perhaps he thought he only meant to shock. But Haffner was never coarse. If he shocked the general public, it was always because of a sincere misalignment in relation to the orthodox. So that even though I am not sure, as he said it, how much Haffner believed in this, it contained – perhaps unknown to Haffner – its own inverted logic, which was Haffner's deepest unexplored motif. He didn't really admire Caligula for the purity of his cruelty: he might have wanted his audience to think this, but Haffner was rarely sincere to his audience. No, Caligula was to be admired for his publicity. Haffner loved him, if he loved him, for the lack of shame.

No one understood the emperors. No one saw how humble they were – free from the deeper vanity of concealing one's own vanity – like Haffner before his family, refusing the illusion of maturity.

Haffner Soothed

1

As Haffner arrived back at the hotel, intent on his newly discovered decisiveness, like an infant intent on the helium balloon
clutched in a tight hand, a man emerged from an inner sanctum
behind the reception desk. He was in a bright white T-shirt and
blue tracksuit with silken sheen – his upper lip stained by a black
and inadequate moustache. This was his masseur! the receptionist
told Haffner, excitedly.

Haffner eyed his masseur, utterly indifferent. The helium balloon
of his decisiveness floated up into the empty air.

Haffner allowed himself to be led downstairs, to the candlelit,
scented day spa: and there, prone on the massage table, his face
ensconced in its padded lasso – wrapped in tissue paper, to absorb
the unguents of Haffner – he lay down.

As he did so, a montage of previous Haffners lay down with him.

2

There were the Kodaks of Haffner reclining on towelled beds in
his sports clubs, then the black-and-white photos of his white
body on a black bench in his army barracks. But the film stopped

on the image of him in New York, at the Russian Bath House on Avenue B. He used to go there with Morton. The steam secluded them. They would sit there: heating up – on the steps of the sauna, as if awaiting some spectral performance, some senatorial oratory. Cleansed, they would go to a bar in the Village – the name escaped Haffner's stuttering memory. Not often, but sometimes. And, in this bar, they would continue their discussion of the Jews and the Blacks. This was why Haffner settled on this image, as he relaxed from his struggle in the committee rooms. He was het up with the century's usual argument. But there it was. Haffner loved the Blacks, and Morton loved the Jews. Enough of this! Haffner would say. Enough of this sectarian rubbish. The race was unimportant. He could go further: there were people with charm, and people without. That was the only division one ever needed to contemplate.

Maybe to him, Morton replied. Maybe to him.

Morton put down his bottle of beer. It rested there, in front of Haffner's tired eyes. A bubble stretched, a condom, over its rim.

He didn't understand, said Haffner. He didn't get what Morton was implying.

—You've made it, said Morton. So you're cool.

—I'm cool, said Haffner.

—Not literally, said Morton. I'd never say you were cool in the real sense of this word. No. But yeah, you're cool. You've won your fight. So you don't care.

Haffner wondered if this was fair. Certainly, he could see the accusation's force. Catholic only in his hatred of all Protestants, all splinter groups – to which Haffner preferred the international art of business: an art to which he felt a strong allegiance, an art of which his central principle had been his insistence, in the wreckage of 1950s Europe, that one could not capitalise, as it were, if an economy wanted to remain national. The future was international. That was all he believed. He warmed to cosmopolitans, like Cesare.

—Is he Jewish? Haffner had asked Livia once, about an acquaintance at their tennis club.

—Oh, interrupted Cesare. Did you not know that the whole concept of the non-Jew is strictly inapplicable?

He had always admired Cesare. Always been fond of him. Cesare, in Haffner's opinion, lived up to his name.

—I mean it, continued Cesare. Every time I meet someone new, I discover they are Jewish. It's true what they say: the Jews are everywhere. It's a problem for the anti-Semites. Everyone hates the Jews; but then everyone *is* a Jew. It's a dilemma.

And Haffner called that fine.

3

In his padded lasso, Haffner began to talk to his masseur. His name, it turned out, was Viko. It was really Viktor, he said: but everyone called him Viko.

—Niko? said Haffner.

—Viko, said Viko.

As if he were Niko's twin

—Your name, it is like you are Hugh Hefner! said the masseur, delighted.

—You think you're the first person to make that joke? said Haffner, grimly.

—You know him? asked the masseur, undeterred. Relation?

It had been an exhausting morning, a very stressful morning, said Haffner. He could feel it, said Viko. There was much tension in him. But Haffner, as he always did, chose to turn the conversation away from his internal tensions.

He supposed, Haffner therefore observed, that it was a very difficult thing, to live in this country after the Communists had wrecked everything. And before Viko could reply, Haffner began to tell him a story about the Communists, which was a story about his brother-in-law: Cesare.

But maybe this was still a way of Haffner talking about Haffner.

Cesare, after the war, and his degree at Cambridge, had eventually decided to return to Italy, where he worked for the next two decades as a professor in sociology. The anecdote might interest Viko, said Haffner – raising himself up, patted back down. He was a Communist, Cesare: a Party man. But to understand this story, one also had to understand, said Haffner – talking into his lasso, to Viko's bright new trainers – that this man had a cold streak. He was hard. But there it was. In Italy, he began an affair with a girl whose name, Haffner tended to think, was Simonetta. Perhaps Simonetta. When it began, she was twenty-five. So Cesare must have been in his forties, in his fifties.

And Haffner suddenly noticed how this disparity in age, which had always struck him as tinged with a Hollywood seediness, was nothing when compared to the disparity between his age and Zinka's.

For Cesare, he said to Viko, it was everything he wanted. This girl of his wore leather; she rode a Honda bike. She was an assistant lecturer at the university. Could anything be more alluring? At the time, Cesare was editing a journal of revolutionary sociology. He made Simonetta his deputy editor. Cesare was a man of the world, said Haffner. A Communist, yes: but a Communist who loved the shops in the Quadrilatero d'Oro. A Communist who bought himself handstitched shirts, or shoes made from a single piece of leather. He loved his life. He was happy.

Then this girl wanted a baby. It made Cesare pause.

—I would love one, he said, absolutely love one. But first I must divorce my wife.

Dutifully, Viko chuckled.

In revenge, continued Haffner, unbeknown to Cesare, she stopped taking the Pill, and got pregnant. But Cesare didn't care about this difficulty. He simply got her sacked from her deputy editorship of the journal; and also from her job at the university. But then, a year later, when Cesare was in the process of manoeuvring for the university rectorship, the Italian Communist Party issued a list of approved yet not affiliated intellectuals. These were the kosher ones, though not confirmed. Cesare was duly admitted as being ideologically pure. But Simonetta campaigned. Using her contacts in the women's section of the Communist Party, she held meetings, she published denouncements.

Of all the intellectuals duly nominated by the Communists, said Haffner, only Cesare failed in his bid for election.

But the greatest moment of all, he concluded, was when Cesare told this story to his mentor at the university in Rome – who, on being told by a mournful Cesare the full dossier of the facts over a lavish dinner at a restaurant in a side street off the Spanish Steps, asked him if this was really how it would be from now on. Were they, said his mentor, to be ruled now by their mistresses?

Haffner! So sure that he was charming! So intent on making conversation – even though, of course, Viko was not interested in his anecdotes about Communism. He didn't care about Haffner's urbane distaste for all the politics.

The anecdote, therefore, did not receive the applause which Haffner thought it was due. A little shocked, perhaps, he tried another conclusion.

That, said Haffner, was the best he could say for Communism. But before Haffner could gratify himself with a murmured smile – as he remembered Cesare ruefully saying that the whole adventure had at least produced one benefit, because his wife, having found out, had finally made him a free man – Haffner felt a moment of alarm. It felt to Haffner's worried senses that Viko might be going too far.

The range of Haffner's body available to massage seemed to be becoming more expansive.

4

Haffner was lying on his stomach: a warm towel over his back. He was naked. At first, he had toyed with the idea of wearing the briefs he usually swam in. But then had thought that really he should not care. They were hardly the most comfortable of items. The important thing, he always thought, was a comprehensive massage. As if he needed to be worried about his modesty! No, not here, not with a man.

But now, he felt Viko let his hands splay and drift with the oil further up his thighs. At first, as Haffner chatted, he had interpreted this as invigorating. Then he began to wonder. But he was too confused to make a sign, to tense his thigh muscles in the ordinary mute gesture of irritation. He could not be sure how European this was – how much to do with the health spa, and how much to do with something else entirely.

His penis was trapped there, under his thigh, its squashed head protruding under his testicles.

And then he felt the man's hand flicker on to the head of his penis. He really could not be sure if this were still an accident. These accidents, felt Haffner, were becoming so much less accidental than he had first imagined.

5

He was rarely successful in his active search for what he considered to be bohemian. Whenever Haffer metamorphosed into the bohemian, it tended to be the result of someone else's choice. He strayed into it. He had understood the streets in Soho – but he had never felt quite at home on Wardour Street, or Frith Street. He went to the French House sometimes. But not the Colony Room, not the Gargoyle Club. Never had the wisecracking hostess Muriel Belcher eyed him from behind the bar, admiringly, as he went promiscuous with a male prostitute who came from the satellite towns around Glasgow. Nor had he drunk with Francis Bacon, vomiting into the gutter, each supporting the other's bent body, wildly applauding.

No, thought Haffner: bohemia, when it came to Haffner, always came in such strangely bourgeois costumes: a moustached man in a tracksuit, say, surrounded by candles.

This confusion was one instinct which he had inherited from Papa. Early on in Haffner's career, in Haffner's marriage, they had sat in the rose garden, in the pale sunshine, a police siren tumescing and detumescing in the background, and Papa had expounded on life. The thing was, a man could either waste his life or live his life. And in the end it was better to live it than to waste it. Did he understand this? Haffner answered that he thought he did. But what was wasting, and what was living? Was it Livia, or not Livia? A marriage, or not a marriage? It was hardly as if Papa had been an expert in distinguishing the living from the wasting – in knowing what was a place of safety, and what was a place of harm. In Haffner's opinion, these terms had a habit of turning themselves upside down. He seemed isolated in this uncertainty. The only other person who shared his bewilderment, in the end, was Livia herself. More often, it led to arguments like the one which had occurred the day of Livia's funeral: sitting in his kitchen with his daughter and her husband, Esmond.

He was, Esther told him, simply impossible. Haffner tried to disagree. She interrupted him. He was impossible. Like an infant. Haffner did not try to disagree.

He cared for nothing, said Esther. And angrily Haffner had replied that in fact it was he, her father, who was the only person in this family to think about other people. Yes, let him speak.

No one was more conceited than Haffner, said his daughter. No one cared more about himself. Did he know what Mama used to say? She had married a Greek god, and had left a Roman emperor. A monster of ego.

—Humble! roared Haffner. I am the humblest person I know.

No one could think what to say next. The chutzpah of it dazzled them. So no one spoke. Haffner simply glared at Esmond. Esmond silently glared back.

It amazed him, thought Haffner, how vanquished this man was: the absolute son-in-law.

Esmond wore the steel rectangular spectacles sported by fundamentalist spokesmen and the vice presidents of Midwestern software companies; but Esmond was neither a vice president nor a fundamentalist.

He admired Esmond for only one thing, did Haffner: his hair. This, he conceded, was splendid – the way it flowed and oozed, a miracle of liquidity. But nothing else. Not the liberal moral certainties; nor the obsession with football borrowed from the newspapers. Yet this was the man who had made Haffner's daughter into a meek provider: who had seduced her into the temptations of Orthodoxy. This was the man who had made his grandson rabbinical.

He still saw no reason, said Esmond, why that other woman should have presumed to come. Barbra, Haffner interrupted, was a very dear friend. Esmond ignored this statement. If that was what Haffner wanted, then he was welcome to continue this friendship, he said. He looked at Esther. She was arranging the cutlery in front of her – which had been laid for a breakfast no one, now, except Haffner, would eat: the rustic basket of *pains au chocolat* before him, the snorting coffee machine on the counter behind him. But there was no reason, Esmond said, for them to have to witness this. He saw no reason why they should have to deal with Haffner's, with his – but Esmond had no word for Haffner's delinquency.

And for a moment, Haffner, on his massage bed, felt a rare tenderness for Esmond. He understood the difficulty – since this was how Haffner had felt too, when trying to contemplate the moral life of Papa.

History, thought Haffner, was simply a playground of repetition. It really did amaze him how limited were its motifs.

Hurt as Haffner was by Papa's reckless behaviour, with the women, and the money, he tried to understand his impulses. Papa was terrified of waste. It was the only lesson he had ever learned; the only one he could ever impart. Haffner thought he understood, therefore, why his father had acted with such theatrical self-pity when selling off the only other inheritance with which Haffner had been involved. Papa had been the greatest collector of cricketana the world had ever seen: he bought engravings, handkerchiefs printed with the laws of the game, mugs, memoirs, the technical manuals. In cricket, Papa found his reason for being. It made him safe. He compiled bibliographies, small monographs on centenary tankards. Haffner had inherited this love – a love he had passed on to Benjamin, his grandson and heir. Then, before Papa died, in what Haffner regarded with tacit admiration as an act of grand malevolence, but which was interpreted by everyone else as an act of petty and vindictive spite, he auctioned the entire collection. So that in the course of Haffner's life, in random provincial museums, he would observe a small typewritten card marked neatly in a bottom corner with his ancestral name.

When Haffner's mother died, no one expected his father to be sad. Only Haffner. It didn't amaze Haffner to receive a noble letter from his father in which Solomon told him that had he never known his wife, that grief would have been even greater than the grief he now felt at this temporary separation imposed on them. And maybe this was not so wrong. Maybe this was the only way in which Solomon Haffner could have loved his wife, in this exorbitant way – writing to posterity. Whereas Haffner's love for his mother had been different. It was all nostalgic. Whenever he remembered her, it was only as an idyll.

But then maybe every idyll is remembered: maybe memory is a condition of the idyllic.

So Haffner had sat there, his father's letter beside him, and remembered how his mother used to lay the lemon meringue pie on the stone floor of the larder, so that it could set.

6

The previous section, dear reader, as Haffner is lost in his memories, is a way of describing Raphael Haffner asleep.

For although to Haffner's dismay his penis had begun to burgeon towards Viko's hand, thus creating, in Haffner's opinion, a situation of the utmost delicacy, he couldn't think what to do. The solutions seemed absent. Previously, when faced by situations which disturbed him, Haffner had consulted his mental library of exempla. So now, desperate, with his face down, Haffner tried to consider his mentors. But, once more, the external forces which tended to disrupt the straight line of Haffner's life overtook him.

Worried, Haffner fell asleep. He relaxed. He drifted into a place of absence, emptiness. Drifting further, his legs spread slightly more apart, in a gesture which was unmistakably flirtatious, thought Viko.

Viko was used to these situations. They occurred often, in his candlelit basement. They followed an ordinary pattern.

Viko, poised above Haffner's back, couldn't see that Haffner's eyes were closed. He assumed that the greater deepness of Haffner's breathing meant only one thing: the masseur's skill at finding individual ways to please the gratified client. He continued to move his hands around Haffner's thighs, the tops of his thighs, brushing his penis and testicles with slow abandon. All the signs were there.

The fact that Haffner had made no protest; the fact that he had positioned his penis deliberately so that its tip was softly available to Viko's touch; the fact that now he was even moving his legs apart to allow the masseur easier access: these were the ordinary, done thing.

His fingers ran up and down the shaft of Haffner's penis. As Haffner slept, Viko touched him, slid his hand in such a way that Haffner half woke, aroused, descending into thoughts of Livia: the only woman who had ever touched his penis so deftly. Who, even before their wedding in the Abbey Road Synagogue, as Haffner never tired of remembering, slipped her hand beneath the tightness of his waistband, just as she had done before: a gesture which remained the erotic zenith of Haffner's marriage.

7

Haffner's wedding! At this zenith, while Haffner remains there, happily asleep, with his penis in a stranger's hand, I am suddenly reminded of another Haffnerian story.

Haffner used to tell his stories in the car, while he was driving. Haffner drove like they drive in the ancient movies: inexplicably watching his passenger, and not the road. Between rows of parked cars, Haffner drove – as if before a pre-recorded backdrop – courageously oblivious to the malice of wing mirrors.

And, one night, Haffner told me the story of his wedding.

The service had been taken by his rabbi: the Reverend Ephraim Levine. The kindest man in the world, said Haffner. A very fine man. Who in fact, strange as it may seem, became the legal guardian of every Jewish refugee to London from Germany before the war. But that was another story. Yes, that was another story, which involved the story Haffner preferred to forget: of a girl upstairs in a locked bathroom, young Raphael adding up his batting average in the dining room with a pencil stub, its end wrinkled where he sucked it. Whereas a story Haffner always remembered was his father leaving the wedding service and asking for theological guidance.

—Ephie, why do we have two days for Rosh Hashanah?

And the Reverend Ephraim Levine looked at him and said:

—Solly, why do we have five days for Ascot?

It was very fine, said Haffner. Very fine. He was the wittiest of men. You never knew what to expect. And after the wedding, after his mother had by mistake drunk the wine which was meant for the bride, thus causing a dumbshow, a hiatus in the service, there was a tea dance at the Rembrandt Hotel, in Knightsbridge. Haffner's padre from his unit shared a taxi to the reception with the Reverend Levine. And did I know, Haffner asked, what the padre had said to him, astonished, when they returned to the unit? The padre took him aside. The things he had been told, the padre confided in Haffner, afterwards, refusing to enlarge this statement with detail. The things the Reverend Levine had told him. He had been shocked, said the padre: absolutely shocked.

And now, I think, I know what Haffner liked in this anecdote. He liked the revelation that all men were men of this world. Because every story, for Haffner, was the same.

Haffner was an admirer of the classics. He went to the classics for the higher gossip. Haffner, humble Haffner, wanted to understand how everything declined and fell. The history of the classical era was the history of decadence. Curious, Haffner read of Nero and his monstrous appetite – which overruled his reason so comprehensively that Nero devised a pretty game. He was released from a den, dressed in the skins of wild animals, and would then gnaw at the penises and exposed pubic bushes of servile men and women who had been bound naked to stakes. Haffner appreciated the underlying philosophy. For, in the vocabulary of Solomon Haffner, the patriarch of Haffner, to live one's life was the same thing, in the end, as wasting it. This was what the stories taught the gentle reader. Just as the classical, in the end, wasn't really classical: it led for ever to the Goths, to the Picts and the Saxons, the Visigoths and Ostrogoths: all the savage barbarians. The classical only existed in retrospect, when everything was over. You couldn't separate the classic from the decadent. No, the defeat might seem to come from nowhere, but really there was no escape from it: because it was visible, really, all along, from the beginning. So every story was a story of defeat. Even the stories about the victories.

Yes, I think now, as I contemplate the stories of Haffner, this seems true. Victory is only a series of slow defeats. Defeats so slow that for a moment they could seem like a victory.

Or maybe it was only true of Haffner. Maybe this was only the principle of Haffner's exorbitant life.

8

For this was how the farce of Haffner's finale continued. As Viko tended to Haffner's penis, Haffner's phone began to ring, pulsing where it lay – the shrill twin to his penis which was pulsing, contentedly, in Viko's hand. Blearily, his heart pounding with an ill heaviness in his chest, he raised his head and – a gecko   stared at Viko.

Haffner never did anything wrong – not willingly. It was just he was so often trapped by forces which were beyond him. But no one believed him.

The degree to which this scene seemed his fault was debatable. Perhaps Haffner, in some way, was guilty. Usually, the guilt came from women. The list of the women who felt disappointed by Haffner was one which Haffner usually preferred to ignore. At its head, there was Barbra, who had given up, she said, so much for him: but then there were all the others – Cynthia, with freckled hands; Joan, who only drank champagne; Hyacinth, who cried whenever Haffner called her; and Pilar, who was happily married, she said, happily married. But Haffner would never join this resigned lament. When it came to guilt, Haffner was immune.

This wasn't to say he regretted nothing. Not at all. Naturally, there were things he regretted. Regret was the territory. But regret, he wanted to assure the absent gods, the cartoon gods, was not responsibility.

Once more, he tried to convince the world that the world was a menace for Haffner. Hazily, he explained to Viko that he had just dropped off there. He had no idea, really. To which Viko, a professional of politesse, simply replied that but of course.

There was a pause of awkwardness.

—I should take this, said Haffner – pointing to the telephone: relieved in relation to the masseur; depressed in relation to the fact that, once more, it was Benjamin.

—This is the third time I'm calling you, said Benjamin.

—Really? said Haffner.

—I'm just saying, said Benjamin. You could at least be polite.

—I don't think, Benjamin, said Haffner, that you should be lecturing others on how to live their lives.

Haffner's opinion of Benjamin had once been more forgiving. When Benji had been into sports, Haffner had adored him.

Like Haffner before him, Benji was a goalkeeper. Haffner would watch him from the touchline, in the Jewish soccer leagues. Benji possessed poise. He had the weight. He was noted for his bravery. As colossal boys jinked and trampled towards him, Benjamin didn't hang back. He didn't remain stymied on the goal line. No, he closed down the angle. He tumbled down at their dangerous feet. Haffner applauded. Benjamin pretended not to be pleased. Mimicking the great goalkeepers of the past, he pretended to care only about his team. Having gathered the ball, he would ferociously bowl it to a free player on the wing, or kick it back into the opposing half. With the back of his gloved hand, Benjamin would smear the mud across his sweating forehead. Then, silhouetted at the far end of the pitch, in splendid isolation, Benjamin leaned against a goalpost. He observed the flow of play. He lined up the fingers of his padded gloves on each hand, as if in prayer.

At the weekends, when Benji was meant to be learning the piano, studying some piece by Mendelssohn, with a bordered cream cover, Haffner read the paper. In the adjoining study – called so boyishly and pathetically his den – Esmond looked at X-rays in his lightbox. As soon as Esmond wandered away, then Haffner began with the weighty discussion of sports.

Then, a few years later, a change occurred. Or not so much a change in Benji's character: just a change in the objects of its affection. The reasons for this affection had always been the same. There he was, on the outskirts of London, in the northern suburbs, and Benjamin discovered drugs. Not the terrifying, working-class drugs: not the crack and the glue and the marker pens. Instead, he discovered the recreational drugs, the ones with intellectual pedigree. Benjamin discovered the lure of cool. It upset Haffner, but he coped. It was, at least, a pastime he could understand. Now, even that had changed too. Now, for reasons which Haffner could not understand – in fact, he did not believe there was any actual reason – Benjamin had adopted his race's religion. He had adopted it, said Haffner, with a vengeance. And this vengeance, thought Haffner, was continuing.

—It's not me, said Benjamin. I'm not lecturing anyone.

—You tell me this, said Haffner. Is it really a way to live your life, to do what you're doing out there? With your missiles and your lunatics.

He hadn't phoned, said Benjamin, to have this conversation. He wasn't having this conversation. They'd had this conversation.

—Are you ever going to tell me how things are going? said Benji. Are things fixed yet?

—No, said Haffner. They're not.

—I really think, said Benjamin, if you're having so many problems, then I should come and see if I can help.

Haffner considered Frau Tummel, and Zinka, and felt alarmed.

He couldn't bear it. Youth, he thought, was the spirit of the petit bourgeois. Of course, thought Haffner, the young needed their myth of adolescence, their myth of '68 – of course they needed the romantic movements. Without the romantic movements, the young would have to see themselves for what they were: always the most punitive, the most envious, the quickest to judge. So Haffner, as he lay prone, on the massage table, opted to ignore Benjamin's proposal of a friendly visit. Instead, Haffner asked Benji if he'd ever heard of the celebrated Peter Ustinov. Benjamin said that he hadn't.

—He's never heard of Peter Ustinov! said Haffner: possibly to Viko, but almost definitely to himself.

—Now, let me tell you something, continued Haffner. Peter Ustinov possessed a quality which is in very short supply nowadays. In very short supply.

—And what's that? asked Benjamin.

—Charm, said Haffner. Now listen, old chap, I have to go.

—This is ridiculous, said Benjamin, and continued the conversation: in which he told Haffner that he could get a flight that day. He really thought he should. He could be with him by tomorrow. But Haffner never heard this conversation, nor Benjamin's frustrated squawk when he realised that Haffner was no longer listening, because he had hung up.

Haffner turned to the masseur. Suddenly, he felt naked. But he felt calm.

—Thank you, said Haffner.

—*Mais merci*, smiled the masseur.

—Absolutely, said Haffner.

A change seemed to happen within Viko: a ripple, a sigh. He turned away. He seemed to be smiling to himself. Haffner questioned him on this. He denied that he was smiling.

Sitting on the table, Haffner gave Viko all the money in his wallet. It was not much. It seemed ungrateful.

Not for the first time, Haffner felt overtaken by an exhaustion. He looked at the chair beside the massage table, at the arms of his tracksuit top, helplessly hanging down. Clutching his towel to his waist, Haffner gathered up his clothes – a hunchback. And then Haffner – who so wanted sleep, and rest – shyly shuffled out of Viko's salon.

9

There could be courage in retreat. Think, pacific reader, about Napoleon. The wars of Napoleon led to a million bushels of bones being taken from the plains of Waterloo, Austerlitz and Leipzig, then shipped to Hull, there to be sent to Yorkshire bone-grinders and converted into fertiliser for farmers. Haffner knew this. But he also knew the greatest bon mot ever, when Napoleon, recounting to the Polish ambassador the story of his retreat from Moscow on a sledge, observed that from the sublime to the ridiculous was only a step. No experience, after all, could not be transfigured by the telling. No retreat, therefore, was always shameful.

Yes, to Haffner, who admired the war books, the manuals on strategy, Napoleon was not so much the emperor of Europe, but more an expert on an empire's inevitable decline and fall.

Many years ago, on the French Riviera, when he was there for the jazz festival at Juan-les-Pins, Haffner had seen a waistcoat of Napoleon's, worn in exile on St Helena: it had charmed Haffner with its miniature size. Everything he loved in Napoleon was embodied in this waistcoat: he understood the littleness of things. Napoleon: the man who, at the Battle of Borodino, stayed in and issued orders from his tent. Yes, that man knew about the tactics of withdrawal: just as Bradman, another of Haffner's imaginary mentors, when faced with batting on a disintegrating wet pitch at Melbourne, in 1937, sent in his batting order entirely reversed, so that by the time Bradman went in at number seven the pitch had dried out, and he made a double century and won the match. That was the action of a true genius of victory: a man who was an expert in the mechanics of timing, a connoisseur of retreat.

With these reflections, Haffner returned to the hoped-for safety of his room, where he discovered a chambermaid, in an abattoir of her own devising: surrounded by the intestines of the Hoover cabling; the wet towels on the floor, like tripe.

And so Haffner, homeless, retreated further: he turned round and walked away, searching for somewhere to sleep.

Haffner Timeless

1

Haffner went out on to the veranda. Finally alone, Haffner lay in a lounger and looked at the mountains. He saw nothing which might interest him. Should he go so far as to say that he was exhausted? Yes, Haffner was exhausted. The sun was softening. And Haffner only wanted rest. For what a night it had been! What a morning! In the distance, the dogs in the village were yelping. He willed them to be quiet. Just as he had often willed Livia's pets to be silent: the moody schnauzer, the bulimic borzoi.

A tree was leafing through itself, anxiously.

Into a doze went Haffner. He drifted and looped as if through a dream of an endless sky. In his sleep he could rest and then fall, fall further, rest and then fall. His doze was a dream of diving.

Peace for Haffner! Let him rest!

While Haffner falls asleep in the midst of the afternoon, maybe I should let him be – reclining in my invisible deckchair, my imaginary lounger.

Haffner's sense of time was often subject to odd absences. Now that he was older, his time spans had lengthened. Benji, for instance, felt grand when he thought in terms of months. Haffner was used to thinking in decades: the decades seemed more accurate to the nature of the facts. They were the more useful unit of measurement. But here, in the mountains, these problems with time involved new proportions entirely. At moments, and this was one of them, he could not tell how long he had been in this spa town, in this hotel. Everything up here had become timeless. The usual co-ordinates were lost.

At what point had Haffner been innocent? Haffner, who could still remember with more vividness than he experienced many other things how on his eighteenth birthday, during the Scarborough Cricket Festival in 1938, Papa had invited the greatest opening batsman in England, Herbert Sutcliffe – a Yorkshireman, and a professional – to dine with his wife in the Grand Hotel. He was the first professional ever to be invited to dine, during the Cricket Festival, at the Grand Hotel. Before Papa's invitation, it had been strictly reserved for the amateurs. But Papa could not be denied. For Papa believed in cricket more than he believed in class. So into the dining room of the Grand Hotel walked Papa, followed by his wife and son, behind whom came Herbert Sutcliffe, with his wife, Emmy. Haffner danced the Lambeth Walk with Emmy. And around nine months later Sutcliffe phoned up to ask Solomon Haffner if he remembered that evening in the Grand Hotel, and Emmy and the champagne?

—Well today, said Herbert Sutcliffe, Emmy presented me with a son. And Sutcliffe started to laugh.

This was how Haffner's soul functioned – through these anecdotes which everyone else had forgotten, which no one else had noticed: like the ballet of electrified shrugs and ripples given off by the fringe of a beach umbrella, on a terrace, at midday, while every-one lies there sunbathing, with their eyes closed against the light.

There were two methods for the historian to record the history of Haffner. The obvious way was to follow the chronology: the annals of Haffner. But then there was the more philosophic way, which happened to coincide with the way Haffner really thought about it: with events overlapping, grouping themselves into themes. In his privacy, suspended in the fluid of his memories, Haffner approached the philosophical himself: a medium of total objectivity.

So it was only right, perhaps, that he should perform his finale up here, in the mountains, where everything seemed turned upside down: in the endless light of midsummer. Up here, as Haffner would have read if he had begun the novel beside his bed – but he had not, because he cared too much about the lives of the Caesars – life is only serious down below. Up here, all the being ill, all the dying and recuperating, all the endless and serious work at the spa was just weightless: life was just another way of wasting time.

He was not who he was! Not an aged patriarch. No, Haffner was so much younger than he looked – and he looked younger than he was. With Morton, as they sat and steamed, he used to turn the conversation to the women. at what point, he asked Morton, did he think they would lose their right to try it on with the women? At what point did Morton think the lust would leave the body of Raphael Haffner? Morton only looked at him, with an infinite amused pity in his eyes. He pointed out that one thing he loved Haffner for, indeed he would go so far as to say it was definitely what he loved him for, was that Haffner always thought there was so much more to Haffner than anyone else ever thought. He had the arrogance of potential. He was a romantic, said Morton.

It didn't seem so unreasonable. What was down was up, and what was up was down: so that Haffner, who boyishly soared above the hills in his usual dream of flight – the sky turned underwater, with dolphins in the trees – was really this aged Haffner, in a lounger, as the sun declined and the clouds bunched and pooled together, while Zinka – the dream of Haffner's youth – approached his horizontal form, accompanied by Niko.

Haffner was never left alone by the world for long.

Zinka nudged him, then nudged him again, until he spluttered himself awake. With depression, he realised that he was still so very tired. With elation, he realised he was looking at Zinka.

And then, to Haffner's startled gaze, Zinka said to him, with a grin, that this man of hers was refusing to chaperone her that night. It was always like this with him – impossible. Haffner nodded, slowly. He tried to understand his role in the conversation; but he could not.

So, said Zinka: he knew what he could do. Haffner smiled, benignly. Think about it, bonza. Haffner tried. He still could not.

He could ask her to dinner himself, said Zinka. Haffner looked at Niko. His face betrayed no expression. He shrugged. Haffner looked at Zinka. Was it dinner time? he asked her, wonderingly. She tenderly smiled.

Was this a dream? thought Haffner. He could not tell. Carefully, Haffner considered his options. His adagio was over. This seemed obvious. There would never be a period, he worried, when adagio would exist again. His options seemed limited to one.

Prestissimo, Haffner said yes.

3

The maître d' ushered Haffner to his table, where Haffner's bottle of wine from the night before was settled in a shallow silver salver, the cork stuffed in at a jaunty angle. Swiftly, declining to express his inner smile, his inner shock at seeing Haffner so publicly tend to Zinka, he then gathered an extra chair.

Haffner began to talk to the waiter, offering Zinka an aquavit. No, she interrupted. It would be better if she took care of this.

He must, for instance, try the cuisines of the region. And Haffner, as she conversed with the serious waiter, the marvelling waiter, took the opportunity to wonder about this continuation of his syncopated adventure with Zinka.

There had been the incident of the wardrobe, then the incident of the lake. Neither of these episodes, he thought, had enabled Haffner's true charm to shine. But now, here she was – opposite him in the elegance of a dining room. This was Haffner's more usual backdrop. He considered Zinka: in the residual glow of his amazement. The persistent, grand desire for her disturbed him. And yet, he sadly considered, he could not think for a moment that Zinka desired him. He possessed no liberating craziness about his erotic attraction. He knew that Zinka represented the unattainable. Even if, he wanted to add, there had been the improvised escapade with the wardrobe. This, surely, was not without some kind of wordless flirtation? Although, he corrected himself, it could so easily have not involved any wordless flirtation. She had been talking to him about his wife, all the melancholy reasons why he was here, in this spa town where everyone, she said, was so unhappy. Haffner was drinking some kind of grappa. And, as normal with the women, Haffner asked the intimate questions: because he was always intent, with women, on understanding their hidden sadnesses, the depth of their secrets. Which he perhaps inherited from all the imprecise conversations with Mama. And Zinka told him about her love life, and together in this conversation they knitted and clothed a rag doll of Zinka – unfulfilled, sarcastic, mischievous. So it had seemed somehow natural for her to lean in and propose – in English so accented and asyntactical that Haffner worried he had utterly misunderstood – that Haffner should conceal himself in a wardrobe and see how brutishly Niko treated her. If he wanted. And Raphael Haffner very much wanted indeed.

No, thought Haffner, the episode was not about him. And there he paused, because he had no wish to spoil this image of the two of them there – dining together: this image of the old and the young entranced. He didn't want to do anything which might disturb this dream of Haffner.

He discovered that Zinka was already involved in conversation. In Zagreb, she told him, she had trained as a ballet dancer. This he knew. Evenings, she used to practise trapeze. The trapeze was what she really loved.

Haffner mentioned that all the same he thought he would order an aquavit for himself.

Patiently, she explained to Haffner the various terms – the French vocabulary: the *croix*, or crucifix; the *grenouilles*, or candlesticks; the *soleil avant*, which in English was the skinner; the *chutes*, the drops. The *tour du monde*. And then the important *sorties* – as you extricated yourself from the tangle of movement.

Haffner, concealing his excitement at this vision, these outlined movements, asked her if it weren't dangerous. Zinka said no. Not at all, on the flying trapeze? Haffner had always imagined . . .

—Not the flying trapeze, said Zinka. Just trapeze.

There was a pause.

—I was on the stage once, said Haffner.

4

It was towards the beginning of the war, in 1939 or '40. In Haffner's battalion there were many actors. Since he was in a London regiment. Many famous actors. And one day the actors said that they ought to get the whole battalion together and put on a variety show. Did she understand? She thought so. And they put it up to the second lieutenant – who went on, added Haffner, to become a very eminent newspaper editor, as it happened – who agreed, and so they put on this show which couldn't have been put on at the Palladium. No. There was Max Miller, and. And. No, Haffner had forgotten.

—How can you be a name-dropper, wondered Haffner, if you can't remember anyone's names?

He looked out of the windows at the sky: out of the grand windows at the grand sky.

There was Enid Stamp Taylor, Renée Houston, Oliver Wakefield, Guy Middleton, Stanley Holloway, Hugh 'Tam' Williams. These names probably meant nothing to anyone now. These chaps were putting on their own little sketch. And one of them, who was a well-known producer, Wallace Douglas, fell ill and Guy Middleton came up to Haffner and said that Wallace Douglas was unwell and he wanted Haffner to take his part.

Should Haffner tell this story?

In this sketch Middleton was a colonel and Haffner was a subaltern. And all that happened was that Middleton would ask Haffner where he had got his breeches. And all Haffner had to reply was that he had got them in a shop in the Strand, sir.

No, thought Haffner. He should not.

He was so old, so woebegone, thought Zinka. She felt a tenderness for him. Tenderly, she tried to retrieve the conversation.

—You were in the war? asked Zinka.

I was in the war, said Haffner. Of course. Everyone was.

He paused. He looked at her.

Zinka was wearing a grey boiler short-suit, with black tights and rouge noir fingernails. Her hair was brown and her eyes were blue. The style was beyond Haffner: he had no idea, any longer, whether this was a style at all. He no longer cared. She was so utterly and completely beautiful, thought Haffner. So absolute in her body.

Then Zinka took hold of his hands, and looked at his palms.

Haffner, amazed, asked her if she was reading his palm. Meditatively, ignoring Haffner's scepticism, Zinka said that he was intelligent.

—Unintelligent? misheard Haffner, depressed.

He shouldn't have been shocked. The women he wanted were so often unhurt by a feminine self-hatred. Instead, they were happily confident in describing how Haffner could fail.

—Intelligent, repeated Zinka.

A paper flower of relief unfolded itself in the solution of Haffner's soul. He smiled at her, as she continued to read from his hand. But, she added, sombrely, he was unlucky.

—Unlucky? repeated Haffner.

—Well, said Zinka, trying to reconsider. Yes. Unlucky. I am sorry. I tell things as they are.

Haffner looked round, in an effort to find comfort in the view. But the view had disappeared. All that was visible was human. There, as usual, were the usual diners. At the table by the opposite window sat Frau Tummel, and her husband. They sat silently, in their marriage of silence. So Haffner turned back to Zinka.

—You do not wish you were eating with her? said Zinka.

—Her? said Haffner. No no.

—I am glad, said Zinka.

He knew his place in the art of love: the comic figure, for ever grasping after the women who fled him. Just like Silenus, whose comically old flesh concealed the youth of the lust within.

He tended to see himself in poses. This was true. But I saw him as something else. Like the hero of every legend – you had to gnaw on him, like on a bone, to discover the richness, the inner meaning. So I preferred my private image. Haffner was his own *matrioshka*: concealing within himself the other, diminutive dolls of Haffner's infinite possibility.

5

Zinka used to live in a village with her grandmother. Haffner considered if he could think of any questions about this arrangement. He paused. So, asked Haffner, were her parents dead? Not at all, replied

Zinka. She described their characters for him. Her mother was hysterical. Her father was calm. That was all he needed to know. Haffner paused again. In this pause, Zinka asked if he believed in God. Did she? asked Haffner, avoiding the question. She replied that she believed in an energy. And Haffner? He did not believe, said Haffner.

—I will tell you what you are, said Zinka. You are realistic, but also a dreamer. I think you are easy to melancholy. Is this true?

—Oh it's true, said Haffner.

—Yes, said Zinka. Now you tell me about myself.

—Oh, said Haffner. I think you are: I think you are tough, but you are not as tough as you want to be. Something softer there.

—Oh, said Zinka, you are fifty per cent true. No. No, you are much closer. Too close perhaps.

Haffner wondered what he was really doing here.

—I have no regrets, said Zinka. People have to live the moment.

Haffner murmured something indistinct.

And because Zinka seemed suddenly sad, Haffner asked her, delicately, if she were sad. Yes, she replied, she was sad. But she did not want to talk about it.

My country, it is destroyed, said Zinka. The baddest country in Europe.

But Haffner had seen worse.

The light outside, as usual, still persisted. It was as if the light went on for ever. In this light, Haffner looked down at his plate. He had to confess, the food here distressed him. He had never been one for the Jewish food, the food of Eastern Europe. He preferred nouvelle cuisine to the heaviness of starch. In a sauce of sour cream and oil lay a dumpling, stuffed with pork. Haffner considered if at this late stage he should return to keeping kosher. It seemed desirable. The dumpling outdid him. First, it had been fried. This fried dumpling had then, surmised Haffner, been boiled. Nothing else could have created this texture, of the softest rubber. He did not understand it. In the sauce of sour cream and oil, small moments of bacon were visible.

In what way, thought Haffner, could this hotel be said to care about health? What was the point of the massages, the waters, the sauna?

He looked across at Frau Tummel. She was staring at him, angrily; and Herr Tummel was staring at his wife. He also seemed to be angry.

There had been a woman in love with her in Zagreb, Zinka was telling him. Did he understand this? He did, he assured her, he did. But why should she seem so proud of this fact, thought Haffner. It wasn't so strange, to fall in love. It just needed, in the end, someone else to be there. Oh Zinka was so tired of love, she said. And Haffner raised an eyebrow: a self-interested, altruistic eyebrow. He mentioned, for instance, Niko. Yes, she said: but Haffner knew Niko too. That boy. She was not sure he understood her. But no. She did not want to talk about this.

—No? said Haffner.

He began to worry that she wanted to mention the wardrobe, and all the pleasures which Haffner had seen. On this subject, he worried, he had no conversation.

No, she said. There were things it was good not to talk about. The matters of the heart. It was complicated. He did not want to hear this. Haffner tried to assure her that he did.

—No, she said. Not now.

The sex scene which was not a sex scene: this was the recent story of Niko and Zinka. The idyllic scene in the hotel room had been only theatre, after all. They were absent from each other. They coupled only in disguise, in the dark.

How could Haffner know this? Was it Haffner's fault, dear reader, if he did not know the inner history of Zinka?

6

No, Haffner wasn't free. Unlike the transparent and liberated reader, he couldn't be everywhere, like the bright encompassing air.

For these were the nights of Zinka. The concrete balcony to her apartment was covered by an advert, a scrim hung down ten floors from the roof. The scrim was printed with a woman on a cell phone, in some countryside, surrounded by birds. On Zinka's balcony, therefore, the reverse of a savage, eight-foot swallow looked in on her – observing the television in its mahogany hutch; a garden chair, for ever folded, in a corner; the reproductions of Impressionist paintings, from the era when leisure was invented. In the apartment block opposite hers, the forgetful cleaner – who returned home on the buses, disliking the organic smell of her shoes, the chemical smell of her hands – would leave random lights on, illuminating the darkness for the potential spectator. But there were no other spectators. Except for Zinka's books – an illustrated translation of Pushkin, a novel in Russian by Dovlatov, a history of ballet – which looked down on her and Niko in their bed.

And Niko would touch Zinka's thigh, gently – which began their new game. In response to Niko's roughness, Zinka now never gave him permission. He could do what he wanted, she said: just so long as he expected her to do nothing.

And so, sadly, Niko did.

7

Perhaps this, then, was one reason for her silence. Perhaps this was one reason why she said to Haffner that she didn't want to talk about herself. Instead, she wanted him to tell her about Haffner's war.

And she looked up at Haffner.

So Haffner began where he always began, with the long night of

Haffner's spring in Italy: in the foothills around Anzio. Haffner got there on Valentine's Day. They were in the woods, on the flat ground, and the Germans, with the Ukrainians, were on the Alban Hills outside Rome. So they could see everything. There was nowhere you could escape. Everything was bound to hit something. The Germans had one wonderful gun – an 80 mm. Much better than anything the British had. They were sending over these great big heavies called Anzio Annies. Going for the docks. But it was much worse when they came over at night with the cluster bombs. On the whole, said Haffner, the British were very well dug in. But just about the time that Haffner got there, on Valentine's Day, was when the Germans made their one last big effort. They couldn't use their armour in that sort of mud. He didn't know it at the time. He didn't realise that those four or five days were the Germans' last chance to push the British and the Americans into the sea. They put everything into it. The noise, said Haffner. The noise. Their artillery was very good. The British had some destroyers outside the docks who were firing as well. And years later, on holiday in Madeira with his wife, he met a naval chap, who said: it was him. He was helping them. So there it was. Things got better when they began to see their own planes.

It was amazing, thought Haffner, how you settled down to a life: truly amazing. The chaps in the front were machine-gunned, killed in hand-to-hand fighting. And yet soon this seemed like a *façon de vivre*. His job as the second in command was to take up all the rations and things. And there was really only one way, which the Germans knew about: an alley.

Haffner paused. He considered himself. What could he tell her about Haffner's war? It seemed indescribable.

He remembered the yard in a town outside Alexandria, where he had enjoyed the greatest shrimp of his life, its flesh a white fluff inside the charred shell: there was a concrete reservoir, and a wind pump pumping water into it, clacking as it turned, casting a flickering shadow on the house.

This was all he could really tell her.

The problem about catastrophe, he had learned from the silences in his conversations with Papa, and then had learned for himself, from the silences in his own conversations with other people, was the incomprehension. There was the incomprehension of those who had seen nothing; and then there was the incomprehension of those who had seen everything.

Everyone persisted in the safety of flippancy. But maybe the flippancy was right.

At home, when the war was over, Livia would ask him why he was so private. She used to ask him this as if it were a fault, remembered Haffner – only idly noticing the fact that Frau Tummel was suddenly talking with animation to her husband. Livia expected Haffner to behave like a hero – to revel in his war stories. But Haffner never felt like a hero; not when he was being heroic. It had only bred in him a certain humour: a wit which could enjoy the gags of the emperors, like the one who, when a man asked for extension of his sick leave, ordered that this man should have his throat cut – for if the medicine had taken so long to work, then the man needed to be bled. With this humour, Haffner preserved his version of privacy. Livia used to upbraid him for his gaucheness at parties. He was always ready for his tête-à-têtes, she said. So why could he not be charming when there was more than one person present? And Haffner tried to explain that he had never been one for parties: for all the social whirl.

But maybe it was more of a problem that after the war Haffner's sense of humour had been replaced with something no one, really, wanted to know.

In Rome, Haffner had admired the triumphal column on which was carved a panel displaying a German baby being screamingly torn away from the arms of its mother by a stern Roman soldier. But most of all, he admired the Roman talent for the comic. Because – wrote a scholar in a booklet which Cesare bought and then translated out

113

loud for Haffner, over a coffee in Piazza Navona – although a modern viewer might see this panel as deeply affecting, for the Romans it would have been amusing. It would have been sitcom.

And maybe Haffner and his Romans had it right. A war as a farce: this doesn't seem to me to be so implausible – with its mismatched exits and entrances, and its grandly outflanked speeches.

8

No, he hadn't told Livia about certain things. So he was hardly going to be able to do it here, thought Haffner, with a girl he hardly knew.

His anecdotes faded away.

But then Zinka said that her friend, she too had been in a war: the recent war. Haffner nodded. She once told Zinka that she had seen such a horrible thing: she had seen one of her neighbours with his mouth propped open with a piece of wood. Then they made him swallow sewage water. This was the woman who loved her.

—She committed suicide, said Zinka, thoughtfully.

—Who? said Haffner.

—That woman, said Zinka.

—The lesbian? asked Haffner.

—Yes, said Zinka.

—In what way? said Haffner.

—Drinking pills, said Zinka.

—It's easier, said Haffner.

The conversation paused.

This wasn't something that she told people, said Zinka. But she would tell Haffner.

This struck Haffner as strange, but he was feeling so unsure of what was happening that he decided to let this thought go. So intent was he on constructing his own escape, his desertion from his duty, he didn't consider that, for Zinka, Haffner could represent an escape too.

There was one time, said Zinka, when she was walking down the street in Zagreb. And some soldiers were outside an embassy. And she was with her friend. As they approached, the soldiers began to raise their rifles. This was true.

He didn't doubt it, said Haffner.

And this was what she had never forgotten, said Zinka. They were shouting that they were nothing: they were only walking home. And eventually, of course, as he could see, nothing happened. But at the moment when it seemed possible the soldiers would shoot, said Zinka, she stepped behind her friend. And although immediately she stepped back out, level with her, she could never forget this moment of self-betrayal.

There was a pause.

And at this moment, Haffner – timeless – felt everything returning to him.

The beach at Anzio strewn with bodies, as if everyone were sunbathing.

But most of all, in the series of women who had graced the life of Haffner, here, at its zenith, there was Zinka – for whom he felt such absolute adoration. Yes, at this moment, thought Haffner, extravagant through nostalgia, ignorant of Zinka, he could have endured anything, if only she would love him. Even if there was, I feel, little left for Haffner to endure. Yes, this was Haffner's ideology now. Maybe it could even borrow a slogan. *Love me as little as you like* – this was Haffner: *but just love me as long as you can.*

For Haffner believed in coincidence – he saw his life as a system of signs. He scanned each new acquaintance for the meaning they were trying to figure in the everlasting life of Haffner. So here, in his finale, he could only see in Zinka a kindred spirit, the twin for whom he had been searching all his life. The twin whom Haffner tried to align as closely as possible to himself.

—Oh but that was nothing, said Haffner.

There were so many ways, he said, that you could feel ashamed. Not just the obvious betrayal. In Anzio, he said, at night, they had to leave the bodies on the beach: it was too dangerous to go back for anyone. So Haffner had to lie there. And a boy was calling, quietly: Mama Mama Mama.

—Mama Mama Mama, said Haffner.

All he wanted, said Haffner, was for this boy to bloody shut up.

It was only some years later that he realised how much he was like his father – when Esther reminded him of the story her grandfather had once told her. He described to her the wailing you could hear from no-man's-land, at night. At this point, he recalled, Papa would begin to shout. Because Papa was still angry at the disparity between this wailing and the official British telegrams, informing the anguished families that their heroes had died instantly, from a bullet in the heart.

—Sometimes, Haffner said to Zinka, one has conversations which are impossible with one's wife.

—But you're not married, said Zinka. Your wife, she is dead.

—It's the principle, he said.

And Haffner smiled.

—She's still alive in spirit, said Haffner.

And Zinka smiled too.

And in the sudden pause of their understanding, Haffner could still not prevent himself remembering the first time he had used this line about impossible conversations. It was one of his ordinary lines: in the Travelodge, at the business convention. Each time he used it, even now, even though he could remember all the times he had used it insincerely, he believed in it as true.

9

As if to celebrate this moment of Haffner's glory, the small jazz band serenading the hotel's residents began a melody from the oeuvre of Haffner's hero, Artie Shaw; and, cushioned by this melody, Frau Tummel descended on him, as if from the highest clouds.

Haffner looked to Zinka. Zinka looked away, staring at the indifferent mountains, as if finding in their indifference some kind of solace.

Frau Tummel was simply here, she said, to have the smallest word with Haffner. She beamed at Zinka. She did not want to interrupt.

He was all ears, said Haffner. She was sorry? said Frau Tummel. He was listening, said Haffner.

But this was not entirely true. The melody began to bother Haffner. He couldn't remember the title. Even as Frau Tummel stood in front of him. It suddenly seemed important. And maybe this wasn't just a ruse of Haffner's. For his only dates left were the songs. The songs in which dead people sang about their immortal love. As soon as he heard a song, then everything came back to him. With the songs, he could happily wallow in the wreckage of Haffner.

She just wanted to check that they still had their arrangement for the next day, said Frau Tummel. And Haffner nodded: a toy dog.

That was wonderful, exclaimed Frau Tummel. Because if he didn't want to, then he only needed to say.

It was a conversation Haffner was practised in. Of course he wanted to see her, he said, fluent and abstract with flattery.

In that case, said Frau Tummel, she would leave them be. Or perhaps, she added, she could take a glass of aquavit with them – glancing over at her husband making pencilled notes in his guidebook.

Zinka sighed. Haffner was silent. Encouraged, Frau Tummel motioned to the distant waiter. She pointed to Haffner's glass of aquavit. She mimed her desire for another. Then no, she reconsidered: she called the waiter over and ordered a glass of dry white wine.

—The aquavit, she explained to Haffner and Zinka, it is not for me.

She smiled, at Zinka, who did not smile back.

Frau Tummel, thought Haffner, was the absolute bourgeois. She embodied strength: the statuesque matronly repression. There was nothing, thought Haffner, which Frau Tummel could not sublimate. And perhaps this, if he were honest with himself, was also why Frau Tummel so appealed to him. He liked the effort of her strength. Her strength enchanted him. Yes, he realised, for Frau Tummel he felt a spreading tenderness, welling under Haffner's soul, like a bruise.

Frau Tummel was talking about her husband. She was playing the part of the wife. One never knew, she said, how much one was doing the right thing.

—Perhaps, said Frau Tummel, I am not the right woman for him.

—Come now, said Haffner. Of course you are!

And perhaps if he had thought more precisely or extensively he might have decided that this was not exactly the right tone; that seduced as he may have been by Frau Tummel's calm he should still have understood its fragility. He should still have expected that his pity was not what Frau Tummel wanted.

He really didn't need to talk to her like this, she said. It was hardly elegant. To this accusation, Haffner made some kind of noise. In this noise, he hoped to register a charming protestation. Frau Tummel regarded him. He was useless, she observed.

—No denying it! said Haffner, cheekily. He opened out his arms in a happy gesture of surrender.

And in her irritation at Haffner's refusal to offer her even the most minimal affection, Frau Tummel informed Haffner that she really should be returning to her husband, and so rose swiftly from her chair, thus colliding with the waiter who – as if he and Frau Tummel were a carefully rehearsed double act, a famous pair of clowns – tipped the wine gently over Zinka, as if in benediction.

Frau Tummel, in a flurry of mortification, tried to apologise to Zinka, who waved her irritably away, pressing her napkin to her top. Haffner looked out of the window, at the sunset, at the inexpertly murdered sky.

He scanned the horizon – like isolated Crusoe, with the craziest beard, wishing for a rescue which he never, now, expected.

10

Haffner was timeless. Perhaps this moment where Haffner scanned the horizon was one small proof. As he watched, he wondered to himself how far this scene was his fault. He searched the scene for hidden motives. And as he did so, all the previous allegations against Haffner fluently returned to him – trapped on his stage, in his follow spot, the ripples of a sequinned backdrop behind him, facing the disdain of his miniature audience: one couple waiting for another act, the manager himself, the confused splinter group of a stag party, one baffled drunk soldier on leave. In Haffner's lone state, Frau Tummel multiplied into the other women – like Barbra, or Esther – who had found Haffner so disappointing.

His efforts were rarely enough, thought Haffner – as he stood up with a superfluous napkin which he held out to Zinka, who did not see it, occupied as she was in preventing Frau Tummel from offering advice, while wiping off the sticky sheen of alcohol from her skin. It was so often the same, he thought – picking up his own glass, correcting himself, putting it gently down: like the confrontation with Livia, after the Allied liberation of Rome, who was wild with jealousy, having been sent a photo of the Colosseum.

It was not the usual tourist cliché.

In the centre of the photo was a jeep, on which an Allied soldier was sitting, at the wheel: a white carnation was a badge in his beret. A suntanned woman in a navy dress, with large sunglasses up on her blonde hair, was showing something to this Allied officer, which was making him contentedly smile. While beside them an assortment of elegantly coiffed, sunglassed Italians were clapping.

Haffner had always denied that this was Haffner.

The photo had been sent to Livia – whom Haffner had at that time not seen for two years, not since he had been mobilised straight after their marriage in 1942 – by a so-called friend of hers who had seen it in the newspapers. She was jealous, said Haffner. She was mad with jealousy. It was a spiteful thing to do.

It was true that there was some ambiguity. The man in the photograph was looking down, in profile: so there was room for doubt. And this doubt also left room for Haffner to escape the accusations. When, fifty years later, Benjamin discovered this photograph too, going through a pile of Haffner's things, Haffner repeated his excuses again. Why then, thought Benji, had Haffner kept this photograph for fifty years, if it wasn't of him? Why would you preserve the triumph of another man?

But I thought I knew. I tried to tell Benji; but Benji was unconvinced. For I was the only one who believed in Haffner's innocence.

This photograph marked Haffner's jazz. His ultimate in pure freedom. It represented every moment in which Haffner had escaped, momentarily, from the observing world.

Like the riffs he had heard played on Artie Shaw's masterpiece 'Nightmare', in the rundown clubs of the Via Margutta. At some point, after all, you lost your moral compass. This was true. But it was difficult to know where. The borders of the bourgeoisie and bohemia were so hard to identify – like the manic jazz tune of Artie Shaw's which was now returning to Haffner, as he sat there in the dining room, flanked by two gilt mirrors so that an infinite regress of Haffners looked with joyful affection at Zinka: her wet hair slicked to one side, like all the androgynous fashions of Haffner's century: the flappers and the *nouvelle vague*, the *movida* after Franco, the perverse and civilised *dolce vita* of the Fascists and the Communists in Rome.

11

Zinka stood up, and said that he could follow her. And Haffner, who wanted no fuss in his public life, who wanted no attention to be drawn to him, followed mutely after Zinka, nodding adieu to Frau Tummel.

The air above Zinka smelled of florals and herbs: the intoxicating warm forest contained in the wine she had been doused in. Safely alone, in the hotel foyer, she contemplated her ruined hair, the map of stains forming on her dress. And Zinka said to Haffner that perhaps he could escort her to his room, so that she could wash.

Oh Zinka! Haffner would have bathed her himself. He would have prepared baths of asses' milk, vials of perfumes. He was an old man still piqued by lust, by love. Of this, Haffner had no illusions.

He had so often believed in the counterlife, the myth of Haffner's excess. A Haffner untrammelled by his marriage, his Atlantic existence. Haffner unencumbered! Like the most distant tropical sunset, reached by regal Concorde, supersonic – its front wheel propped under its chin, like the solid goatee of a monumental pharaoh. But his escapes were always so fleeting. A night with a girl, a night at the opera: these were Haffner's *Cinco de Mayo*; his risorgimento: the Parisian *événements* of Haffner's savage uprising.

These were the new life which Haffner dreamed of – but it always needed, he felt, someone to take him there. And no one, in the end, had really wanted to go.

So maybe, Haffner thought, he understood. The problem had been that he always wanted an elopee. Which meant that the problem, really, was Haffner. He could conjure with time as much as he liked, but the anecdotes only proved one thing. They were a strip cartoon which always involved the same dogged character: a Haffneriad. For the metamorphoses which lust invented in Haffner were never permanent. The glimpses of other Haffners – Haffner the New Yorker, Haffner the Roman, Haffner the free – did not transform him: just like Silberman, in Palestine, in 1944. Haffner had been told to do something with a couple of the other Jewish soldiers in his platoon. Surely something could be done to tone them down? Which Haffner contested. For nothing could be done with Silberman – disguised as a non-Jew with his clever costume of yarmulke, tefillin, and the extraordinary rapidity with which he entered arguments in Hebrew at roadside cafés frequented only by Russian Zionists and the occasional Zionist mule. Now, fifty years too late, Haffner had some sympathy for Silberman: disguised only in the guise of himself.

Haffner Roman

1

After Haffner had located the key – with its tasselled mane – Zinka immediately made for Haffner's bathroom. She went in, slammed the door. From within the bathroom, then came the sound of running water.

Haffner sat on the edge of the bed; took off his shoes; discovered the *Lives of the Caesars*, in paperback, underneath the scalloped valance; placed the book on the bedside table, beside his edition of Gibbon; and he sighed.

Three eras, he decided, marked any possible grandeur he might have ever had, the eras when he was most true to himself: there was the war; then the glorious 1970s; and maybe, he considered, now. At this coda to his life – as if his life had been extended, in a moment of grace, just slightly too long.

Zinka had a mole on her left cheek, tusked with twin hairs. It was the same mole, with the same tusks of hair, as the one which had belonged to a girl whom Haffner had met when the war in North Africa was over. This was 1942, or thereabouts. The regiment had gone to Bone, a lovely little place. And there it was, somehow, that he had met a lovely Jewish family who gave two or three of them a dinner. Haffner often wondered what happened to those nice people in North Africa, after the war was over. He always remembered the girl, with the darkest skin Haffner had ever seen, playing 'Invitation to the Waltz' on the piano. The next day the family arranged for them to be called up to read a portion of the Torah at the synagogue.

An echo in the bathroom, Zinka asked him if he wanted to come in.

He didn't think that this was his right – this openness which women so often displayed towards him. He never felt so confident as that. It was why the women loved him: his inherent modesty. He knew that this was happening by a grace which was beyond him.

Joyful, as he stepped into the bathroom, on stockinged feet, he paused at his window – where the sky was now one single shade of red, like a colour sample.

2

And Haffner was transported.

For just as the sky was now a painting of paint, to Haffner's distracted eyes, so he remembered how, in 1973, he had seen an exhibition of pure colour: at MoMA in New York. The exhibition was of paintings which were simply called *Colors*. The trip, on this Sunday afternoon, was Livia's idea. Haffner, always eager to discover new maps of his cultural ignorance, happily agreed.

Thin slabs of colour were laid next to each other: like in a paint catalogue. There seemed no genius, thought Haffner, no sublime. It was the absence of hyperbole – but precisely at this point Haffner found himself warming to this painting. Yes, this – so Haffner once told me – was the only art which he had ever liked. Livia had expected him to act with his normal grumpy chutzpah in the face of the masterpieces of modernism. But Haffner was transfixed. He was transfigured.

Long after Livia had left him for the cafeteria, where she sat with a filter coffee and three shrugs of sugar, Haffner still stood there, gazing into colour.

Such freedom! Although Haffner also enjoyed trying to trace the patterns in the grid – trying to work out if the repetitions of the yellow or the red could be predicted. He wasn't sure they could. So he let his eyes go endless.

Livia had disliked this abstract art: this most abstract of abstract art. It seemed emotionless, she thought. It was cold. This was what she told Haffner in the leather nook of a banquette at the Plaza, in the Oak Room. It had nothing to do with the real world. And Haffner had discovered a tirade within himself: that what the fuck did she care about the real world; that as far as Haffner was concerned there was no such thing as the real world; that this painting – to which, he reminded her, she herself had taken him, it wasn't Haffner's idea – this painting was as real as anything else; that in fact it seemed to Haffner an accurate portrayal of the real world in its clarity, its order; that quite frankly he saw little difference between the world which Livia called real and the world of colour in the grid on a wall at MoMA.

In the colours, Haffner found something he loved. He didn't understand it. But he knew that he admired it. This world beyond the world: where everything was pure.

3

There in her bath, Zinka was a vision of bubbles. Haffner knew the word for this. It was a fantasia. The vision of Walt Disney, the master of cartoons.

From the costume of her bubbles, Zinka said that first he must blindfold himself. Haffner queried this. Yes, she said. If he wanted to stay. He could take that stocking from over there. Haffner looked: a sliver of black pantyhose was slumped under her dress. He looked back at her. She nodded. That was the condition, she said.

These were the trials, thought Haffner. He was happy with the trials. Yes, for pleasure, Haffner could undergo anything.

With clumsy hands, Haffner tied the stocking limply over his eyes: a robber baron. But Haffner didn't care. He could still see: cloudy, in black and white. The peep shows of his maturity.

Haffner transformed by lust! Haffner crowned with the head of an ass!

If Haffner wanted, she said, he could now come and help to wash her. Would he like that? If he wanted, he could take that sponge and wash her back. Just so long as he was careful.

The fragrances from the water overtook Haffner. He stood over her. He wished he could have seen more. There her outline was, like the coyest vision of Hollywood, submerged by infinite foam. Her hair was done up in a hazy bun. One hand was leaning over the rim of the bath. She was looking up at him.

She told him to tighten the stocking. Haffner obeyed.

Then he took off his jacket, pushed the cuffs of his sweatshirt up – a bad imitation of his father, whose billowing sleeves were always secured with two silver bands, like the neat cuffs for napkins. He took a sponge, and dunked it: then expressed the water in warm rivulets over the curve of her back, with its peeling patches of foam.

An incubus, Haffner hunkered over Zinka. Perhaps this was another image which Haffner thought he should have minded. Haffner, however, never minded the embarrassments in his pursuit of pleasure. The embarrassments were just the acknowledged debt one owed.

Just below the disintegrating level of foam, he could see – through the thin blindfold – the momentary beginning of Zinka's breasts. He could see the side of her left breast, but the slope was something else. Pretending not to look, he tried to notice as much as he could: to preserve it for the playground of his memory, while Zinka told him that he was being very kind. He was quite the gentleman.

Haffner wondered how long he could maintain a courtly conversation with a woman while blindfolded with her stocking. Its scent was odd: a mixture of must and shoe leather and the faintest last echo of her perfume.

Yes really, she said. He was a civilised man, and she liked that.

She flattered him. As Haffner had been flattered all his life, by the women. The women loved to flatter him: they loved to exercise his ego. He was cosseted. Not every woman, obviously. Not, most importantly, Livia. But the women Haffner went for in his secret life, his private life, were images of his mother. They told him how wonderful he was. They wrapped presents for him, surprises. On his sixtieth birthday, a woman for whom Haffner had only the most vestigial of passions privately presented him with a giant trunk of presents: sixty, each wrapped inside the other. A present of presents for the birthday boy. But maybe Livia had praised him like this, at the beginning. Maybe she simply got tired of his demands for flattery: or simply realised the untruth of all her praise – the practised way in which he enticed her with his vulnerability.

But there was another explanation. Her love was quieter because it was more true. Unlike everyone else, she trusted in Haffner's love. She would never, she once whispered to him, be loved by anyone else in the way that Haffner loved her. So how could she refuse him?

Zinka looked at Haffner's hand on her shoulder, drowning it in droplets. It was a girlish hand, she said. And Haffner wondered if at this late stage in his life he should waste himself in exercising his vanity on this kind of phrase. He decided that he had no choice. How could he invert the habits of a lifetime? He was not up to it.

So Haffner felt silently annoyed, silently exercised on behalf of his masculine hands.

Zinka asked if he were satisfied. He repeated the word to her: a question. Was he happy? she asked. But of course, replied Haffner, with a delirious grin. Then he paused. But maybe. Maybe what?

she asked him. No, it was nothing, said Haffner. But he had to tell her, said Zinka. Well then, maybe, Haffner wondered, he might be allowed to kiss her.

4

Now that, said Zinka, would be a very improper request. And Haffner, downcast, agreed. But, he added, contemplating how far down the path of humiliation Haffner might be prepared to walk, it would make him very happy.

He discovered that the path of humiliation had unexpectedly scenic views.

For although Zinka eventually said, from the depths of her silence, that yes, he could kiss her, it was not the kiss which Haffner was expecting.

She raised her left knee so that it rose from the water, crested with scintillating foam.

—You may kiss me on the knee, said Zinka.

Haffner considered Zinka's knee. At its tip, there was a small scar, translucent. A blurred and miniature map of France.

His own knees hurt him, cramped there on the bathroom tiles. He tried to ignore this. He bent his head to Zinka, hoping to see beyond the clouding bubbles: to the dark crevices of Zinka. He could not.

And Haffner kissed her.

His mouth filled with a froth of foam. It gilded his upper lip with a stray moustache. It embittered his mouth with chemicals.

How pleasurable was this? Haffner asked himself. Was it enough? For her part, Zinka thought it was. But Haffner wanted to lick her until her true smell returned: the delicious bare smell of her skin. Not the sterility of artificial foam. He asked if he could kiss her again. She said no. She was going to wash now. It was time for him to go back into the bedroom.

128

Haffner tried to stand up. He could not. Like some immovable sphinx, with buried paws. He could only turn his head away. He tried to explain this to Zinka, with the utmost maintenance of his dignity. In that case, said Zinka, she would just get out and dry herself. He must not look, she said. He promised this? Haffner promised. He turned his head.

There was a surge of water beside him. He tried to wrench the stocking away. Too late, he gazed at Zinka, with her back to him, wrapping herself in the softness of Haffner's towels: a Roman matron, in her flowing toga.

5

Sourly, he tasted the foam in his mouth. There was no doubt, thought Haffner, that his dignity was in danger. And yet, he was discovering, he seemed curiously avid for this degradation. It seemed, this ruin of Haffner, to be a kind of triumph too.

This wasn't a new motif in the life of Raphael Haffner.

In Rome, after the liberation, while Haffner waited for an infinitely postponed decision on his regiment's movements, he used to go up to the Pincio Gardens, and smoke his traded cigarettes, dropping the butts in the sand. Even up there, the smell from the sewage was heavy. The cigarettes, among other things, were Haffner's improvised pomander.

The light up there was pulverised; it was dust. The Tiber below Haffner was sluggish mud. A breeze made the leaves on the poplars silver themselves. Their pollen floated whitely on to the ground.

And Haffner looked down on the ruined, eternal city. It was the ruins, considered Haffner, which were precisely what was eternal.

Yes, this seemed to be Haffner's pattern.

Up from Anzio, before they reached Rome, they had ended up sleeping in the grounds of Ninfa. At that time, Haffner had not been horticultural. He had not admired the romantic unkempt wilderness. Kept awake by mosquitoes, Haffner instead found himself oppressed by the death of kings.

The gardens of Ninfa were built on the ruins of Ninfa – a town which had been sacked by its neighbours in the thirteenth century. The basilica had once held the coronation of a pope: now it was a dismantled heap of stones. Then, in the twentieth century, the town had been made into a true romantic garden: a meditation on the ruins of time. But Haffner had been troubled. There was no romance for him in ruins. They made him sad. Although this sympathy could so easily have been a more inward form of sympathy: Haffner's empathy for himself. In these cities' destruction, he only saw the futility of Haffner. The hollowness of Haffner.

—I will be remembered, he once told me, for my after-dinner speeches.

And then he paused.

—But that's worth nothing, he said.

And then Haffner smiled, glorious in the knowledge of his defeat.

6

Awkwardly, Haffner unfolded himself upright, via the rim of the bath, then the rim of the basin. He looked around – at the emptying swirl of the water, the deliquescent towels on the soaked mat. His masculine cologne was sitting on the shelf, its bottle embossed with a white tear of toothpaste foam. The toothpaste itself lay there, its tail twisted like a comma – like a fortune-telling miracle fish: its red plastic curled into the sign for passion, for jealousy, for sadness. The scenes of pleasure usually ended up this wasted, like the hotel in Venice where Haffner and the girl who had chosen him from his perch at the bar proceeded to order a feast of room service, one bottle and dish at a time, delighted by the maid's growing confusion between curiosity and distaste.

You should be happy for the things you get, Mama had said. No man should think he could have more than the Lord intended. So Haffner was humble. For at least the worship of women was a brave and noble aim.

Methodically, he laid out the full range of his medicines, in preparation for the night ahead. They included pills to combat the intensity of his blood pressure, pills to lower the ratio of bad cholesterol to good, antidepressants. Then the more soothing medicines: the ones to relieve Haffner's body of pain; the ones to make him sleep.

He picked up the wet towels, scented with Zinka's body. Then she appeared in the doorway.

Did he want to walk her home? asked a clothed and beautiful version of Zinka. To which a reduced version of Haffner wailed in response that the idea that he should ever be parted from her oppressed him with an absolute melancholy. If this miniature Haffner were to be allowed to rule reality, they would never be parted.

So Haffner said yes; and went out with his chaperone into the midsummer night.

Haffner Buoyant

1

To kiss a girl's knee, while on one's own knees, might have seemed, to the outside observer, a little pitiable, thought Haffner. To the outside observer, it might well have seemed to indicate some incipient breakdown. But Haffner tended to disagree. He admired the effects. The sound and light. The softly spattered fireworks above the ruined chateau: the fading and luminous palm fronds, thistles, water lilies in the sky.

For Haffner was in love.

They had left the lake behind; and the park, with its watchful factories. In what looked, to Haffner's bourgeois eye, like a shanty town, a tzigane was carrying a blue gas canister and a gold can of beer, following the dug-out route of a possible but phantom pipeline. Then they found themselves in another, less private park. It was a shortcut, said Zinka. At the centre of this park was a boating lake, embossed with a fountain, a fraying plume of foam. The rowing boats by the side of the lake crossed their arms neatly; the pedalos were chained together, clopping. Yes, there they were, at midnight: with the monuments to the source of the river; the monument to the unknown soldier. All the angels in stone, their wings in imitation of the earthly wings of pigeons.

Haffner's knees, aching from their bathtime antics, made walking difficult for Haffner. As they passed a sinuous bench, he asked if they could sit down, just for a moment.

—Not yet, she said. Not yet.

He was so old. And Zinka was so young. These facts were undeniable. But Haffner did not care. He looked at her, she smiled and Haffner did not care if this girl were using him; if she looked on him as an old fool. He was an old fool. There was no shame in that.

—How old am I? asked Zinka.

—Thirty? hazarded Haffner, baffled utterly.

—So old? said Zinka, disappointed.

—I was wrong? asked Haffner.

—A little, said Zinka.

And she, beckoning to tired Haffner, began to climb some small and artificial hill. Wincing, Haffner followed her. They sat for a while, to ease Haffner's legs, in the bandstand. But no band could stand this bandstand – thought Haffner. Dejectedly he regarded the signs of a struggle, a flight in haste: two condoms; a cigarette packet and its scattered assortment of butts, some blushing with lipstick, some not; a bottle of beer, without any beer. He looked out over the landscape.

From this point, perched on an artificial mound, Haffner saw the fields outside the city: the yellow rape fields, now blue in the dark, against which were dabbed the cypresses' black Japanese brushmarks.

From here, Zinka told him, she was fine. She was just in that apartment block – the one he could see, on the other side of the park. Haffner slowly nodded. She kissed him goodbye on his cheek.

Around him clouded his life: its particles – as usual – suspended, motionless. He hardly knew where he was: or to whom he belonged.

2

But no, just right now, I'm not quite in the mood for Haffner, and his confusions. Instead, I am into the different confusions of Zinka.

For Haffner suspected that to Zinka it was simply a matter of the usual story: an old man being used by a young girl. But this, I think, was not fair to the complicated romance of Zinka.

He was, thought Zinka, the first man she had ever met who enjoyed it when she teased him. He did not mind when one praised him for the smallness of his hands. He did not mind when you asked him to follow you, when you refused him the kisses you knew he wanted from you.

To Zinka, Haffner represented freedom. He had a politesse which she admired. This would have seemed unlikely to the women who had known the previous incarnations of Haffner: the forgetter of birthdays and anniversaries, the man incapable of returning a phone call. But maybe Zinka was not so wrong.

In front of her apartment block there was a water feature which she had never seen working: in its trough lay a ready-made of garbage. So she looked up instead, at the giant advert covering her balcony: the manic woman, the manic birds.

He didn't need his pride. This, she thought, was why she liked him. At last, she had discovered a relationship which could be improvised by Zinka.

And as Zinka went into the kitchen, to find some food – emerging with a packet of crisps – above her hovered the moon, the clouds in a cirrus formation which watched over the buildings with their scaffolding, their satellite dishes and air-conditioning units, the adverts (*Heineken: Meet You There*), the raised blinds and the shut blinds: all the domestic paraphernalia.

She turned back the two folding doors to the television. She switched on some form of American TV. A baseball star was showing the camera crew round his house. They were approaching the bedroom.

He was going to say, thought Zinka, that this was where the magic happened.

She reached in the packet for some crisps; her fingers emerged empty, but dandruff'd with salt.

—This is where the magic happens, said the baseball star.

And Zinka marvelled, silently, looking out at the suburbs by night, through the advert's gauze: wishing she could have told someone. First, she thought of Niko. But she wasn't sure Niko would understand any humour, let alone hers. And then she thought of Haffner.

And there she paused.

On the packet of her paprika crisps, a slice of potato with arms and legs beckoned to her with delirious eyes.

3

Alone in the midsummer night, Haffner had wandered off towards the hotel – on a road marked only by stray houses, then a Service Auto, beside a shop which seemed to sell the million varieties of cigarette, displayed behind glass cases, like extinct species of insect. Then a pizza place. And then a strip joint.

The twenty-four-hour bar (*Service Non-stop!*) into which Haffner descended, down a steep flight of stairs, was apparently in its busiest period. A group of possibly Polish truckers and a couple of policemen off duty made up the front row. Behind them, amphitheatrically, were ranged an assortment of men.

Haffner, however, wasn't here for the men.

He watched the women extend their legs around a stainless steel pole. He observed the way their breasts fell forward, elongated pyramids, as they leaned over – touching their toes in some strange imitation of an eighties aerobics routine, without the pink leg warmers, the turquoise sweatbands.

Then, in the crowd, Haffner recognised Niko: Zinka's boyfriend. He felt a descending qualm, a chime inside his chest. Niko gestured to him, warmly. He wanted him, it seemed, to join Niko's group. Haffner wondered about this.

He decided he had no choice.

—You all speak English? said Haffner to Niko.

—Of course we speak English. Fuck you, said Niko.

—That's a good accent you've got, said Haffner.

—*Merci*, said Niko.

It was the world of men.

—This man, said Niko, he look after my mad girl tonight. She bored you?

—No no, said Haffner, brightly.

—Yes, she bored you, said Niko. It's OK. We all understand.

And everyone, including wistful Haffner, laughed.

—You want to play a trust game? said Niko. It is what we are doing. You can zip the person next to you – zip zip. Only zap the person across from you.

—No, said Haffner.

—Zap, said Niko.

—You mean zip, said Haffner.

—Yes, said Niko.

—Can we stop this? asked Haffner.

On stage, a girl was now entirely naked, apart from a pair of translucent platform heels, on which she was balancing with a grace and ease which charmed old Haffner's heart. But not Niko's. She lacked flair, he argued. If, however, Haffner wanted her . . . He indicated that he had not finished his sentence. Haffner, however, was beyond the innuendos now. The masculine, and its zest for the tight-lipped, no longer charmed him.

He sadly nodded no.

—This is what you are here for? asked Niko.

Wearily, Haffner explained that, in fact, it was not why he was here. Or not officially. Nor primarily. Haffner was in this town to secure his heritage, his inheritance. He was here to do honour to his wife.

Angrily, he began a tirade against the state. He could not understand it. The bureaucracy bewildered him. It demeaned the human spirit. Why did no one seem to care? What, he asked Niko, did you have to do in this country to get anything done? He only wanted what was his due. He was hardly demanding the moon.

—You know, said Niko, I like you.

—I like you too, said Haffner.

—Yes, I like you, said Niko, then wandered off, leaving Haffner with Niko's friends, who did not seem to share his pure love of Haffner.

4

Ignored, listening to Niko's friends talk freely about him in a language he could not understand, Haffner sat and watched the women. If these men wanted to mock him, then so be it. He could do abasement. The silent pattern of his life had been delicately training him, thought Haffner, for these moments of humiliation. Like the time when he came home to discover that his father had sold all his bar mitzvah presents, arguing that they only took up space in the house, declining to discuss the possibility that he was going to use the money for some selfish gain. Yes, Raphael Haffner was used to the destruction of his hopes.

Then Niko came back.

—You want this place? said Niko. Maybe we can do this for you. But it costs.

—I'm sorry? said Haffner.

—You want this place? said Niko.

—I don't understand, said Haffner.

He understood, of course, that Niko had a proposal. It wasn't the deal which was beyond him. It was the fact that Niko seemed to think he could effect such a deal: this was beyond the limits of Haffner's scepticism.

—Simple, said Niko.

He began to explain. It all depended on knowing the right people; and Niko knew the right man. It was not so difficult. It all depended on the right things getting into the right hands.

—You are not from here, said Niko.

This was just the way things were. Everyone knew how this worked. Either you could go through the ordinary ways of doing things, or you could enter the speed road. It was just a question of speed. Then the papers could get handed over, and the villa would belong to Haffner. The wheels would be oiled.

—No questions ask, said Niko.

There was a pause. In this pause, Haffner considered the perfect bodies of imperfect women.

—I am your patron, said Niko.

—Cash? asked Haffner, suspicious.

—Cash, said Niko. You crazy or what?

Niko didn't really understand, he said, why Haffner needed any more detail at all. He only needed to know this. If he was so impatient.

—I'm not impatient, said Haffner.

If he were so impatient, said Niko, then things could be worked out. He had seen this problem before. He knew how to fix it.

Haffner had to understand, said Niko, that it was still the same people in charge. Yes, Niko knew what had happened. Haffner's papers would be sitting there, ignored, in someone's office. Just waiting for a reason to be dealt with.

—Let me think about it, said Haffner.

And as he tried to balance his doubts as to Niko's efficacy – his general untrustworthiness, the danger of relying too much on a man whom he had spied on only the night before, and whose girl-friend had so recently been soaping herself in Haffner's bath – against the obvious benefit of having, as he used to say, a man on the ground, Haffner excused himself: desperate to find a toilet, a cubicle where Haffner could think.

But reality continued to pursue him. He took a few steps, into a corridor which bore graffiti, torn posters, an exhibition of faulty plumbing. Then all the lights went out.

And Haffner was in the dark.

5

Practical, Haffner told himself that he mustn't get this wrong: he didn't want to lose his way. To his surprise, in a basement, in a bar, in a wasteland, he found himself wishing he had the practical wisdom of Frau Tummel. He stopped. He considered this thought.

To whom was Haffner loyal? It seemed unsolvable. There seemed so many ways for Haffner to demonstrate his disloyalty. Livia, the obvious candidate, was so fluently replaced by all her avatars, her rivals.

In the dark, Haffner edged his way along the wall – his hand extended, palm flat: directing invisible traffic. Distant whoops of masculine joy reached him from the main area, whoops which were tinged, now, for Haffner, with a poignancy. It seemed unlikely he would ever see humans again. Then suddenly the wall gave way, as it transformed itself into a door. Haffner peered into the black. Soothing plashings from what he thought could be urinals echoed throughout the room. Was this a bathroom? wondered Haffner. He could not be sure. It might have been, for instance, the hideout of the janitor.

Then he discovered one tiled wall. It decided Haffner on the question of a bathroom. Where else did one find ceramic? He ignored, for instance, the possibilities of storerooms, the opportunities of kitchens. Facing this wall, Haffner stood, unbuttoned his fly, and began the lengthy process of unburdening himself – telling himself that, after all, it wasn't as if Haffner disliked the dark. Bourgeois he may have been, but Haffner wasn't spoiled. He started working at Warburg's in the winter of 1946: the nightmarish winter, when the electrics failed and everyone in the City worked by candlelight. The clerks sat with their feet encased in typewriter covers stuffed with newspaper – gigantic and ineffectual slippers, improvised snowshoes. That spring, the streets were still a mess of rubble sprouting woodland plants – ragwort, groundsel. The dark had nothing on Haffner.

When he emerged, the lights were still not on. Now, however, a selection of torches had been discovered, and lighters, and solitary candles. A man was savagely strumming an acoustic guitar.

—Like a refugee camp? Niko breathed into Haffner's startled ear.

Haffner stared at him.

—So wonderful, no? said Niko.

Haffner looked around. In chiaroscuro, a girl was holding a flashlight above her head, like a handheld shower. In the sway of its light, she was dancing. As the light swayed, her breasts swayed with it. Another girl was on all fours, while a man mimicked the act of whipping her: his whip ascending in flourishes, an undulant lasso. The shadows made momentary blindfolds on the man's face; or the girls acquired sudden grimaces, as if from the painted masks of Venice, which Haffner had looked at, in wonder, in 1952, at the carnival with Livia – while she began to cry beside him, describing the carnivals she had seen before the war. Which seemed so long ago, she said. And already, at this point, Haffner had considered if he could ever leave Livia – because this was how he tested all his affections, by imagining him leaving them behind – and had realised that, for him, it was unimaginable. She was the only person he would never leave.

—Vodka? asked Niko.

—Perhaps not, said Haffner.

—Maybe you prefer tea? asked Niko. It is more British?

—A double vodka, said Haffner.

Returning with a plastic cup awash with vodka, Niko asked Haffner if he knew that they had all survived radiation. Or survived as much as they could. Oh yes, many years ago, when they were children, a factory had blown up a hundred kilometres south of here, but the distance was nothing, said Niko. The radiation was everywhere, all over the countryside.

—The motherfuckers, they killed us. Fucked us, said Niko.

His sister, he told Haffner, was born with only four fingers on her left hand. He moved closer to Haffner. He understood this? Only four fingers. On her left hand.

Unwillingly, Haffner inhaled the alcohol of Niko's breath. He drank a gulp of vodka, for equilibrium.

Haffner, said Haffner, understood.

It wasn't as if Haffner hadn't seen the horrors: he had seen the rule book torture – the forced standing for twenty-four hours, so that the prisoner's ankles swelled up, blisters developed on the soles of the feet, the kidneys shut down. In one village in Italy, the soldiers had just gone mad. They dressed up in women's clothes. They hung clothes in the trees. They went through the houses. Soon, there was nothing left to eat. Once, on the edge of the desert, they came across a food truck, carrying fruit. The people inside were crushed. Haffner and his unit stopped. They wiped the fuel and blood off, and started to eat the peaches, the heavy grapes. They hadn't eaten for a day. There was a girl there who had a dress but no legs. This was one of the women to whom Haffner felt closest. At a checkpoint in Syria, a kid was in an abandoned truck, cowering. He went to help her. He picked her up. Her head slumped off the neck on to his arm, heavy, like a pumpkin.

It wasn't then that Haffner threw up. It was ten minutes later, after he had buried her. After he had buried her just there, by the side of the road – because what fool would wander off to find a place to bury the dead? Just as what fool went off to seek his necessary privacy if he wanted to shit? The sniper fire on the way out; the friendly fire on the way back. Instead, you squatted there, in front of everyone, discussing the imaginary world of sports.

And Haffner discovered in this moment with Niko its secret twin, which already existed in the story of Haffner.

In another blackout, the universal blackout of 1977 – the summer Haffner came back to New York after being away for three years – he had argued with Goldfaden about sport. They were in Chinatown. Goldfaden had just outlined his theory that genetically the Jewish race was programmed to adore Chinese food. And Haffner felt no urge to disagree. He was happy. Before him, sat a plate of crispy shredded beef: a pile of orange twigs – which was Haffner's most reliable delight.

Then the lights went out. And Haffner found the conversation turning to sports.

It was escapism, said Goldfaden. There was nothing wrong with this, he wanted to add. He believed that everyone, at some time, needed a way of escaping. For Goldfaden, it was love. For Haffner, it was sports. Where, then, was the argument?

The argument, thought Haffner, was precisely in this idea that anything could be imaginary. Nothing was imaginary. This was Haffner's idea. So often accused of being divorced from real life, Haffner always maintained that – on the contrary – he would love to be divorced from real life, but the divorce was impossible. There was no counterlife.

As waiters began to scurry round for candles, Haffner talked.

The accusation of escapism was not a new one. Normally, however, this was seen as a bad thing. Esther used to accuse him of a lack of seriousness. Sport wasn't, said Esther, real life. She asked her new husband to agree with her. And Esmond did. But Haffner now maintained, in front of Goldfaden, in the dark, that there was no difference between a sport and real life: how, he wondered, could there be? In what way was real life suspended by the act of kicking a football, that would not mean that the act of sipping a coffee also represented a suspension of real life? The theory was ridiculous. What escapism was it to be battered by emotion, scarred by defeat, elated in victory? In Haffner's opinion, this proved a further and deeper truth: there was no such thing as escapism. No, never. How could you escape? Where did Goldfaden think he could go?

Well, said Goldfaden: he supposed he was much more of a romantic than Haffner.

Did he really want to talk about football? said Haffner, ignoring this comparison. Because he could. The Norwegians, for instance, who refused to play Nazi football. So the quislings watched each other in desolate stadiums. How was that not real life? So OK, said Goldfaden. But Haffner wasn't finished. Let us not, said Haffner, forget the Viennese genius Matthias Sindelar, known as The Wafer, who was said to have brains in his legs, and many unexpected ideas occurred to them while they were running. For instance, said Haffner, there was the last ever match between Austria and Germany, a month after the Nazis had annexed Austria in 1938. Everyone knew that Sindelar had been told not to score. For the whole first half, therefore, he pushed the ball a little wide of each post, sarcastically. And then, in the second half, he couldn't stop himself: so Sindelar scored. And then another man scored a free kick, thus sealing the game, and Sindelar, because he had ideas in his legs, went to celebrate by dancing in front of the Nazi direc tors' box.

That, said Haffner, was sport. It could never be an escape from life. Life was everywhere.

No, there was no such thing as a counterlife, Haffner wanted to argue. Just as there was no such thing as a real metamorphosis. In the end, you only had yourself to work with. Wherever you went, it was still you.

While around them, the city of New York was looted. Though whether this proved or disproved Haffner, in his imaginary nostalgic lecture hall, he didn't know.

He carried on looking at the girls. In Italy they had called them *segnorini* – the girls who went with the Allied soldiers: they mispronounced them, *a l'inglese*.

When she bent down, you could see the neat fur between her legs.

Behind him, the light of a candle flickered. A girl was standing beside him. She was tall, she had straight black hair, she was what the world would consider the pornographic ideal. Whatever her breasts were made of, Haffner liked it. She told Haffner her name. He could not hear it. She told him again. She thanked him for buying her a drink. He raised an eyebrow. Behind her, Niko raised a glass, gaily.

—You have a drink? she asked Haffner.

Haffner had a drink.

—So, she said, you are good to go.

He couldn't deny it. Like one of Benji's wind-up toys, which could unleash its skittering movements wherever it was placed: on the neat chevrons of blond parquet in a country-house museum or the linoleum of a kitchen floor – with damp stains, starry splashes of coffee, and one irrevocably non-matching square of concrete, where the lino had given out.

The girl who now thought of herself as Haffner's – or who thought of Haffner as her own – led him into what seemed a cave, or tunnel. It ventured into the underground. She told Haffner to sit – on a crate, or possibly an upturned bucket. It was difficult to tell. Haffner only knew that it had some kind of rim. It hurt him.

Haffner had never been into the pornography, nor the pubs to which his City friends used to go: where angry women undressed and despised their spectators. All his pleasure was more traditional. He disliked the obscenity of modern film, the sexual glee of modern literature. There were things which shouldn't be written down, said Haffner. There were certain forms to be observed. Pleasure was all about privacy, he thought: the burden of the boudoir.

And even if I disagreed, I still agreed with Haffner's motive – it wasn't from primness that he thought this, but from a wish to preserve the erotic as a secret which one kept from other people. This didn't seem unreasonable.

But now, in this unstaged intimacy, Haffner could still not discover in himself any obvious erotic surge. He should have done, he knew this. And perhaps, even recently, he would have done – but no longer. Now, Haffner was more in love with love.

This love was partly visible in the way his thoughts were tending to Zinka, in her bubble bath. But it was also visible in the way Haffner kept thinking of Livia. He sat on an upturned crate or bucket and told himself that he should simply do this so that Niko would still admire him. Because Niko was his ally. Niko was the friend who would restore Haffner to his heritage.

8

In his blackout basement, Haffner conversed urbanely with his girl. Her name, she told him, was Katya. A nice name, Haffner assured her. It was not her real name, she replied. Who needed real names? Not in here. Tonight, she said, she wanted sex, and she wanted vodka. And she had the vodka already, she said – raising the smudged plastic glass to Haffner's worried gaze. So only one thing was missing.

As usual, the god Priapus harried Haffner: with his cloven hooves, his staff entangled in ivy. His entire being a pulsing penis.

An arm was twined around Haffner's neck. He felt his lips being kissed. Then he realised that the small bikini top which Katya had been wearing was now slipping, weightless, on to his arm, then on to the floor – where it rested, invisible, unknown to Haffner, on his foot. She lifted a candle to her torso: her breasts were there, in the magical light. Katya told him that he could touch. If he were gentle.

He belonged to an older world. The older he got, the more he believed in it. Here, in the centre of Europe, in a town which was so nearly modern, and yet had been already so melancholically superseded by other fashions, Haffner believed in romance: the candle-lit dinner, the car ride home, the kiss on the cheek. This routine to be repeated, with variations.

He tried to explain to Katya that he really did not want to touch her. If she didn't mind. He wondered if perhaps they should rejoin the others.

But he was in such a rush, said Katya, sadly. Did she not please him?

He tried to look for Niko, and could see nobody. He was alone with her, in this back room. Of course, he replied, she pleased him.

Visually, it was inarguable.

Then he felt her press her breasts against him. Softly they gave against the protrusion of Haffner's nose. The rough nipples rubbed against the harsher roughness of Haffner's cheeks.

But no, it wasn't Haffner's thing. He tried to explain this to her. Really, she had been very kind, but he ought to be going. And to his unsurprised dismay, Katya seemed to feel wronged by his explanations. Angrily, she upbraided him. Never, she said, had she met such a man.

Helpless Haffner bent his head.

Did he think she really wanted him? she asked Haffner. Dumbly, Haffner shook his head. Did he think that this was her idea of love?

—You're nodding when you're not supposed to be nodding, she said.

—Ah yes, said Haffner.

—You're still doing it, she said.

They were everywhere, thought Haffner: the experts in what was real; the people who wanted to begin, or complete, his education.

Look at him! said Katya. The man was dressed in a cagoule. She could not understand how stupid he was.

And Haffner wanted to assure her that he was capable of stupidity so gigantic that she would hardly comprehend it.

Maybe, thought Haffner, he was going off sex. Once, a Texan friend of his had told him a Dallas proverb. Every time you find yourself not thinking about sex, so ran the proverb, then your mind is wandering. And this had been Haffner's philosophy, in so far as the man could have a philosophy.

My squalid Don Quixote: avid for the higher things. The higher things which Haffner looked for in the lower things: in the lust, and the vanity, and the shame.

The point was, said Katya, that she at least needed to be paid.

It was the second time that day, considered Haffner, amazed emptying the pockets of his cagoule, presenting her with all the notes he found – when he had paid for sexual services he had never wanted. But Haffner was flexible.

He should never forget his favourite item of vocabulary. When he was in Brazil, when they were leaving the theatre, laughing to themselves at the disconcerted policemen, his counterpart in the Rio bank had tried to explain how one survived in these great times. You could do it, sure, by going underground and becoming a hero. But then you died. Or you could do it by offering up your politics to whatever came along. You preserved yourself through sacrificing your ideals. They had a word for this, he said. It was trampolinability. And this immediately became Haffner's favourite word. He could trampoline. Yes, this seemed possible.

To trampoline: the only form of maturity which Haffner ever recognised.

9

Rising back into the air, buoyant against gravity, Haffner made for the exit – where Niko was waiting for him. Was Niko not good to him? asked Niko. Haffner replied that Niko was very very good to him. So what, asked Niko, did Haffner think?

Haffner promised him that yes: why not? If Niko thought he could help. He didn't see why not. And Niko said that this was very good. He had perhaps said this before, but he liked Haffner very much. Now then: the practicals. He knew the snooker club? Of course, said Haffner, he didn't know the snooker club. Well then, said Niko. Well then. They would sort something out. Niko himself would take him there.

Whatever suited him, said Haffner, simply wanting to end the evening: and he walked out into the benighted dawn.

And carelessly, without thinking, the hand of fate or the world-soul nearly placed a man in a bowler hat, Haffner's twin, his arms by his side, like a sentry, at the end of Haffner's day, as Haffner turned the corner into the town's main square. But luckily this world-soul managed to arrange it so that Haffner changed his mind, did not proceed briskly back home, but lingered, looking in the window of a shop which sold domestic cleaning products, ironing boards, Hoovers, dog baskets, plastic and multicoloured clothes pegs; then the window of an adjoining lingerie shop in which was fixed a row of disembodied and cocked legs, like the Platonic ideal of a cancan.

Finally, Haffner reached the hotel. He ignored the greeting of the woken receptionist – clutching a paperback and a serrated freshly burning plastic cup of coffee – walked into the lift, and pressed the wrong button, so that when he turned as normal to the left and tried to move his key in the lock, it would not work. Finally, after three minutes, he realised his mistake – oblivious to the scene he had left behind the door: a man in pyjamas, wielding an umbrella; a woman whimpering in the bed; a marriage teetering.

Haffner went to sleep, dressed in the tracksuit which now doubled as his pyjamas. Commas of white chest hair nestled in the gap above the jacket's open zip. He wanted to talk to Livia. He wanted to tell her about that conversation he had had in Chinatown, twenty years earlier, with Goldfaden. The conversation about sports. And she would turn to him, sleepy in her velvet nightgown, and tell him that of course Goldfaden was wrong. He knew that. For Livia, like Haffner, understood the majesty of sport.

Yes, it was Livia who had watched the 1980 Wimbledon tennis final with Haffner one weekend, in the early morning, in Florida – where they had gone for a summer break: featuring the American kid with the curls, and the Swedish man with the blue-eyed stare. And it was Livia who had pointed out to Haffner the obvious symbolism of the fight: the two versions of machismo. And which one, did Haffner think, was him? He thought, he said, that he was possibly the kid with the curls. And which one, asked Livia, did he think that she would go for?

The likeable kid with the curls? asked Haffner, hopefully.

No, unfortunately for Haffner, Livia's preference was instead for the resourceful and quiet man: whose machismo needed no theatricality. Even though as she said it Livia kissed him on the cheek, and grinned at him. And Haffner was glad that as he looked at her blouse – one button wrongly fastened so that the fabric bunched out and Haffner could see the beginning of a breast, the lace florets of her bra – his lust was unabated.

But Haffner's audience was gone. So Haffner lay there, on his left side, then shifted, to give solace to his heart, so placating the superstitious aspect of his soul. The aspect of his soul which believed in a soul at all.

PART THREE

Haffner Interrupted

1

The next morning, Haffner woke up late, to hear Benji in conversation outside his door.

Perhaps it was a bad dream. He tried to wake up further.

He couldn't. The dream was real.

2

—Me, Benji used to say, to his friends, his admirers, I have the greatest breasts of anyone I know. If I were a woman, said Benji, I'd want me. I mean yeah. I mean absolutely.

Yes, Benji was huge.

The hugeness had caused so many miniature aspects of Benji. It was, for example, one reason why he hadn't really had girlfriends. His emotions were distractedly doodled with shyness. Self-consciousness possessed him. This was also a reason why Benjamin was beauty-obsessed. He was always a sucker for the grand beauty. When it came to female beauty, his standards were strict. And finally, the size was why he had been forced to teach himself survival through wit.

—You want to know something? Benji said to our mutual friend Ezekiel: Ezekiel, known as Zeek.

—They look at my penis in the urinals, continued Benjamin, and they can't see it. It's like I'm pissing from my belly, you know?

—You shouldn't be too hard on yourself, said Zeek. It's not so bad. I mean, you're not circumcised, are you?

—No, said Benji.

—So you've never tried to masturbate when you're circumcised? said Zeek.

—How could I try it? said Benji.

—So then. The thing is this, said Zeek. It needs a lot of Vaseline.

—Vaseline? asked Benji.

—Or something similar, said Zeek.

—I don't need Vaseline, said Benjamin.

—But you're not circumcised, said Zeek.

—Yes, I know, said Benjamin. I told you that.

In the grey dawns after parties, we would sit out in the garden and talk: while in the living rooms, the bedrooms, the girls dozed in each other's arms, the junkies talked to themselves.

The issue of circumcision used to worry Benjamin. Once, Benjamin had talked to a girl whom he dearly wanted to kiss. As so often in the imperfectly Jewish life of Benjamin, the conversation had turned to penises, and their foreskins. She really did think, she said, that circumcised penises were preferable. They lasted longer, she smiled at him. And Benjamin, with his yarmulke, his deep knowledge of archaic law, wondered if by this she meant to flirt with him. It was possible. Come on, kid, it was possible, he said grimly, to himself. Even if, as only he knew, her hope was utterly misguided. He had to be honest. Sadly, Benjamin admitted to the intact nature of his penis, its shroud of flesh: its headscarf. It was the only way in which Esther had resisted Esmond's Orthodoxy: the practice of circumcision, she used to say, was barbaric. She couldn't countenance it for her darling son. But of course, Benji's girl then added, the circumcised penis had its own charm too. She looked at Benjamin. Confused, he looked back at her, and was quiet.

This was the boy whom Haffner could hear outside his room: while Haffner struggled to extricate himself from the placid dreams of his sleep, into the more unnatural dreams of Haffner's Alpine existence.

3

Haffner picked up the phone. He was sorry, said the receptionist to this newly bedraggled version of Haffner: his whitely blond hair awry, uncombed; his beard sprouting. Haffner asked him what he was sorry for: the receptionist explained that his grandson had said that his grandfather should be expecting him.

—No problem, said Haffner, exhausted. No problem.

And it was nearly lunchtime, added the receptionist, pedantically.

It could hardly get worse, thought Haffner. But then, as he struggled with the sheets, his shoes, the elongated dimensions of his washing routine in the bathroom, he was interrupted by the realisation that it was, in fact, worse. Benjamin, Haffner suddenly realised, was not talking to himself. Though why he had thought the boy would be talking to himself, he didn't know. No, there wasn't just Benjamin. There was also Frau Tummel. They were engaged in conversation outside his door.

And why not? thought Haffner, in dismal jubilation. Why wouldn't Frau Tummel be here as well?

It was as if the farce of his life were repeating itself, just on a diminishing scale. The interruptions of the real – the unwelcome real – which had marked his life continued even here, when Haffner was nowhere.

In the corridor, Frau Tummel was telling Benjamin that such devotion to a grandfather was rare in his generation. It was admirable, she said.

—Uhhuh, said Benjamin.

He had just arrived from the airport. And as he made himself known to reception, he had been interrupted by this woman whose appearance Benjamin felt he knew all too well, from the mothers of his schoolfriends: she was stern, and extravagant, simultaneously. When she discovered who Benjamin was, she was delighted, she said. She was ravished. She knew his grandfather, she assured him, very well. She was just on her way to see him.

He would never understand what the women still saw in his grandfather, thought Benjamin, resigned. No, he wouldn't even try. There was no point. It was part of the whole mystery of sex: a mystery which he felt was way beyond him. Though why the mystery of sex was not by now beyond his grandfather seemed an injustice too cosmic to be contemplated.

Frau Tummel asked him if he was here for a holiday as well, like his grandfather. He replied that sort of. Yes? she said. He was more here on business, said Benji. Like his grandfather.

He really did look very like his grandfather, she said. Absolutely handsome.

Benjamin simpered.

If only, thought Benjamin, she were about thirty years younger. It was always like this. If only women said this whom Benjamin thought of as girls.

Frau Tummel thought that he must admire his grandfather very much. And Benjamin replied ruefully that he could be quite different at home. Frau Tummel queried this. No, said Benjamin: it was true.

In the window, the Alpine mountains were blankly beautiful.

Well, said Frau Tummel, she had to admit that maybe there was something in what he was saying. Herr Haffner had his complications. This she would admit. But that, she said flirtatiously, smiling at Benjamin, was, after all, the signature of a man! She had no idea, said Benjamin sadly, how difficult he could be. Difficult didn't cover it.

But he did not expand on this to Frau Tummel. No, Benji was loyal. He did not tell her what he was now remembering – how once they had discovered Haffner on the island of Malta. He was with a dancer from a cruise ship. Another time, in Florence, Haffner simply wandered off; and was found two days later, in a bar on the south side of the river.

She could not believe it was true, said Frau Tummel. She had not seen this difficulty in Herr Haffner. Herr Haffner, she would at least accept, was a man with his own sense of himself, said Frau Tummel. That was one of the problems, agreed Benjamin. But there were others.

Benjamin was an expert on his grandfather. Observations of his grandfather had formed his education. Once, he had idolised him. Now, perhaps, his idolisation had become inverted: a strange form of love, which was inseparable from dislike.

5

Haffner opened his door.

—You're here? said Haffner to Benji. How?

—Surprised? asked Benji.

—Not really, said Haffner.

It was true. Nothing surprised him when it came to the decisions of his grandson, the wayward passions to which he was subject.

—Shouldn't you be in school? asked Haffner. Shouldn't you be learning something? The cultivation of forelocks? The possibility of prayer?

—You see? said Benjamin to Frau Tummel.

Anyway, said Benjamin: he had told him. Haffner questioned this.

—On the phone? said Benjamin, with his American fall and rise.

—You never told me, said Haffner.

They paused, in this silence of disagreement.

—Are you really wearing that? said Benjamin.

Yes, said Haffner, he was: refusing to explain this unusual wardrobe choice of pink hiking T-shirt and his familiar sky-blue tracksuit.

There was another pause.

—It is so wonderful, the devotion! exclaimed Frau Tummel, beaming on Haffner.

Haffner looked at her, then at Benji. He could do, thought Haffner, curtly, with losing some of that weight. But there it was. He had always been spoiled: by Esther, and then by Livia. Who always cooked the kid steak. Who made hand-cut, hand-fried fries: a treat which Haffner, in fifty years of marriage, never got for himself.

—You had breakfast? Haffner asked his grandson.

—On the plane, said Benji. Plane food.

—Hungry? asked Haffner.

—I'm hungry, said Benjamin.

Haffner's appetites were catholic. Benji's appetite had been for food. Now, unknown to Haffner, he was concerned to broaden the range of his appetites. But it was his appetite for food on which Haffner and his grandson had forged their friendship.

—You know what's happening in the cricket? asked Haffner.

—No, said Benjamin.

—Blowing a gale? said Haffner, cryptically, with an intimate smile.

Benjamin looked embarrassed. And this saddened Haffner. Mutely, he went in search of the long-lost time when Haffner had taught Benjamin his favourite routine from the movies – dialogue which they had then so often recited by heart – where a man stranded in a mountain hotel phones home to find out the cricket score.

Now Haffner had to quote to himself, in silence, the next lines in his adored dialogue – *You don't know? You can't be in England and not know the test score* – grimly thinking as he did so that it was only natural that this was how his century should end: with everyone having lost their sense of humour.

—I will leave you two boys together, said Frau Tummel.

She would meet Haffner back here, she said to Haffner: to talk. For a moment, she looked darkly at Haffner. And then, smiling more benignly at Benjamin, she left.

Haffner turned to Benjamin, and he sighed.

6

Precocious, in the heyday of his teenage years, Benjamin had listened to the hip hop from New York, the ragga from Jamaica. His favourite thing was the Los Angeles hip-hop artist, the modern saint: 2pac. Everyone loved 2pac, true. But in this love, Benji was unusual. He didn't care about the drugs, nor the women. Nor about the gold and diamanté T round 2pac's neck, a cartoon crucifix. No, for Benjamin, 2pac was an example of pure romance. His favourite song – which he played on repeat – was 2pac's elegy 'Life Goes On'. Have a party at his funeral, let every rapper rock it, sang 2pac, rapped 2pac. Let the hos that he used to know from way before kiss him from his head to his toe. Give him a paper and pen so he could write about his life of sin, a couple of bottles of gin in case he didn't get in.

The swagger had Benji entranced.

He'd be lying, continued 2pac, if he told him that he never thought of death. My nigger, they were the last ones left. But life went on.

It was so cool, thought Benjamin. Once, he tried to explain this to Haffner. Haffner tried to listen. This presented some problems: practical (the fitting of the earphones, the working of the portable

CD player); and aesthetic (the understanding of this noise as music, rather than noise).

As a teenager, Benji's ideal habitat was the urban sprawl of Los Angeles: the gang warfare, the misogyny. He spent his life in thrall to the foreign, in thrall to images to which he had no right.

This was the younger Benji – the boy whom Haffner still admired.

A hint of the devastating problem which was to ensue occurred when Benjamin, aged fifteen, decided that, while everyone else went on holiday with their youth groups to Israel – to meet girls, and sleep on beaches – instead he wanted to stay in a Buddhist monastery. This monastery was located in the countryside outside London: in Hertfordshire. It was his spiritual goal. He arrived with a smuggled packet of cigarettes, and a biography of Arthur Rimbaud. For Benji, at fifteen, was a rebel, and philosopher. But when he was confronted by the bell at five the next morning, the meditation for two hours before breakfast, the unidentified and unidentifiable breakfast itself, the work in the fields, by the afternoon he was too depressed to carry on. He couldn't even tell the men apart from the women. He went into the room of the Head Monk and asked to leave. The Head Monk looked at him. He implored him, having made the important break from the temptations of the city, to persevere in his difficult task. The worst was over, he said. But Benji was not so persuaded. There was a skull on the Head Monk's desk; and Benji did not want to be confronted by memento mori. He could not tell, in fact, why it was he was here at all. He had simply liked the idea of it – a man above the temptations of beaches, and girls.

Two hours later, Esther had arrived to take him home.

He had at least learned something, Benjamin told everyone. He'd discovered how deeply he believed in food.

And Haffner loved him for this. The boy was independent! He understood how much more important the senses were than a sense of the serious. But the let-down came soon afterwards. Benji, after all, was in a crisis of faith. He had gone through hip hop, drugs and Buddhism. And now he returned to the most basic, the least loved. Benjamin returned to the religion of his forefathers: a lineage which began with his father, if one missed out his grandfather.

That was why, at university, he spent his vacations in the Promised Land. That was why, after university, he had entered the summer school of a rabbinical seminary.

But then, Benjamin's Jewishness, like all his other crazes, was really a form of romance. He wanted a past: he wanted a past which was more torn apart by history than the history of his happy family.

In Tel Aviv, Benjamin had met a girl who came from a family of Jewish-Algerian intellectuals. Somewhere in the Sahara, she said, there was a tribe which bore her surname. Benji wished that this girl's past were his. He didn't know what he might do with it – but he was sure that this was the missing piece of Benjamin's jigsaw, lost in another jigsaw box, abandoned underneath a sofa.

His forefathers! Who else was more like Benjamin than Haffner? Like his grandfather before him, Benji was a sucker for bohemia.

7

Haffner, however, only saw in Benjamin an exponent of the Law. He was constantly depressed by the cowl of seriousness with which Benjamin so often insulated himself: the easy *tristesse* of history which enticed him.

This judgement was true, in a way. Benjamin dearly wanted the reassuring safety of the righteous, the morally certain. But this was no reason, perhaps, to dislike him, to think that he was prim. He wanted order because he was so often overtaken by compulsions he could not understand.

His first craze was soccer. On the white gloss of his bedroom cupboards, whose moulding was painted dark blue, in imitation of the Tottenham Hotspur soccer strip, Benjamin had arranged stickers produced by Panini for the 1986 World Cup. His favourite stickers were the Brazilians – with their pineapple T-shirts, their one-word names (Socrates!), their impossible hair. Benjamin had arranged Brazil, and Paraguay, and England, gently overlapping, following the blue line of gloss along his cupboards.

Benjamin, in the youth of his youth, didn't have ripped-out pictures of film stars, or porn stars, on his ceiling. No nipples, or even bikinis, in black and white or colour, were visible in his room. True, he did possess one photocopy of a pornographic image. This picture had been given to him, as a special favour, by Ezekiel. A girl with thick, if indistinctly printed, nipples was raising a sailor-suit top towards her chin. A sailor's hat was cocked, coquettish, on her white-blonde permed hair. How innocent he was! In Benjamin's special dreams, he would touch her nipples, curiously – like tuning a radio. But this image was not public. He had simply tucked his pornographic possession, neatly folded, between pages 305 and 306 of his book which contained 1001 facts about the French Revolution, with its glossy laminated boards.

Instead of sex, Benjamin had crazes. There had been the soccer, then the drugs, and the hip hop, and the Buddhism. Then the Orthodox Jewishness. And now, finally, Benji had been disturbed by the true sexual furore – inspired by his Jewish and Algerian and French girl in Tel Aviv. With this girl, finally, Benjamin had lost his virginity. She was hairless between the legs, except for a black tuft, so that when he touched her all he felt was a slick softness. He nearly swooned. For this, thought Benji, was love.

It wasn't love, of course. Over various phone calls, Zeek tried to explain this to him. But Benji didn't care. Instead, he simply retreated into the burrow of his feelings. He told Zeek what he had not told her: that when he left her, the next morning, after they had slept together, in the taxi, he wrote in the dawn, on the back of a receipt, that this was true desire, a true passion. And passions were so rare.

This was why Benjamin was here, in the spa town. He needed an escape from the summer school, the regalia of his religion – and he needed to talk to the man who was his only authority when it came to women. The man who was his – faulty, despaired-of authority as an adult.

But I think there was a further complication. Benji was here because he wanted permission to leave the summer school: he wanted to replace his respect for his religion with a more freestyle interest in his girl. This was true. But in his amatory crisis the family's inheritance had therefore acquired more significance than it might, perhaps, have had. For Benjamin felt guilty at his wish to abandon his religion. The villa was therefore his chance for redress: his chance to show his family and forefathers that he had not abandoned them entirely.

The villa was an excuse.

Which was, perhaps, one way in which Benji differed from his grandfather.

8

He should really stop looking at women like that, said Benjamin. Haffner said he would look where he liked. And believe him, he wasn't looking. Benjamin said that it just wasn't right.

Again, the lethargy which Haffner felt when contemplating his adventure with Frau Tummel transformed into something so much more protective. So much more like love. Such sadness which Haffner felt for the bodies of women! Such sadness which transformed into a pity of the flesh!

She was, said Haffner, a very handsome woman.

—Whatever! exclaimed Benjamin. Whatever.

Benji was here for business. So skip the breakfast, said Benji, skip the lunch: surprising even himself. They were going to sort this whole thing with the villa today. It was why he was here.

He knew, as he said this, that his motives were mixed. He knew how much he was fleeing from his summer school. He knew what a convenient excuse the story of the family villa was to him. But surely, thought Benji, the fact that he was in panicking flight should not mean he could not solve a practical problem. At least the villa was a problem whose solution was obvious.

—Not so simple, said Haffner.

—It's simple, said Benjamin.

—Believe me, said Haffner. If anything were simple, this isn't it.

Would the young not give this up? wondered Haffner. When would they learn to talk precisely? He wanted to be done with trying to bring them up. Or, maybe more precisely, he wanted to educate them out of their attempts to bring him up.

Why did no one want to believe him when he said that he had done all he could? But then, he was forced to concede, it was hardly surprising: this scepticism, this doubt in Haffner. He could understand the disappointment. As if Haffner were the omnipotent yet constantly underachieving god of the Christians and the Muslims and the Jews.

9

—I don't think you realise, said Haffner, sitting with Pfeffer, on Haffner's return to London, when the family had first discovered the existence of Barbra, the problems of living with a beautiful woman. I mean an apparition. You think it's easy?

—I don't think anything, said Pfeffer. Well maybe. I think it's easy living with the woman you love.

But no, said Haffner. Pfeffer, with his utter confidence, could never understand the problems of living with such a woman as Livia. The endless problems of self-worth. Think about it, he urged Pfeffer. You woke up every day with this noble profile. You looked across at the elegance of her face and it destroyed you. It was no way to treat a man: to emphasise the bags under his eyes, the marbled skin. It wasn't a sexual success. It was a crisis.

Pfeffer raised a philosophic eyebrow.

He wasn't blaming him, Pfeffer had said, but it didn't look good. That was all he was saying.

Only Pfeffer had tried to disabuse him of his guilt, only Pfeffer – with his retractable gold Biros and pots made for him by his children – pots of beaten bronze with enamel detailing, and mahogany lids. And maybe this was a surprise. Only Pfeffer, the family man, tried to persuade Haffner that his guilt remained unproven.

They had been to school together, at prep school. Pfeffer was the man Haffner's father wanted him to be, or as close to it as possible – ever since Haffner betrayed his family by refusing to enter the family law firm. Pfeffer was a libel lawyer. He knew the secrets of showbiz. Which meant, thought Haffner, that he knew the secrets of everything, since everything was showbiz. Pfeffer lived in St John's Wood, in the largest apartment known to Haffner, with drawing rooms, and living rooms, and multiple bathrooms with multiple basins. A redundant triumph of the plural. It had always amazed Haffner, the sleek animal adaptability of these humans he grew up with: how Pfeffer, the kid he had known since prep school, who was so docile, who wore grey flannel shorts when everyone else had understood the only cool thing was trousers, could morph into this maven of luxury, silken in his deskchair. A chair in which he wallowed, his small hands neat and hairless on his blotter – whose corners were curtailed by leather bands, into an octagon.

But I don't feel like sketching Pfeffer's form. He can remain there, an outline in black, transparent against all the background colours – like some minor figure in a painting by Dufy.

Haffner was unshaven; he was in a summer suit. Beside him was a plate of biscuits brought to him by Pfeffer's secretary, a secretary whom Haffner always suspected of harbouring designs on Pfeffer. He was wearing the panama which Livia hated. It came rolled up in a metal tube. He liked to think it made him rakish.

But hey, Pfeffer added. He was the last person to be advising anyone on a marriage. What was he meant to do? His wife was in therapy. His daughter was in love with some Greek entrepreneur. Or possibly a Turk. How was Pfeffer an expert in the family? He was as much a natural family man as Artie Shaw. Or Goebbels.

And Haffner had to admit, at that moment, that he loved Pfeffer, whose idea of fun was crossword puzzles, Scrabble, memory games. The man who saw the world as a perpetual acrostic. He spent his conversations, Haffner remembered, reconfiguring each sentence backwards. Otherwise, he told Haffner, it could become boring for him. This produced no obvious vacancy in his expression, or concentration. Sometimes, just backwards was not enough. Sometimes, he had to reverse according to gaps of two or three. He was toying with implementing logarithms.

He just thought, he said, that Haffner should explain what was going on.

But what could anyone else know about the marriage of Haffner and Livia? It was a world with only two inhabitants.

When the time was coming for war, but they didn't know when, Haffner and Livia had a code – for Haffner, like every soldier, was banned from giving any prior information about his movements. He had a rich and rather unpleasant uncle, called Uncle Jonas. And the code was that if Uncle Jonas were very fit and well, everything was fine. If the prospects for Haffner to be mobilised were doubtful, then his health was not too good: and then the time came when Haffner knew he was to go abroad, and he said that he was sorry to tell her, darling, but Uncle Jonas had passed away. He was at Basingstoke at this time, in a telephone booth. It was April, and curiously cold. They had embarked from the docks in the west of

Scotland. He didn't quite know where. He didn't really know what a dock was, if he were honest.

A marriage, thought Haffner, was the invention of a code.

No one knew the secrets of a marriage: maybe this was true. Just as Haffner didn't know the secrets of his grandson, the conundrum of his grandson, standing there in front of him: confused, like his grandfather, by the monstrous state of love.

Haffner Banished

1

The villa which belonged to Livia's family was out on the outskirts of the town, above a slope which ran down to the river. Across from its veranda was the range of snowy mountains.

In 1929, the universal crash had meant that her father took a loan from his cousin's bank in Trieste. Seven years later, his talent for money had been so adroitly employed that he had earned enough to buy this villa.

Here, Livia used to argue with her father: a nationalist when considering the Italian state, an anti-nationalist when considering the Zionist cause. He was a businessman who imported coal from Britain. Through the quiet rise of wealth, the steady progress of business, he wanted his nation to be great again.

Her father had become a Fascist after fighting in the Great War. Then, in 1922, leaving behind his daughter in her blankets and her cradle, leaving behind his pregnant wife, her father had taken part in Mussolini's March on Rome: his pedestrian coup. Her mother had cut out clippings from the newspapers. They featured grand vocative apostrophes (*O Rome!*) written in a rhetoric which even then seemed obscure (*O ship launched toward World Empire that emerges from the flux of time!*). She kept them in an album for her husband.

He believed in Italy. It was a refuge – his family's final escape from the misery of politics.

Even if this escape was a politics too.

Cesare was duly made to join the youth movements. He wore the uniform, scowling. In retaliation, he decided that when he grew up he would be a Communist. If, that is, he ever grew up. As for Livia, she also wore her black pleated skirts, white piqué blouse, long white stockings, her black cape and beret. This was her Fascist youth.

Her father believed in discipline. Neither Cesare nor Livia was allowed to rest a wrist on the table when they were eating. She was told to hold two napkins under her armpits, so that she might achieve the correct deportment. His ideas of order were immutable.

She was too melancholic, her father told her, when they argued. Always on the dark side of the moon. She didn't have a positive concept of the reality of life. In reply, she would quote the Romantics to him. What else was this life but a failure? It lacked beauty. She looked forward to the one radiant light, bathed in which humanity would come together in perfect union.

In the café in the main square, Livia, when she was sixteen, had been asked to dance by a man whose eyebrows and teeth she distrusted. She had looked at Mama. And Mama had nodded her head. Her mother had never done this before. Normally, every dance was forbidden to Livia. And when she asked her mother, afterwards, why she had made her dance with that horrible man, Mama had simply said that it was because she had to: the man was a director of the secret police.

When Livia told Haffner this story, one day in 1953, he smiled at her. And did she, he wanted to know, tread on the man's toes?

—*Naturalmente*, said Livia. And she kissed him, her mischievous boy.

There had been a swing on the cherry tree outside the villa, stranded on an island of grass in the drive. They used to go looking for mushrooms and blackberries. In the early summer they would go to the seaside, on the Adriatic. And in August they would come up here into the mountains. That was their life.

And once, when the Buffalo Bill circus arrived in the town, Livia's mother told her that this would be the greatest night of her life. But when she told Haffner about this, forty years later, as they passed a sign for a travelling circus on the outskirts of London, following some visit to see their grandson, she did not remember the trapeze, nor the spectacle: all that had remained with her was an inarticulate concern for the living conditions of the elephants.

This, then, was what Haffner was now due to inherit: the occluded history of Livia.

2

—If you had only not been so impatient, said the Head of the Committee on Spatial Planning, perhaps I help you. Not now. Now the matter is closed.

—What do you mean closed? said Haffner.

—You think this is not something I understand? said his opponent. This is something I perfectly understand.

—Really? said Haffner.

—Aggressing my staff, said the Head of the Committee.

To Haffner's surprise, within ten minutes of entering the building, they had secured an interview with the Head of the Committee on Spatial Planning. It had been to his surprise, but also to his mild irritation, giving as it did an unfortunately fluent appearance to Benjamin of the Committee's workings. This irritation, however, had been mollified when they discovered that the Head of the Committee, having dismissed Isabella as unnecessary, spoke an English which was accurate but so heavily accented that they found it difficult to follow him.

This linguistic confusion, however, was possibly irrelevant. The case, it appeared, was closed.

—First place, said the Head of the Committee, you come here earlier, much earlier. Now the window is over. Occasion gone. Doubly, I cannot do nothing for you.

—So that's it? said Haffner, banished from his estates.

—I will make to you a concession, said the Head of the Committee.

—A concession? asked Haffner, eagerly.

Yes, said the man. I am sorry for you, I really am. But my hands are tired.

—I'm sorry? said Haffner.

—Yes, said the Head of the Committee. Tired. It is a pity for you.

—That's your concession? said Haffner. In what way does that represent a concession?

—He means confession, said Benjamin.

—What? said Haffner.

There was no goodwill. Haffner knew that. But he hoped to be surprised. And so often he was duly let down.

He indicated to the Head of the Committee that he strongly intended to pursue the matter further. In Haffner's experience of offices, this phrase was usually potent. For Haffner's threats were real. It seemed less potent now.

The Head of the Committee was blowing away the flakes of an eraser, which he had been vigorously rubbing against a mistake in his calligraphy. It was music to his ears, he said. Music to his ears. And never, thought Haffner, would he trust a man again who used this phrase. All his sense of style was outraged.

But nothing in this room was stylish.

It was situated on the first floor of a building which once housed Hapsburg bureaucrats, and had then been gutted to service the administration of Communist aristocrats. From its ground-floor windows lolled the coiled tubes of the air-conditioning units, like elephant trunks. The office looked out on to a garden, with a sparse alley of plane trees which were sickly with dust, their leaves patchy with psoriasis. A poster on the wall implored Haffner not to smoke.

Haffner had no intention of smoking. Instead, he chose escalation. His last descendant beside him, fighting for his lineage, Haffner chose defiance. Yes, Haffner began to plead and rage, while beneath the stern poster – a man palming away a proffered packet of cigarettes – the Head of the Committee smoked from his collection of Marlboro Reds: ten of them in a bleak row.

3

—How can we have a conversation, cried Haffner, reasonably, when there is no goodwill? What kind of justice is this?

In the corner of the office, there was a bucket of soapy water: a soufflé of foam disintegrating above its rim.

—Judge you? said the Head of the Committee. What else do you expect?

Once more Haffner fought against the prejudices of the ages.

After all, insinuated the Head of the Committee, it had taken him a very long time, no? To bring this suit? When it didn't seem so difficult. Haffner conceded this point. Perhaps he now thought there was money in it, said the Head of the Committee. Given his backdrop. To which Haffner replied that he didn't understand. Did he mean his British backdrop? Background?

—No, said the Head of the Committee.

But, he added, it was obvious that he was not from Britain. Haffner asked him what he meant. One only needed to look, said the Head of the Committee. Just one's eyes.

He understood. Yes, Haffner understood. Blond and blue-eyed among the Jews: and Jewish to everyone else. But just because he understood didn't mean he wasn't bewildered. Haffner wasn't used to fighting the prejudices of Central Europe. He had grown up happily in the pleasures of north London. He wasn't used to regarding himself as part of a race, rather than a nation. He was just a Haffner, not a Jewish Haffner. As he had tried to tell his driver, on their way from Haifa to Cairo – but that was another story. As he continued to try to tell various taxi drivers and financial wives, in London and New York. The cricketing taxi drivers of New York and the intellectual financial wives of London. The pattern of it, perhaps, should have made him pause. But Haffner rarely paused.

Just as he should perhaps have paused on the fact that he still possessed a *News Letter to the Forces*, dated Chanukah 5705, which he kept, he always said, not for its ethical stance but because on the back of this sheet of paper were adverts for Elco watches, from Hatton Garden; the Grodzinski chain of modern bakeries; and Lloyd Rakusen's Delicious Wheaten Crackers. He went for its nostalgia, maintained Haffner. He did not preserve it because this newsletter announced the triple burden of the continuing fight against the menace of Fascism and Nazism, the effort to rescue as many as they could of the remnants of their brethren left in Europe, and the refusal to relinquish one iota of their just claims to Eretz Israel as the Land of Israel belonging to the People of Israel. But I am not so sure. Maybe Haffner had never quite resolved the problem of his loyalties.

Was he saying, said Haffner, pounding the desk, like the grandest businessman of all time, that this Committee was refusing to help him because he and his wife were Jewish? Was that the missing word? And as he did so he believed that surely now this man would retreat: surely this man would not have the temerity to disagree with Haffner. But no, even now this man preserved his calm. Of course, he said, he had not said that. He was merely observing.

But Haffner was unbowed. As Benjamin glowed with mortified pride beside him, Haffner gave a speech. He was noted for his speeches, and Haffner gave the speech that he had always dreamed of making: where the audience quails beneath the shaking fist, the pointing finger; where the righteous man can demand of the wicked man that the truth be finally told.

—These are the things you always say, said the Head of the Committee. That everyone is against you.

—Me? said Haffner. I just met you.

—Not just you, he said. All of you. That you are always prosecuted.

—Persecuted, corrected Haffner, haughty.

The secretaries, Haffner fancied, were crowding at the door. One, perhaps, was being hoisted by a sturdy palm to the rim of the door, where a crack allowed the earnest spectator to get a glimpse of Haffner in his finale: rising now, pushing back his chair, and demanding that the Head of the Committee offer him an explanation.

—Let me put a question for you, said the Head of the Committee. You think you have nothing to do with us? You think you can take what you want?

Haffner wondered what he was asking him. Was he now to take on the guilt of the entire Soviet empire? Because he and his wife were Jewish? Were the very Communists who had stolen his wife's home now to be seen as Haffner's fault?

This was Haffner's twentieth century – where the history of London was also the history of Warsaw; and the history of Tel Aviv was also the history of Paris. And so on, and so on: in the endless history of the geography. All the separate national histories were universal, if you looked from far enough away. So how could Haffner escape?

4

The Head of the Committee motioned to a man who was no doubt an assistant, an apparatchik – who had been sitting in the shadows of this vast room all along – to show these gentlemen out. He was sorry, but he really must cut short their appointment. Naturally, he said, a decision would come in due course.

Unexpectedly, as he rose passionate from his chair, Haffner discovered that he was leaving with a sense of triumph. A sense of triumph accompanied by a worry that he had rather lost the upper hand, by making such a scene – but a triumph, nevertheless, that he had been so free with his fury. He had reached a place of poetry.

He was hoping so much, thought Haffner, that Livia was watching. He had never believed in ghosts before. They had seemed gothically unnecessary. But now they seemed the only just solution to the difficult problem of death.

For Haffner was furious with loyalty. His history was Livia's too. He couldn't deny it. He had thought for so long that this villa was just a chore. And it was a chore. But it meant more to him than that. It was suddenly, he understood, all to do with Livia.

And Livia, he thought, would appreciate this fight for her cosmopolitan history. She would appreciate, above all, Haffner's unorthodox methods. For, as he confided to an astonished and worried Benjamin, he had another plan as well. To Benjamin he offered an edited version of his conversation with Niko. He perhaps exaggerated Niko's authority. He did not mention the locale where he had conducted these negotiations. But Benjamin still protested. Was he going to do something so illegal? No, Benji couldn't believe it. He mustn't do anything of the sort.

They paused outside the entrace to a jazz café in a garden – its walls graffiti'd with red and black unicorns: the arpeggios scaling the heights of the trees. They considered it; they walked on.

Maybe all of Benjamin's anxiety was his fault, thought Haffner. Maybe this was the natural consequence of Haffner: he had bequeathed accidentally to his grandson this exorbitant need for rules. In Benji's wish to be the opposite of his grandfather. Walking towards the hotel with Benjamin – as, still feeling exhausted, after two dramatic nights, Haffner dreamed of a possible nap, since exhaustion was becoming his natural state – he wondered if it was somehow in opposition to the ghost of Haffner that Benji had inherited this absolute anxiety about the feelings of others: a total timidity.

And it seemed that Haffner was right.

Only when they reached the doors to the hotel did Benjamin finally begin to talk about the fact that Benji was now in love. Yes, he said, he had met a girl whose gorgeousness transcended everything of which Benji had thought the world capable. But, wondered Benji, could he really know she liked him?

—Have you kissed this girl? said Haffner.

That wasn't the question, said Benjamin. The question was: did she want him to do this again? She seemed so cool. It was, said Haffner, an easy question to answer. He should simply see what happened next. He should kiss her again. What harm could that do? And Benjamin replied that, well, he just didn't know how much he wanted the burden of it. He didn't know if he wanted the relationship. And if he didn't want that, then he thought it was better to do nothing.

Which made him more mature than Haffner, thought Haffner. It was not a position he had so far reached himself.

—That's fine of you, said Haffner. That's very fine.

He didn't know that Benji was not quite telling him the truth. He did not know that Benji was not quite telling himself the truth. Benji's struggle against his senses was Benji's mute interior.

He needed to sleep, said Haffner. He needed to lie down, old boy. And Benji, in a gentle gesture of goodbye, kissed him on the forehead.

Innocence and experience! But which was which? The old young or the young old? Haffner wept for the things he thought he would no longer have; Benjamin for the things he thought he would never have. Both of them possessed their own comedy.

Both of them were banished.

When Livia was ill once, long before the end of their marriage, she had promised Haffner that if she died, she would come back and talk to him. He would know of the existence of an afterlife from the fact of this return; or the fact of a non-return. When she finally died and she did not, as Haffner hoped, come back to comfort him, he was not so astonished. After all, they had rarely seen each other in the two years preceding her death. Then a graver thought began to trouble him – that this was no proof of a lack of afterlife; it was only proof that she had not been able to come back. He was haunted by this idea of her trying to communicate with him, pressed to his ear, to his eyes, and Haffner unable to hear her, unable to see her. Or then an even graver and more plausible interpretation presented itself: it was only proof that she had not wanted to come back. She had decided against it.

He had mourned alone in the empty house, like the tearful queen mourning that schmuck Aeneas, as she gazed at her abandoned couch.

5

In the summer of 1938 – when Haffner was away, playing for the Old Boys cricket team of his school – Livia's father was reading, in silence, the Manifesto of the Racist Scientists. In the dining room, Cesare, who was sixteen, and believed in the greatness of his talent, was engaged on his great ceiling painting: *The Dream*, he said, *of Europa*. It featured three semi-nude women. No one was convinced of the mythological provenance: no one believed that the seriousness of the gods could compensate for Cesare's shaky technique. The pipe in his father's mouth was making him grin as he let the smoke dissolve in slow small clouds: a few smoke rings disappearing into other smoke rings. Outside, someone was beating a rug on the sill of the steps. And Livia's father was reading that Jews, according to the ninth section of the manifesto, did not belong to the Italian race.

He laid his pipe down.

At first, Livia's father, an honourable Fascist, was one of the discriminati: those discriminated from discrimination. Very soon, however, it was all over. His clients were forbidden to trade with him; his salesmen were banned from negotiating for his list. He decided to send his children to Britain, to stay with friends of his in the paint industry. They required a passport and a transit visa through France. He went to the Fascist chief of police – whose wedding anniversary he had recently celebrated at a small dinner party in town – and he said to him: either he arranged this, or he would break the law. He would buy the papers on the black market. Surely the police chief didn't want him to break the law?

The Fascist chief of police agreed that he should not break the law. So Cesare and Livia went to Britain.

Haffner still owned a photograph of Livia's mother – taken in 1915, to give to her fiancé when he went to war – dressed in a Japanese kimono. Her father owned a black Fascist fez with a silken fringe. Indignantly, he would tell her the shameful story of the Dreyfus case – from the time when Europe was imperial. And yet, on the other hand, the blue-and-white collection boxes for the nascent state of Israel: these he ignored. As if it was nothing to do with him. There was no need, he argued – unlike, perhaps, in racist France – for such drastic measures.

Yes, Livia's father believed in order. It was possible, he thought, for there to be an end of history: a utopia. But Italy, Livia wanted to say, was still Europe. Nowhere was safe from the stupidity of inheritance.

But he believed in the nineteenth century, and its bourgeoisie. The year before, in 1937, Ettore Ovazza – who was Fascist, and Jewish, and saw no contradiction in this position – wrote his reply to Paolo Orano's pamphlet which had maintained that in fact these positions were indeed contradictory. Livia's father had agreed with Ovazza. If one wanted to express one's sympathy with one's suffering fellow Jews in Germany, this didn't mean one wanted to found a second Fatherland, in the contested lands of Palestine. No, this was precisely what it meant to him to be Italian. Italy was the Fatherland for which so many of the purest heroes of Jewish blood had died.

Later, Livia always used to berate her dead and absent father. Why hadn't he understood? Why hadn't they all left sooner? And Haffner would always reply that it was difficult to leave. Who knew when the right time was to flee? It was so difficult, abandoning the things you loved. It was difficult enough, said Haffner, abandoning the things you hated.

Haffner Delinquent

1

In his bedroom, finally, Haffner drifted into what he hoped would be the greatest of all restorative sleeps.

For a moment this was true. Then he was transformed into a baby Haffner, playing with the other children while in the next room sat Frau Tummel, taking tea, with all the other adults. Although, when he considered this, some minutes later, when Haffner had been woken up, it struck him as unusual: for Frau Tummel was nearly thirty years his junior. So what was his unconscious doing?

But really, Haffner wasn't often worried by his unconscious: nightly, his dreams were delinquent, involving all life forms, all birds of prey. He had grown used to ignoring the signs. He no more wanted Frau Tummel to mother him than he wanted Zinka to be his daughter.

Enough of the family! Let the eternal couples unite!

But Haffner was only thinking this because, as he was playing on the floor of his imaginary playpen, there came a knock at the door: this knock was then repeated. And when Haffner finally dragged his body – with patches of sweat on his back, scored creases on his cheek – to the door, he found the real Frau Tummel, who wished so urgently to speak with him.

2

So many things had been running through her head, said Frau Tummel. So many sad thoughts. Haffner murmured: as he had always murmured when confronted by the sadness of women. To see him there, talking with that woman: to see him with that girl. She knew that she was imagining things. And Haffner assured her that yes, absolutely: she was imagining things. What relationship could Haffner have with a girl so young? It was ridiculous.

—Yes, agreed Frau Tummel: ridiculous.

This disturbed Haffner's vanity.

Perhaps she understood, said Frau Tummel. It was as if Haffner would not trust himself, she said. What was wrong, she said, with the passion? Why always run away from it?

There was nothing, thought Haffner, that he could say to this. It seemed so obviously true, in the abstract. As a statement it had its accuracy. But not to his friendship with Frau Tummel. Only to his friendship with Zinka.

And he stood there, rummaging through his brain, like a man searching in his pockets, in his bag, for the ticket which might finally allow him entrance to the airplane which will take him away from all this misery, but finding nothing: just three coins, a key, an obediently switched-off cell phone – none of which, when proffered in a gesture of goodwill, convince the air hostess that he possesses the authority to board the plane and leave.

In this pause, Frau Tummel lit a cigarette: she only managed to light half its tip. She inhaled deeply, until the whole circumference fiercely glowed.

She appeared to change the subject. What a wonderful grandson Benjamin must be, she said: what a solace – as she busied herself with tidying Haffner's bedroom, opening the curtains, neatly folding his tracksuit jacket: its arms pinned behind itself – a straitjacket.

Perhaps, thought Haffner, he was not so wrong to dream of Frau Tummel as his mother. She represented all the domestic he had ever known, a sinful heaven of supervision. And Haffner liked to feel that he was supervised. It was how he had lived in the family home – where at Pesach the cockney maid fell into the dining room, closely followed by the cook, who had been listening in amazed curiosity at the door: a door which had been flung open by Papa in hopeful if theatrical expectation of Elijah.

But surely, thought Haffner, he wasn't here, in exile, banished, to find a second version of a mother. It couldn't be that. Haffner was here to find a house, not a family: not a mother or a wife.

Yet Haffner was still so easily won over by those who tried to care for him. Those who sacrificed themselves for Haffner! Like Barbra, the delight of his New York years, who used to keep a selection of his clothes freshly ironed in her wardrobe. The secret of a marriage? Haffner once argued with Morton. He wanted to know the secret of a marriage? You had to find someone who agreed to be the slave. Somebody had to give up. That was the only solution. Two people in love with their pride, then everything was over. Maybe not immediately, but in the end. The only successful marriages involved someone giving up on their life.

He did not tell Morton who, in the marriage of Livia and Haffner, was the masochist, and who was not.

But it wasn't just marriage. It seemed, thought Haffner, to be the secret of everything. At a certain point, you just gave up on the infantile wish to be an emperor. You stopped complaining that people were changing their clothes beside your marble statue, or carrying a coin stamped with your counterfeit face into a bathroom, or a brothel. Those were the crazy edicts of Augustus. And Haffner, now, was beyond them.

Frau Tummel stubbed her cigarette, half smoked, into Haffner's ceramic ashtray, engraved with a view of a mountain whose name Haffner did not know. Then, slowly, Frau Tummel began to undress.

—We don't want to talk, after all, she said.

What was the point in all these arguments? They loved each other; that was all that mattered. Her husband, he was talking to her all day. His health, it was so up and down. He planned walks in the mountains which he would never take. And to think that she was contemplating leaving him! So much strain she was under! But what could she do?

She wanted the sex. And this might have suited Haffner, but the sex was wasted on him, because she wanted to make the sex love. It wasn't that he couldn't have the two together at any point, but with Frau Tummel it was impossible. He didn't love her. The dramatics bored him. With Frau Tummel, he just wanted the purity of pure dirt. The kind of dirt Frau Tummel could have been into as well, with her lavish breasts, the tired lilt of her belly, if only she had been less in love.

She reclined: as normal, her bra still on

—There might be no more beauty, said Frau Tummel, observing herself, but there can be a little grace.

And although this forgivable vanity touched Haffner with a remote tenderness, he still felt nothing. Yes, at this point, Haffner suddenly discovered that not only did he not love her, but he didn't even want her. It struck him as strange.

Would he put her on her stomach? Frau Tummel asked him.

He wished he could; he wished that he wanted to do this for Frau Tummel; but he could not see his way to it. Kneeling on the bed, he toyed with her bra. She looked up at him, breathing heavily.

Then there was a knock at the door.

Saved! thought Haffner. Saved!

He dreamed of the receptionist, of Viko, of the waiter in the dining room: joyfully, he considered how it could only be someone who was here to help him, to release him from this agony of politesse and sadness.

No voice came. Haffner asked who it was. Still no one replied. Frau Tummel looked at him: startled.

—My husband! she exclaimed, in a whisper.

To his surprise, Haffner discovered that he was enjoying himself. The male competition of it appealed to him. Anything, so long as Frau Tummel was returned to her own life: a life which had no place for Raphael Haffner.

Did she think so? he whispered back to her. She was sure. Who else could it be? It could be anyone, he argued. Absolutely anyone from the hotel. Or even Benjamin, he argued. Whispering, she shouted at him that this was no time for argument. It was obvious who it was. They needed a plan.

Haffner had no plan. Haffner had no plan.

They looked around the room: at the desk, the window, the elegant armchair, the veranda and its view, the door to the bathroom.

Five seconds later, Haffner confdently opened the door, to discover Zinka: in her sunglasses – twin beige lenses, flat against the hollowed angles of her cheeks.

4

Haffner could understand the icons of the Orthodox Church, with their mournful expressions: the deep sadness of distance inscribed in their high cheekbones, almond eyes, the nose which Haffner always found alluring: dense with bone, its line an asymmetrical quiver.

Perhaps it was true that he had momentarily abandoned the quest for Zinka in his quest for the villa. He would admit so much. But that was no argument against the sincerity of his desire. The true desire, as Haffner was discovering – as Haffner had so often discovered – was returning. Just as it had returned when he first met Barbra, in his office on a twilit morning in November in Manhattan: a story which Haffner cherished. Just as it had recovered when he had met a woman called Olga, in an executive box at the World Series, who said she was with the Dow Jones, and who so wanted to write about his career, who would appreciate just a few moments with him in private: a story which Haffner, when questioned by his colleagues, had always denied.

Zinka stood there in front of him. She had just come because she had a message from Niko. That he would meet Haffner in the car park: after dinner. It was OK with Haffner? He understood? It was OK, said Haffner.

—So OK, she said.

Haffner did not shut the door. She noticed this. She did not move.

She observed that they seemed to get along. And Haffner agreed. So she had nothing to do now, she said: she was just here to tell him the message.

Haffner thanked her. He told her to thank Niko.

—Maybe, said Zinka, I can come in?

Panicking, considering Frau Tummel in the bathroom, a recording booth, Haffner asked her if she wanted to get a coffee. It seemed the better option: to lock Frau Tummel in, rather than let her hear who was now replacing her – in Haffner's room, in Haffner's desire. But Zinka said that no, why did they need to go anywhere else? He wasn't sure, said Haffner, if he had the facilities for making coffee.

—But whatever, said Zinka, elongating past him. And Haffner paused, anguished by indecision.

185

But, too late, Zinka had walked towards the window, where her silhouette asked him if she might change into her yoga things in Haffner's room. There was no way, thought Haffner, in which he could answer this with anything approaching the correct decorum. So Haffner only nodded. And as, delirious, he nodded, Haffner considered Frau Tummel, in the bathroom. Transfixed in the fluorescent light. He considered this in a different delirium to the delirium with which he looked at Zinka: a delirium of pensive concern.

Somehow, he considered, without him meaning it to happen, his actions became cruel in their effects.

And Haffner was not cruel. The emperors, of course, were not like him. The great dictators enjoyed their torture: but it was never Haffner's way – to throw a party for a father, to make his son's execution go that much more sociably.

Haffner looked at the wood of the bathroom door. It was probably just a veneer, thought Haffner: not a solid oak, or trusty beech. Harshly, he judged its inadequate soundproofing. He cursed this country. He cursed the former Communist empire for its inadequate provision of workmanship. Then he cursed the nascent capitalist transition.

On the other hand, if Frau Tummel could hear everything, thought Haffner, could hear that Zinka's was not the voice of her husband, then why had she not come out? This seemed reasonable.

Oh Haffner! He hadn't considered the depth of Frau Tummel's pride. Nor the intricacy of her sadness.

5

Zinka lay there, in no apparent rush to dress herself in the track-suit and vest which formed her sportswear. She lay against the bolster, in a T-shirt, and socks, and panties. She took an apple from the bowl of fruit placed with professional love beside his bed each morning, bit a slim curve out of it, then put it back, on the table. It wobbled; then came to rest. She looked at Haffner.

She hooked a finger under the gusset of her panties. They looked at each other. Then Zinka withdrew her finger, let her gusset move back into place.

In Haffner's memory, this happened with an infinite languor. This was only, perhaps, because the speed of Haffner's thought was now subject to a steep acceleration.

She must like him, thought Haffner. In some way, she must like him. Haffner, after all, did not believe in the maliciousness of reality. This talent allowed him to discover so much solace where other people only saw benightedness, the end of civilisation.

Zinka asked him if he wanted to watch her touch herself.

No, thought Haffner, trying to reason, considering Frau Tummel, considering Benjamin, considering the villa which had led him into this ever more miniature trap: no, if against his better judgement the world was turning itself into a succession of traps, then what did Haffner care? The obvious reasons were there: the many ways in which Zinka might be thinking of repayment. Or she might be acting for reasons which would always remain inscrutable to Haffner. The reasons were beyond him.

And this, I think, was where the story of the villa began to truly become the story of Haffner's finale: at this point, he began to enter a world where all the usual values seemed reversed: a small gymnasium of moral backflips, with the joyful ideas walking on their hands.

He couldn't remember if any woman had ever asked him this at any other point in his history. It startled him with its poise. Usually, the women seemed to expect Haffner to do the action: Haffner was the highest executive, the producer there to give permission to the director in his folding and eponymous chair, with all the lights off and the crew observing him, expectantly, surrounded by vacant lots where the streetlights flickered in their high anxiety. He looked at

Zinka. Frau Tummel, sweating, weeping, did not occur to him, not any more. What he wanted, more than anything else, was to see Zinka touch herself.

Again, Haffner nodded.

Then Zinka flipped over on to her stomach. This was not the position which Haffner had expected: his improvised imagination had been more orthodox, more pornographic. But at this point he was not burdened with the responsibilities of the critic.

Then, he realised, there was a small problem involved in Haffner's own position.

Haffner considered sitting down. He worried this might seem too formal. It might seem rehearsed. So he stood: in the appearance of the casual. As if it were nothing more than an ordinary conversation, this exchange between a hotel guest and his spa assistant.

Standing by his desk, at the foot of the bed, Haffner could see her moving her fingers, the red fingertips emerging where she lay.

And that, Haffner suddenly realised, was it. There was nothing more to see. This moved him. It was, he thought, more intimate like this. He would see nothing, not even her face. Everything was in the noises, the small moans and inhalations, the slow exhalations. Her face was squashed against the pillow. The intimacy was musical. Entranced, Haffner stared.

She rested a cheek on the bedraggled sheet, to look back at him. Her cheek was red, as if she were blushing.

Outside, unknown to Haffner, the sun maintained its fixed decline.

6

Distractedly, Haffner saw once more the *Lives of the Caesars*, there on his bedside table. Even if this was not quite despotic, it was the closest he had really come, thought Haffner, to feeling imperial. This was Dacia, and Dalmatia. He could understand the euphoria.

No wonder they set about erecting columns, thought Haffner: the camels and the trumpets. No wonder they wanted to parade their spoils, in triumph – the chariots drawn by panthers on their padded paws. No arch, no column, was grand enough to commemorate the few grand moments of desire in a life, the even fewer moments of possession.

Yes, there had been twelve Caesars: and now here was the thirteenth – Haffner Augustus: whose image, if there were any justice in this world, should be carved on a marble tomb, its panels chased with Haffner in profile, leading his jungly train – the leopards, the chubby satyrs – to some screwed-up festival of Bacchus.

7

The lamps, in their shades, observed Haffner, delinquent.

And Haffner forgot himself. All the characters of his recent history Frau Tummel, Niko, Benjamin – dissolved like the swoon of a television's closedown. There was only Haffner, in his second best tracksuit: and this figure in front of him, a resting contortionist.

For Haffner was beginning to understand.

That people tended to make other people up, that friendships tended to be formed between two imaginary people: Haffner knew this. What struck him as more poignant and more touching in the friendship of Zinka and Haffner was that it was so much less imaginary than he might ever have predicted. In ways which rather tended to be beyond him, Haffner seemed to offer her some kind of playfulness. And this version of Haffner, he thought, was the truest, the most profound.

When Esther was very young, she used to play with Haffner and their schnauzer. Livia would be in the kitchen, or the garden. In this way, the three of them formed a diminishing series: for Esther would only play so long as Haffner was there, a minor role. Just as

Haffner was only happy when he knew that Livia was there, some-where close, if out of sight. With Haffner in attendance, occasion-ally called on to settle some argument, or adjudicate some game, Esther played with her seven imaginary friends, while pensively chewing on the blonde curling tips of her hair.

Haffner wondered whether this resemblance perturbed him – between his daughter playing and a girl on his bed. He concluded that it did not. At that moment, he realised, he would accept what-ever conditions were imposed, whatever distortions might be demanded. He would do anything: just so long as he could be there, in the sunlit room, with Zinka.

He was interrupted momentarily from this glow of happiness by Zinka reaching a conclusion which Haffner only wished might be a little softer, a little less of a crescendo. And then there was a pause in which the world, sadly, began to right itself. Finally, Zinka sighed, began to move, and then turned round and sat there, on the bed, looking at him, a leg tucked under her waist: a seductive yogi.

She should probably go, said Zinka: Haffner agreed that yes, she probably should. So, then, she said. And he sat down, by the desk, marvelling – a vague state which meant that her dressing and smiling at Haffner, then leaving the room, then the door shutting with its slow delayed click all seemed to happen in a miracle of speed, without Haffner noticing.

She was the only woman he had ever met – apart from Livia, apart from Livia – marked by such self-possession.

But Haffner had no time to consider the line of his life: its line of beauty. Out of the bathroom, in an adagio of sadness, emerged the judgement of Haffner.

Haffner Guilty

1

As in the horror films of Haffner's silent youth, the door to the bathroom swung open, and no one emerged. There was silence: except, thought Haffner, for the liquid, aquatic soundtrack of the bathroom. Then Haffner understood that he was listening to the profound whisper of Frau Tummel's exhalations, the soughing of her inhalations. She had been standing there, staring into the mirror, her profile against the door. For a perturbed exalted moment, Haffner wondered if what he could hear was maybe the after-effect of a simultaneous Tummelian orgasm: still transcendent, cascading.

It was not.

Frau Tummel emerged from her oubliette. She made hungrily for her handbag and discovered her package of cigarettes. She lit one, then relaxed into the usual minimalist rhythm, standing at the window, grinning against the light. To the mountains, the unending sky, she said that she had never been so much made mock of. She was a wife, she was a mother. Everything she had, she had offered to Haffner. And this was how he treated her. He had let her say so many things. He had told her so many untruths.

He was like a boy, she said. This monster of immaturity! Even an adolescent would be more careful with love.

2

—But, argued Haffner, standing uneasily in the middle of the room.

At this point in his intricate reasoning, Frau Tummel interrupted.

She could not understand it. Was he rational? When he had done what he had just done? This man who had just shut her in a bathroom, while he entertained a woman in a way which she, Frau Tummel, could not explain. No, she could not understand it. A man who was dressed, as ever, in a variant on the shell suit.

Haffner only wanted to say, he began again. Again, he was forced to pause.

And although I am Haffner's historian, I can observe Frau Tummel too. He only wanted to mock her, she thought. He must have staged the whole thing. She was feeling so suddenly desolate. Now, she had no one. It was clear enough, she thought, that Haffner would never want her in the way that she wanted him to want her; and yet she did not want her husband, not quite, in the way that she wanted to want him either – a man who was so delicate, so unlike the ideal of Frau Tummel's youth.

Why, she said, must there be so much vulgarity with Haffner? Why this obscenity? Her voice accelerated into the upper registers. What beauty was there in his behaviour? Why the dirt, Raphael? Why this dirt?

And Haffner, still in the cloud of happiness produced by Zinka – illuminated, looking down on the pitiful world of humans – did not know what to say.

But of course, continued Frau Tummel, let everything descend to his level. Because he didn't understand the higher emotions. Haffner tried to remonstrate with her. When, said Haffner, had he ever? Whereas for her, continued Frau Tummel, fool that she was, it was a fantasy: of course, it was just a romance. If that was how he wanted to describe something eternal, something real.

—You! said Frau Tummel. In your tracksuit.

This point seemed incontrovertible.

—You want, she said, to be with this girl? This teenager? It disgusts me.

Once, this accusation would have seemed just to Haffner, perhaps: but not now. Up here, in the mountains, he had discovered a delighted sense of flippancy: yes, up here, he really could dispense with thinking in terms of the up or the down. As if the healthy were really ill. Or the old were really young.

So what could he say to soothe her? She wanted love to be a refuge: the desert island. But Haffner never thought that anywhere was safe; nowhere was truly deserted. Not even a marriage. It was, he thought, impossible to desert into another country, across the border, in the blue dawn.

It wasn't Haffner's fault, after all, if the moments of love and the moments of sex so rarely coincided.

—So, said Frau Tummel. So.

Haffner wondered what that meant. He wondered if he could ask.

It was always the same, said Frau Tummel. Men would always say they were in love, when all they wanted was the body of a woman; whereas for a woman, said Frau Tummel, it was absolutely opposite. He came from an outside place. But what could this man in front of her know about a true woman?

—But I never said I loved you, said Haffner.

And then he immediately regretted this moment of pointless truth. Suddenly, Frau Tummel stalled in the headlong pursuit of her anger. But then, perhaps this was what she had expected all along: this brutal Haffner.

It didn't mean, however, that Frau Tummel was not in love. It only confirmed her in her feelings all the more. The suffering was no contradiction. It couldn't be love, thought Frau Tummel, without the suffering. It came upon you, unbidden.

She waited for Haffner to say something kind, to tell her that of course he loved her. But Haffner simply stood there, deserted by his politesse: maimed by sincerity.

He refused to agree, said Haffner, with her theory. No, love was not a compulsion. The suffering was not necessary. It was just imagination, he told her. Everyone, said Haffner, chooses if they want to fall in love.

And as he said it, he wasn't sure if it was true. It didn't seem true of his love for Zinka. It had never been true of his love for Livia.

Let me be my own author! This was Haffner's cry. He wanted to be the one who invented his own stories as he went along. Except he hadn't then; and he couldn't now.

3

No, there was nothing masculine about Haffner's desire for Zinka: it did not obey the usual categories of Haffner: pursuit, and then seduction. Instead, it represented a happy passivity, content with whatever it might get.

Perhaps Zinka understood this. She wanted a man who was beyond the normal aggression. She wanted, really, an escape from the men. Whereas Frau Tummel – who craved the masculine – did not.

If Haffner were only allowed to exist in one sentence, it would be this: he was a desire that had outlived its usefulness.

And maybe this was the universal law of the empires: the law of decadence. That was the secret history of history. The very quality that led to an empire was the reason why that very empire would no longer be able to sustain itself. No contemporary, in the words of the great historian, could discover in the public felicity the latent causes of decay and corruption. He was talking about the Roman empire. But he could have been talking about Haffner. The long peace, and the uniform government of the Romans, introduced a slow and secret poison into the vitals of the empire. And so the minds of men were gradually reduced to the same level; everyone sunk into the languid indifference of private life.

Not survival of the fittest, then, but the deeper truth: survival of the weakest. Haffner had been so intent on the pursuit of women. He had always been kind to his desires. And now this very taste for possession had led to his transformation into the greatest of fantasists – the most elegant and whimsical of imaginative artists. Because the desire was still there, but Haffner was no longer in control of where he might act these desires out.

And this reminds me of one story from a more decadent empire than our own.

The emperor Elagabalus was emperor when the empire was disintegrating. As if that wasn't obvious. His reputation as a voluptuary was awesome. It might be possible, recorded Elagabalus's historian, that his vices and follies had been exaggerated; had been adorned in the imagination of his narrators. But even if one only believed those excesses which were performed in public, and attested to by many witnesses, they would still surpass the records of human infamy. Of these excesses, the one which I most admire is the way in which Elagabalus – the instigator of a coup – loved to dress up in women's clothes. He preferred the distaff to the sceptre, and distributed the honours of the empire among his male lovers, including one man who was invested with the authority of the emperor – or, as Elagabalus insisted on being known, the empress's husband.

Laughable, maybe – but man! What possessions one could enter into, when dispossessed to this extent!

4

Perhaps, said Frau Tummel, he simply lacked soul.

This was more than Haffner had expected. Perhaps, she continued, the spirit was beyond him. She was sure that he didn't even know how to cross himself. No, said Haffner, he didn't. This, said a demonstrative Frau Tummel, is how you do it.

Was it only Haffner, he wondered, who was constantly available for education?

Like this? he wondered. No, that was wrong, she said. The forehead first? queried Haffner. The forehead was not important, said Frau Tummel. The forehead was nothing. Why was he worrying about the forehead?

Then there was another knock at the door.

—Don't answer it! cried Frau Tummel.

—Why not? said Haffner, flinging open the door, to reveal a boy bearing a tray.

It was reception, he said. They were sending Haffner complimentary refreshment.

—Why? said Haffner.

—A gift, said the boy.

—From whom? said Haffner.

—I don't know, said the boy.

And he placed on the table an inaccurate planetarium: a galaxy of white chocolates, with seven half-moons of cinnamon biscuits.

Frau Tummel looked at Haffner.

—You mock me, she said.

And, for a moment, he wanted to enfold her in his arms and tell her no, he did not mock her at all.

He was truly a monster, she told him. What right did he think he had?

He could admit, as she said this, that there were ways of finding Haffner guilty. Therefore, maybe it was right that, more and more, his life resembled some bizarre form of punishment, some gonzo idea of karma. But Haffner wasn't one to be abused by ideas of sin. The devil, like all the other gods, was one invention among many, in Haffner's improvised theology: the gods were just decoration; scribbled marginalia. The gods were doodling. He preferred to form the categories himself. If Haffner were pressed, he preferred the more charming and likeable others: the demigods. The infinite fairies: the 33,000 gods of the pagan religions. These were the gods he might have called on when he felt that he was sinning. But the prospect was unlikely, He doubted that, if the gods existed, their concern would be the soul of Raphael Haffner.

—I said I loved you, said Frau Tummel.

She said it, he thought, as if she were in shock.

—It'll be OK, said Haffner. He knew this was not adequate. But there was nothing, he felt, he could say

Naturally, said Frau Tummel, she would have to consider whether to report the girl. It was only right. This seemed unnecessary, said Haffner. No, said Frau Tummel. It was only right. She had to consider what was right. Would there be anything he could do, said Haffner, to persuade her otherwise? Frau Tummel looked at him. She told him that no, there was not.

And she turned and left, theatrically slamming the door. Or, theatrically trying to slam the door: but the door, on its stiff spring-delay, braked, and softly, slowing, slowly, softly closed itself, in silence.

But what else had she expected? He was a monster, absolutely. A chimera, a griffin: a rabid centaur. Nor was this the first appearance of Haffner's multiple personality, his capacity for metamorphosis.

5

The night when Haffner proposed to Livia – just before Haffner was due to ship out – he had gone with some friends to the French Pub in Soho. And at that time he did not realise that the man behind the bar, with the Gallic twin-twirled moustache, was Victor Berlemont, the father of Gaston – Gaston, who after his retirement from the French Pub would play golf with Haffner twenty years later, in the other bohemia of Hendon. A man who understood the problematic species of herbs. With a Pernod in his hand – the first time Haffner had ever drunk this strange and continental liquor – he had talked to a girl about the higher things. Many times, Haffner had considered the uneasy fluctuations of one's sense of beauty. In wartime, he discovered, one could find beautiful most women you met. Because you needed beauty, for the desire to feel rational. Whereas the desire you felt in a war wasn't rational, and there was no beauty. She didn't believe, the girl in the French Pub had told him, that adultery was wrong. It was, let us say, a short story: to the side of the novel. He did not quite understand the analogy; he knew, however, what she meant. But that girl and her analogies dissolved into memory – the steep amphitheatre of Haffner's memory which he looked down on from the great height of his longevity, perched on his seat in the gods, looking down at the rabid lions, the dying Christians.

Haffner had left, and gone to meet Livia at the statue of Eros.

It was always like that, he thought. He wanted to be bohemian, and the bohemian eluded him. He had kissed the girl in the French Pub, and then left, before anything else might happen.

He took Livia for a meal on Shaftesbury Avenue. Then they had gone to some film: of which Haffner only remembered that a man spent a lot of time driving. This was, Haffner remembered, the main reason, it seemed, there had been for making a film: the mania for cars. It was so cool to drive that all any one in Britain wanted to see, all any one in Los Angeles wanted to film, was a man getting in and out of a car. And also, remembered Haffner, smoking a pipe. In and out of a car while smoking a pipe. That was cinema. Afterwards, they were in a taxi round the back of Leicester Square. They were taking Livia home. And did Livia know, asked Haffner, how dangerous it would be for him over there, soon, at the front? Livia made Haffner aware that she did. But perhaps, he continued – wishing he could not remember how the girl in the French Pub had kissed him, the thick dry texture of her lipstick, with its waxy faded rose perfume, like the greasepaint of his recent brief theatrical career, which she then reapplied, open-mouthed, after they had kissed, while Haffner watched the taut ellipse of her mouth – Livia did not quite appreciate the magnitude of the danger. The danger Haffner would be in, over there, at the front.

Haffner touched her on the cheek. He was twenty-two. She was twenty. It was very possible, he said, that he would never see her again. He might never come home. So would she, he said – looking down, bashful – consent to make him happy? It would mean so much to him, he said, to know that someone cared. Livia looked at him: and, as she used to tell Benjamin, and everyone else, for ever after, she did not know what else she could do. It seemed rude to say no. So she said yes and – feeling very fast – cuddled him up, and kissed him.

As Haffner silently and helplessly compared her nervous, gentle, motionless kiss to the inspired kiss of a girl four hours earlier, whose name he would never know.

Haffner Jewish

1

Because Haffner was now in a state of introspection; because his attempt to find Zinka, to warn her about the rages of Frau Tummel, had stalled when, as he leaned casually against the counter at reception, a man sporting a slicked quiff, with a paper rose in his lapel, smiled blankly at him and assured him that Zinka had left the hotel that day; because in any case Frau Tummel was unlikely to draw the hotel's attention to her surveillance of Haffner's bedroom: because of all these reasons, Haffner went walking again. His intention was to sit and reflect on the villa. He was due to meet Niko that evening, in their clandestine arrangement. Before that, he was eating supper with Benjamin. So Haffner now had two intentions. He wanted to sit and reflect, and check that his quest for the villa was being as slickly maintained as possible. And to do this, he intended to find a coffee: the blackest, most acrid, most Mediterranean coffee.

From this search, however, Haffner was sidetracked.

He didn't always know why he did things. He didn't know why, now, he had wandered into a church: first blinded by the darkness, then gradually seeing the light. A shrine on his left was an exhibition of car crash photos: for those who had survived miraculous suffering. A shrine on his right was an exhibition of baby photos, toddlers, foetal scans. The shrine of the miracle births. Haffner sat in a pew, his back straight, his knees aching, and looked up at the crucified God. He looked back down. A woman in a headscarf was shepherding seven bags of shopping. She bent low to worship her Lord.

Just as Livia had bent her head, when she crouched there, on all fours, waiting for the entrance of Haffner. Because she liked to see it, she said. She liked to watch him moving, between her legs.

Haffner looked up. He looked back down. The only prayers he knew were Jewish prayers, and so he tried to say them.

The Jews were, in the end, his people. If Haffner had a people.

Perhaps, then, this was not the digression it appeared to Haffner. Perhaps this was just another way for Haffner to consider his commitment to Livia's inheritance.

—Shema, Yisrael, he said, the Lord our God.

And then he could not remember anything else. Because the way up is the way down and the way left is the way right. He was in a church, and he was Jewishly praying. Did this matter? Was this the sort of action which damned a soul for all eternity? Haffner had no idea.

2

When Livia had died, Benjamin had taken Haffner aside. As if Benjamin were the grandfather. Perhaps, thought Benjamin, Haffner might find solace if he went to shul?

—Shul? said Haffner.

—Shul, said Benjamin.

—Since when, said Haffner, did you give up on the English language?

Haffner disliked the modern trend for Yiddish. It wasn't some recovered purity of the blood that Haffner cared about: instead

Haffner preferred the distinctions of the English language, was learned in the difference between a parvenu and an arriviste, a cad and a bounder.

On the other hand, the linguistics did not exhaust his irritation at Benjamin's suggestion.

Haffner rarely went to synagogue.

—You want to leave the synagogue? the Reverend Levine had said to him. Be my guest. I don't mind which synagogue you don't go to.

And Haffner had riposted with his own.

—Come on, said Haffner, winningly. What is the definition of a British Jew?

—Tell me, Raphael, said the Reverend Levine.

—A person, said Haffner, who instead of no longer going to church, no longer goes to synagogue.

Once, he had felt more allegiance to his religion. At school, he hadn't eaten the bacon, just the eggs; and when there was an exchange, and some German boys came over, he didn't want to speak to them: he had resented them being there. Yet he also went to chapel once a day, and twice on Sundays. He could have, naturally, been excused, but he still went.

—The thing about you, Benji had said to him, during one of their political discussions, is that you're so English. You're luke-warm.

—You're English too, said Haffner. Don't you be forgetting you're English.

—I'm not, said Benji. Well, I'm not English like you're English.

Just as in New York, when Morton persisted in his absolute belief that race was where it was at. That history was where it was at. That no one could be sincere if they tried to deny the world-importance of politics.

In this way, Haffner floated above the Atlantic Ocean, neither European nor American.

During the war, he had disturbed his Jewish friends – particularly Silberman, that comical Jewish soldier – with his unabashed hatred of the Stern Gang: the Zionist Jewish terrorists. With disdain, Haffner quoted from their newspaper, *The Front*, where the crazies argued, crazily, in Haffner's considered opinion, that neither Jewish morality nor Jewish tradition could negate the use of terror as a means of battle.

Haffner didn't care about birth or name or nation. He was not a stickler for such things. He was amused when Hersch Lauterpacht – Goldfaden's new friend – told him, many years after it happened, over dinner, that his nomination to the International Court of Justice had initially been blocked by the Attorney General, on the grounds that a British representative should both be and be seen to be thoroughly British, whereas Lauterpacht could not help the fact that he did not qualify in this way either by birth, by name or by education. Yes, how they had laughed, at Simpson's on the Strand, in 1980. How he had chuckled at this idea that they should in any way be seen as European.

My hero of assimilation! My hero of lightness!

Or so Haffner would have liked his story to be written. But it was not entirely true.

Haffner still treasured his family's stories from the shtetl. Or, more precisely, he treasured the story of their escape. How the final branch of the Haffner family tree to reach England had docked in Sunderland, in the midst of the nineteenth century, with Haffner's great-grandfather, a two-month-old baby, in a box. This was the family romance: the line of the Haffners had only survived the Lithuanian pogroms because of the silence and courage of great-grandfather Haffner, whose name was Isaac – the perfect silent baby. But, thought Haffner, where was the logic in this story? If one needed to hide the baby, surely one would have needed to hide oneself as well? And the chances of a baby remaining silent during a customs investigation, tight in a box, seemed highly unlikely.

So in what way would this ruse dupe an anti-Semite, in Prussia, with his sideburns and the plume of his helmet, the beige snuff stains on the crook of his thumb? But there it was: this story, invented or not, was the beginning of the Haffners' career in polite society. This silent infant generated the family law firm – which Haffner had refused – the house in north London, the servants, the cricket matches, the endless lawn-tennis lessons.

And his mother, his minuscule mother, who fasted every Yom Kippur: who stood on the steps of their synagogue in St John's Wood, asking Raphael to hold her, because she was dizzy.

Haffner thought that with these memories he was avoiding the pressing issue of the villa, the pressing issue of the women who had so invaded his stay here in the mountains. But there was passion in Haffner's indecision. He wanted to be a *flâneur*: he wanted to pretend that he had no engagements, no responsibilities. This ideal Haffner would idle through his memories – flick through them as through the pages of an outdated women's magazine, in the dentist's waiting room, while sitting beside an abandoned playpen made of multicoloured plastic. But this Haffner did not exist. No, the real Haffner was, as always, in the middle of things.

Here, in this church, Haffner tried to disappear from view. As he always tried to do. And he could not.

He was an aristocrat. Could no one understand this? Bourgeois, true, but an aristocrat! He had class. Even as they tried to force him into the Jewish working classes: the ordinary ranks of the Jews. The dispossessed; the heartbroken. No, Haffner had nothing to do with the Yiddish in London. *Koyfts a heft!* they used to cry, in the streets where Haffner was trying to find a cup of tea, after his cricket coaching in the East End. His cousins had set up the first ever mixed Jewish and Christian social club for boys in the East End locale of Bethnal Green, a club whose cricket team Haffner had coached to victory that same summer, the year before he went away to fight in the British army. Buy a pamphlet! they cried, crowding round

Haffner, with their Yiddish literary magazines, their Zionist *cris de coeur*.

Buy, thought Haffner, a fucking pamphlet yourself.

It had seemed so funny then. It seemed less funny now.

3

The aristocracy of Haffner was not a metaphor. A cousin on his mother's side was a viscount.

Yes, Haffner had history.

As a young man, Haffner's viscount had been moved by the plight of the underdog, the abandoned masses in their ghettos. He would go with his father – a liberal politician, a man of principle – to the dilapidated areas out to the east of London, where the less fortunate Jewish people lived, with their impoverished tailoring, cabinet-making, matchbox-making, fur-pulling. Then they would go to the park, to take a stroll, or a ride. The disparity between these two experiences moved the young politician: he wanted to do good. He was so moved that the syntax in his diary became impassioned, inverted. *What are they, dull, short-visioned, who see not the ground shaking beneath their very feet* – wrote the young liberal – *and angry voices, quiet, marvellously refraining yet, that are soon to rise, in ever-swelling clamour?* Later on, when he retired from public life, Haffner's viscount devoted his time to the writing of philosophy. He was, he said, a meliorist. He believed that, with only a small adjustment in our thinking, we would see that this world could indeed become the best of all possible worlds.

Whenever the business of imagining this thing called history came up in Haffner's life – on rare occasions, perhaps when rereading Churchill, or arguing with his grandson, or listening to the stories of Livia's family – he imagined history as a straight line. The line of gravity. The all-encompassing horizontal – its horizon – to which all bodies descended.

It was Haffner's viscount who had argued for the Jewish right of return to Palestine: the Arabs could not forbid the Jews to come back, he had argued, since the Jews were a people whose connection with the country long antedated their own – and especially as it had resulted in events of spiritual and cultural value to mankind in striking contrast with the barren record of the last thousand years. There could be no question, he had told the Prime Minister, Lloyd George, that the best thing for the land would be for it to be reclaimed by the Jews.

He was not dogmatic, however. The rights of the immigrants did not cancel out the rights of the natives: no, the arrival of the Jews must never be marked by hardship, expropriation, injustice of any kind for the people now in the land, whose forebears had tilled the soil and dwelled in the towns for a thousand years.

The viscount possessed the optimism of the romantic.

As the first ever High Commissioner of Palestine, the viscount had sent rare stamps to his philatelic king, painted with Churchill (whose paintings, he noted, were avowedly crude, but nonetheless effective, especially in colouring) and played tennis with Lord Balfour himself. Whose idea – along with that genius Weizmann – the whole country had been in the first place. And it was the viscount who was one half of the most famous anecdote about this country which they still called Palestine. When his predecessor, Chief Administrator Bols, was about to leave office, wrote the viscount, he asked the incoming commissioner to sign a receipt. The viscount asked for what. For Palestine, said Bols. But, replied the viscount, he couldn't do that. He couldn't mean it seriously. Certainly he did, said Major Bols. He had it typed out here. And he produced a slip of paper – *Received from Major-General Sir Louis J. Bols, KCB: one Palestine, complete* – with the date and a space for the viscount's signature. The viscount still demurred, but Bols insisted, so he signed; adding, however, the initials which used often to appear on commercial documents – E & OE, meaning Errors and Omissions Excepted. And Bols had this piece of paper framed, he was so pleased with it.

And when the viscount finally left the country, to further pursue his career back in Britain, he took with him a vision. In his memoir of his time in Palestine, he recorded the wide roads, bordered by little white single-storeyed houses, well spaced out, with creepers over their porches; around them, little gardens of flowers and patches of vegetables, with fields of waving corn and young plantations of trees beyond; groups of men and women in working-clothes, smiling girls and beautiful, healthy, white-dressed children; overhead, the cloudless blue sky. That, he said, was the vision with which he had left.

It wasn't Haffner's vision. Haffner thought it was schmaltz.

But it was with pride that, towards the end of 1942, he had learned in the newspapers of the viscount's speech in the Lords, on the reading of the declaration against German extermination of the Jews. This was not an occasion on which they were expressing sorrow and sympathy to sufferers from some terrible catastrophe due unavoidably to flood or earthquake, or some other convulsion of nature, the viscount had said. These dreadful events were an outcome of quite deliberate, planned, conscious cruelty on the part of human beings. Hear hear, the Lords had murmured. And Haffner with them, in Egypt. Absolutely.

Authority like this was what Haffner was destined for, thought Haffner. It was his inheritance: the natural deference shown to the political classes, the happy comforts of the *Finanzbourgeoisie*. A class to which he naturally belonged, thought happy Haffner, confirmed in this belief by the speech in the newspaper just as much as he was by his first ever deal – at Anzio, when he persuaded some desperate American, a friend of Morton's, just for a cheap bottle of whisky, to part with his regulation, all-terrain, multi-gear jeep.

4

The viscount, however, had still been moved by the ghettos. Whereas Haffner felt more distance from the Jewish underclass. The stories from the ghettos distressed him but they were not his. Partly, this was from a sense that as a cossetted Londoner he could hardly adopt the tragedies of people he never knew. A position which seems calmly moral, precisely modest, to me. But there was also a more complicated distance. The person Haffner knew best, whose stories were ghetto stories, was Goldfaden. With Livia, thought Haffner jealously, Goldfaden possessed a tragic European past. So this meant, I think, that Haffner sometimes exaggerated his haughtiness in regard to history. For Haffner was not without his own sense of racial possessiveness. In Haffner's opinion, there was no reason for the working classes, for the Blacks and the Chinese, to avail themselves of this word *ghetto*. It was a Jewish possession. No one else had suffered like the Jews had suffered. No one else had been persecuted with such universal thoroughness.

In Venice, on holiday with Esther and her family, in the early 1980s, Haffner and Livia wandered away from San Marco: they ended up in what had been, Livia informed him, reading from a guidebook, the original ghetto (—From the sixteenth century! she exclaimed). In the bleak hot sunlight, no one was moving. On the seventh floor of a tenement building, some washing was strung on runners. A wireless was talking to itself.

In this ghetto, Haffner and Livia discussed their recurrent story of the Ghetto: the story of Goldfaden's uncle, Eli, who was now a cameraman in LA.

Eli had not been on the family holiday in London with the Goldfadens. So he was left behind in Warsaw. Before the war, he had been a member of the Bund, the General Jewish Labour Union. He believed in a strange combination of the Yiddish language and culture, and secular Jewish nationalism. Like Livia's father, and Haffner, he was not a Zionist. Unlike them, he expressed this Yiddishly, through his devotion to *doyigkeyt*, to hereness. His family lived on Sienna Street, near the Jewish quarter. And Eli, Goldfaden used to tell Livia, as they reminisced about

Europe – while Haffner glanced at the diary pieces about his financial rivals in the evening papers – Eli was so earnest in his devotion to learning that he even read the novels which were serialised in the newspapers. A man should be prepared, thought Eli. Nothing was alien to him.

In Warsaw, before the revolt in the Ghetto, and before the uprising in the city, but when everything still was bleak, Eli had been told to go with his parents to the main square. This seemed reasonable. Or, at least, not unreasonable. In the square, they were told to walk in single file to the train station, where a train was waiting at each platform. They had asked the rabbi if this seemed advisable. The rabbi, after long deliberation, thought that the best thing to do was obey those in power. Could they really wish them harm? And this, said Goldfaden, was where his cousin became heroic. He came to a decision. No one had ever heard again from those who had got on the trains to the east. Eli knew this. Therefore, concluded Eli, he would run. So what if he were shot in the back, his kidneys torn inside him? He would prefer to stage his own death, rather than sleepwalk into it. And so he ran, and managed to hide out in the rubble of a destroyed apartment block.

Here, in the ghetto in Venice, just before Haffner had retired, Livia had praised Eli once more. But Haffner, this time, had paused. Then he had asked her: what about the others? She had asked him what he meant. They paused and looked at a dark canal. What about the others, the ones the man had left behind? said Haffner. What about his parents? And Livia had replied that they all died. Naturally, they had died. The moral value of Eli's act seemed to Haffner to be complicated by this. He had chosen to abandon his friends. And maybe this was fine, maybe this was unremarkable, but Haffner thought that, at the very least, it was a complication.

She should have known, said Livia, that Haffner would be difficult.

Yes, said Haffner, Haffner would be difficult. Why shouldn't he be difficult?

And perhaps Haffner was right, even if he was only accidentally right, by transforming Eli's story into a story of Haffner: a compromise.

Haffner saw in this anecdote the grand bravery of refusing to act in the way you were supposed to act. In Haffner's rewrite, Eli's escape from the Ghetto was also a desertion.

5

According to Livia, the story of Eli was not a story of a desertion, because a desertion was morally bad. An escape, however, was morally good. But I am not so sure that the two can be so easily divided. People call a flight an escape, only after having been forced to give up the idea that it is moral to remain in a bad situation. So often, people think that if one person is suffering, then everyone else should suffer too. In these cases, if someone takes flight, then their escape is just a desertion.

Yes, the whole vocabulary of flight is puritanical. So every act of desertion is also an act of hedonism.

And maybe the deep reason for this is that no one likes a deserter, an escapee, because it proves the fact that there is always a choice. So often, it is easier to believe that life is a trap. The trap is the image of life's seriousness.

Haffner, however, my hero, did not believe that life was serious. He didn't believe that one must necessarily be faithful to the ordinary, inevitable tragedy of a life. If one could be faithless to anything, Haffner always hoped, surely it would be to one's own past?

But, however much I admire the hope, I am not so sure that this kind of infidelity is possible. And there, in the church, nor was Haffner. Because the story of Eli now made Haffner remember another story which he preferred to keep to himself: how under the patronage of the Reverend Levine, the appointed guardian of Jewish refugees from Germany, a girl stayed in the Haffners' house, in 1938. He didn't remember very much about her: he couldn't remember her name. He knew very little, but he believed that she took her own life. Not when she was staying with them, but eventually.

She must have been about twenty. He didn't remember even trying to talk to her. She must have been with them a very short time, thought Haffner. She was extremely unhappy. Perhaps they couldn't cope with her. Yes, in his mind, he heard that she had taken her own life. But his mind was a bit hazy. He hadn't got involved – but he knew that there was somebody there, upstairs, in the spare room. She was always asleep. He had no idea how it had been organised.

This was what it was to be Jewish in Britain. The East was always making its demands on you: the grief of its history entered your life and so it became your own. You were always being forced back: beyond the pale.

He couldn't remember that girl's name.

He was not sinful: he refused all ideas of sin. But if Haffner had ever sinned, thought Haffner, then this forgetting was it.

6

In the dark church Haffner called on God: —You are the Lord my God, Haffner exclaimed, in silence, in the darkness of this church, and I am a clod of dirt and a worm; dust of the ground and a vessel of shame.

But Haffner didn't need his God for such lavish repentance. The women were enough.

Haffner had used the infidelities within his marriage as the Orthodox used the eruv. They were exercises in invention; the riches of self-blame. His interior life was festooned with sagging squares of string, marking out the permitted areas within the forbidden world. He believed in marriage like the Orthodox believed in God. It was a territory for permitting the unpermitted.

And for testing the soul of Haffner.

Livia had been expert at the put-down. She was, in Haffner's language, a strong woman. This trait had endeared her to him. At the official dinners, the unofficial suppers, Haffner bore with pleased and happy grace her talent to resist Haffner's charm, believing that this public scepticism served to illustrate his moral grandeur, his lack of vanity. It was not an unusual moment in his life when, on the night of the dinner for the City Branch of the Institute of Bankers in 1982, he came into her dressing room while she was in her underwear – blue lace, white frills – and with a crooked finger, its nail tipped with a varnish whose colour Haffner would never be able to name, she pointed out to him the direction of the door. And in his socks he turned around and left.

Retrospectively, however, this moment had acquired a unique weight. For that, thought Haffner, was when he understood that his marriage had in fact been governed by forces which he did not understand or control. That night, after Haffner's speech, after the speeches reciprocating Haffner's speech, as they were driving home in Haffner's Saab – with Livia driving, because Haffner was utterly drunk – Haffner quizzed her on the significance of why he had found her sitting outside the venue, the Butchers' Hall; why he had found her sitting there with Goldfaden, sharing a cigarette while the meat-market traffic began revving and chirring around them and the rinsing smell of meat gusted and retreated: yes, why had he found them there, sitting peaceably, with Goldfaden cupping her hand as he lit her cigarette? And at the time Haffner had not so much minded about the fact that he had never seen her smoking; nor that it was a habit she had excoriated in Haffner: he minded about the casual way in which Goldfaden touched her hand.

Calmly, without malice, Livia had simply told Haffner that it was not as if he could really lecture her. It was not as if he could condemn what she had done, and would continue to do.

Drunk, silenced, Haffner considered this. And what he wanted to say was that the two were incomparable: because when it came to women, Haffner had only ever got whoever came along. They loved him, true – but Haffner never really loved them back. He just amazed them with the strength of his devotion: a devotion which was indistinguishable from the fear that they would leave him. Even if no one did leave Haffner. Whereas Livia had something else. Livia, it seemed, had love.

—Do you love him? asked Haffner.

And Livia, braking gently at the traffic light by the Hampstead pond, said that yes of course: naturally, she said – and she touched Haffner, gently, on the cheek. So Haffner asked her what they were going to do about it now, to which Livia simply replied that she saw no reason to do anything.

Livia didn't believe in an escape.

She parked the car in the drive, went into the house, and Haffner sat there: listening to the rose bushes' gentle crackle in the wind. Just as now, years later, Haffner sat in a church and surveyed the wondrous mistakes of his life: his infidelity to his wife, his infidelity to his race. Or, to put it another way, his infidelity to the women he had slept with – to Barbra, to Pilar and Joan and Laure and all the other names he now could not remember – his infidelity to his nation.

All the nebulous fairies of his history and his politics, dissolving, now, on a midsummer night, in the middle of nowhere.

He was such a klutz, thought Haffner. Then he translated himself out of Goldfaden's language. He was a fool.

It was fitting, really, that one of Goldfaden's favourite party tricks was his riff on the word *dope*. As Goldfaden would explain to you, it was the trickiest word in the language: on the American side, it came from the Dutch for sauce, so meaning any kind of goo, lubricant, liquid, liquor, and hence any kind of narcotic, drug, medicine, adulterating agent, and hence, through the racetracks, and their need to know the inside dope, all esoteric lore, all arcana. And there it met, at its apex, the British derivation, from dupe, meaning the gull, the fool, the absolutely-in-the-dark: and where else were we, Goldfaden would conclude, if not always in the dark, drugged by lack of knowledge, unaware of the systems which eluded us and which invaded us at every moment? This word *dope* was the real thing which bound the British and Americans together: this was the real Atlantic Ocean.

But at this point, with this word *dope*, Haffner had gone as far as he could in the business of self-discussion. Because everything was obvious to him now. Everything had always been to do with Livia. And Haffner had never noticed.

It was so evident, so infinite in its evidence, that Haffner had never known.

7

Haffner stood up: he turned to go – making for the Chinese restaurant where he was meant to eat with Benjamin. In front of the church, where the baroque facade hid the brick barn of a nave, a line of floats was parked, each decorated with a *tableau vivant*. All the actors in these *tableaux* were children. Surrounding them, the adults of the town were taking photographs. Saint Peter was scratching the side of his nose with a translucent wafer, while another boy in white shirt and black trousers kneeled before him, on a plush velvet cusion, with his eyes escaping through the trickle of his fingers.

No, thought Haffner, observing the children. Some things were irreversible. The entropy of Haffner! Not everything could be recuperated. Like Haffner's gilded youth. For how can a man be young, when he is old? He knew enough of the Bible to know that this was difficult.

As Morton would have said, do the math.

Only on the last day in Cairo, in 1946, did Haffner write to Livia as his wife. Throughout their engagement and the early years of their marriage, throughout the war, he had referred to her as his darling girl, his sweetheart. Only now, in the last letter he would write to her from the war, when he was coming home, did Haffner address her as his very darling wife.

—*I only pray that you will find me a better man than when I left you and that I will fulfil all your dreams,* he wrote. *I believe that we can do tremendous things together and that with our lives, with our happiness, we can make others happy. And that is what I think life is for, the real purpose behind it all.* So Haffner wrote to Livia, the night before he sailed back to England, in 1946.

—*Bless you, my beloved girl,* wrote Raphael Haffner, *keep you safe always.*

PART FOUR

Haffner Gastronomic

1

The meals of Haffner and Benjamin were epic. In this gargantuan size, they expressed their love. They went to Bodean's on Poland Street and sucked at the burned ends and ribs of cows – which jutted out forlornly, and unevenly, like organ pipes. They were experts in the cuts of steak: both convinced that the aged hanger steaks of New York were the greatest of them all. Then there were the deep-fried marvels of Japan: the chicken katsu, endowed with its cloudy pot of barbecue sauce. Candy undid them: not the ordinary treats, but the strange, gourmet sugar of internationally local cuisines: nougat, glacé cherries, marzipan fruits, baklava. They invented festivals of junk food: on one famous occasion, they had walked down Oxford Street, eating at every branch of American burger chain they could find. But there was more. This more was the Chinese food.

There was nothing, said Benjamin, more Jewish than this – Haffner's passion for Chinese food. Nothing more emphasised, said Benjamin, his genetic roots to the scattered race.

Haffner looked at him, amazed: his own grandson, with the same weird theory of Chinese food as Goldfaden. Or perhaps he was misremembering. This was, after all, possible.

Underneath a red paper lantern, Benjamin's cheeks were carmine – incandescent. On his face shone a glaze of sweat, echoing the lacquer on the slices of pork belly which lay, unguent, on their bed of shredded iceberg lettuce set before Haffner.

—You ordered the crispy beef, said Benji.

—Yes, I ordered the beef, said Haffner. Of course I ordered the beef. Wait a minute.

Benjamin swivelled round. Or, he swivelled as much as his bulk would allow: an imperfect barn owl.

He saw no one who could help him. He turned back to Haffner.

They continued to argue over whether Haffner should keep his appointment with Niko. Haffner thought it was obvious; Benjamin thought it was less obvious. But he couldn't see, said Haffner, what he had to lose. Could Benjamin explain this to him? He wasn't so proud that he would refuse someone else's help.

It was the principle, said Benjamin. He didn't know these people. How could he trust them?

What kind of principle was that? replied Haffner. It was fear, that was all. And they were hardly, said Haffner, going to rob him – and he exhibited his Nike T-shirt; his flared turquoise track-suit trouser.

Benji swivelled round once more: he still saw no one who could help him.

Sighing, he turned back, and introduced a new topic of conversation.

What, he wanted to know, did Haffner know about hip hop?

—Hip hop? queried Haffner.

—Hip hop, confirmed Benjamin. But not the West Coast hip hop, nor the East Coast hip hop. Instead, his new thing was South Coast: the hip hop of urban and immigrant France.

In this way, Benji combined a former craze, his craze for hip hop, with his new – and, he believed, ultimate – craze for love. In Tel Aviv, he had been introduced by the girl who had deflowered him to the classics of French hip hop: the angry *banlieusards* in the angry *banlieues*.

This was, after all, why he had come to the spa town. Benjamin was in love. He was in love, and was here to receive advice from Haffner.

So he talked about hip hop. To Benji, this seemed logical.

As he ate, Benjamin described the curious fact that his two favourite songs, at this moment, were both about terror: the French hip-hop song called 'Darkness', and the French hip-hop song called 'Mourir 1000 fois', with its dark first line: in which the rapper told his terrified audience about his fears of death, in which the chorus simply stated that existence was punishment. They entranced Benji with their myth of the grand: the imagination of disaster. This was why he so loved the rappers from Marseilles: a city he had never been to; a city which, if he were honest, scared him with its reputation for the brutal.

Everything in Benjamin's life now seemed so fraught with significance. As if, thought Benji, he could destroy his whole life with one wrong decision.

He hazarded this to Haffner. Haffner thought it was unlikely that a life could be destroyed. It would take more than one wrong decision for that. Then he reached for the giant bottle of beer in front of him, and poured an accidentally overfoaming glass.

The restaurant advertised itself as Chinese. In its provenance, the food perhaps tended more towards the Vietnamese than the Chinese. There were moments when it was nothing but Thai. But no one here was concerned with the detail of origins: not the sullen Slavic waiters, the absent owners. Haffner, however, didn't care. So long as the effect was Oriental, then Haffner was happy. It possessed an aquarium in which melancholic fish hid themselves beneath mossy banks, munching sand. It seemed Oriental enough for Haffner.

In this setting, Haffner sat and listened to his grandson: his anxious grandson. He was, thought Haffner, the kind of kid who was so vulnerable to women that he'd probably get aroused just by the naked mannequins in shop windows, their robotic defenceless arms. Their invisible nipples and missing pubic hair, like some statue of Venus found beneath the tarmac of a Roman street.

But I think that Haffner could have gone further than this. There was so much to worry about, when considering the character of Benji.

2

Benji was the solitary only child. At fourteen he threw up in a girl's toilet after an evening of drinking whisky and was pleased at the suavity of his aim until he found out the next day that they had found sick everywhere. He used to listen to Liverpool matches on his clock radio in the dark under his Tottenham Hotspur duvet, for he was fickle. The first girl he kissed frightened him. Aged nine, he used to rehearse cricket strokes with a cricket stump and a practice golf ball in his bedroom, while listening to the classic ballad 'Take My Breath Away' on repeat. Like Haffner, the songs were always his downfall. He listened to 'Bridge Over Troubled Water' when Esmond drove him to the cricket matches.

Nothing in Benjamin's early youth had poise, or cool. Instead of cool, the miniature Benjamin hoarded Haffner's anecdotes. The stories of Haffner formed Benji's inheritance.

He treasured a portable Joe Davis snooker table – made on the Gray's Inn Road, in London, and guaranteed to add a touch of fun to family occasions – which he had found in Haffner's loft. One ball, the pink, was still in the centre right pocket, slung in the netting. It nestled there, solidly. Benjamin studied the faint lines printed on the baize. There were shiny trails of turquoise chalk. There was a line horizontally printed across the table, a little below the top. From this, a semicircle arched and settled. It reminded Benjamin of a soccer pitch. It was like a magnified penalty area. But this was not why Benji loved it. Its instructions, glued to the wooden underframe, were signed, in facsimile, by the great Joe Davis himself. From then on, in bed, with his clock radio beside him, its incensed digital digits flipping luminously and silently, Benjamin would read about Thurston's Billiards Hall in Leicester Square. Because he was romanced. For Haffner was Joe Davis's banker, in the 1950s. One day Joe Davis was in South Africa, at a hotel. He was resting. He was having some time off snooker. But then some guy challenged Joe Davis to a game. This man didn't know Joe Davis was Joe Davis. He thought he was just an ordinary person. It was, Haffner would remind his grandson, before the days of television. Joe Davis tried to refuse. He didn't want to play snooker, on his holiday. But the man was insistent. So Joe Davis played snooker. Naturally, he played with exquisite grace. And his challenger was amazed.

—What are you: Joe Davis or something? he said.

And Joe Davis paused.

—No, he said, but I know the man who sleeps with his missus.

Yes, Benji loved his grandfather: his grand grandfather. He was a romantic. And the romance was all inherited from Haffner.

So Benjamin found himself here: in a Chinese restaurant on the outskirts of a spa town, in the centre of Europe. And because he was here, he could ask Haffner anything.

—Is it true, said Benji, that you once gave away the Mercedes to someone else?

—No, said Haffner. No, it isn't.

—OK, said Benjamin.

He returned to the more familiar ground.

—This food is good, said Benji: piercing the inflated curve of a chicken dumpling with a chopstick. I mean it's exquisite.

Haffner queried this; the food, he thought, verged on the inedible:

like every cuisine in this town. But for a moment Haffner loved him – his progeny with the marvellous appetite.

3

The problem was, Benji told Haffner, how did he know that this wasn't a craze? Because he was prone to crazes, he knew this. It was just that this didn't feel like a craze. It felt true. What else did he feel but love, thought Benji, when looking at the curve of his girl's breasts, matched yearningly by the imitative curve of his penis in his briefs? But, continued Benjamin, even if it was true, how important was this, in the end? It was only desire. It wasn't everything. So maybe he should return to his summer school, and forget all about her.

Haffner raised an eyebrow.

And he considered how, in the more ordered nineteenth century, the ordinary family judgement was the father on the son. This was how Haffner's life had begun – with Solomon Haffner in judgement. Now that the twentieth century was ending, however, it turned out that there could be something different: the judgement of the grandfather on the grandson. But instead of judging him for his lack of restraint, it was the lack of chutzpah which Haffner found wanting in his descendant. He would have to educate him into courage.

—Let me tell you my story about Palestine, said Haffner.

—No, I know this story, said Benji.

—I haven't started, said Haffner.

—Your Jewish story? said Benjamin.

—I will tell you again, said Haffner.

Having missed the major battle of the war in North Africa, then serving in the liberation of Italy, Haffner had been posted to Palestine. He was twenty-four at the time, he reminded Benji. He was – how old was Benjamin? He was about the same age as Benji was now. In fact, Jerusalem was the setting for his twenty-fourth birthday, on which day he announced he was going to drink twenty-four pink gins. And he did.

His battalion was ordered to keep the peace between the Arabs and the Jews: or, more precisely, between the Arabs and the crazy Russian Zionist Jews.

His people! As if those crazies were his people! What did Haffner have to do with the Orthodox, the serious – complete with dyed sidelocks and dyed caftans, the fringes of their prayer shawls ragged around their waists? In Palestine, Haffner had learned one of his very first truths. To be bohemian you had to be an absolute insider. It was the recent immigrants, the suddenly displaced, who most believed in nations and in boundaries. The ones who believed in a people at all.

Benjamin threw a wasabi pea up into the air and, to his profound satisfaction, caught it in the maw of his mouth.

Haffner ignored him.

It turned out, however, that in the eyes of the British war cabinet the crazies were Haffner's people. All members of the Jewish faith, commissioned or uncommisioned, were to leave the battalion in Palestine and travel to Cairo in the next forty-eight hours. This was the order. And yes, Haffner would concede, if discussing the matter with a benign historian, at that time the Jewish underground was conducting tactics not dissimilar to those of the IRA – but the order utterly devastated him. He had been with his battalion for nearly five years and fought through the Battle of Anzio, the only battle – he would remind this now less benign historian – in the World War which, like the Great War, had been fought in the trenches, and here he was to be kicked out because of his faith. He wouldn't stand for it. His faith, not his race. This was the important distinction. Even if Haffner still had a faith at all, which was doubtful.

Haffner was the senior Jewish member of the battalion, so he called all ranks together: about thirty of them. All felt as Haffner did, with one exception. Whose name now eluded him. Haffner went to see the CO, who took him that evening to see the divisional commander in his HQ at Mount Carmel overlooking Haifa. He was a Canadian, who afterwards became Vice Chief of the Imperial General Staff.

At this point in the story, Haffner would put on an accent which he assumed was Canadian (it was not).

—Well, Haffner, I'm a Canadian, and if I were asked to fire on my boys in Montreal, I'd refuse.

—But, Haffner replied, in his own voice, I do not regard the Jews here as my boys. I'm an Englishman and my faith is Jewish.

Benji continued to scan the empty restaurant for a waiter to bring the beef: crispy, shredded. Or the approximation to crispy shredded beef which Benjamin had hoped to see in the fried ripped beef offered to him by the menu's translation: in haphazard italics, and assorted brackets.

—It's a good story, said Benjamin.

—The divisional commander, said Haffner.

—You should do the clubs, said Benji, grinning. I'm amazed you haven't.

The divisional commander, said Haffner, gave him permission to go and see the C.-in-C., Middle East Forces, in Cairo. So Haffner went with his driver, Private Holmes. They travelled 600 miles in twenty-four hours. Across the only little metal road in the desert to Cairo. Put up in a hotel to wait the pleasure. Etc. His driver had sunstroke and went into hospital. But the C.-in-C. had been sent to deal with the Communist threat in Greece. So Haffner was seen by his deputy, who sympathised, but there was nothing he could do. It was a cabinet decision.

A cabinet decision, emphasised Haffner. This was in about November 1945. In June, the war in Europe had come to an end. It was now three years since he had last seen his wife, just after their wedding. For the early married life of Haffner and Livia was an absence: a hiatus. And here he was being questioned about his Jewish loyalty: his Eastern heritage.

—No really, like Lenny Bruce, said Benjamin.

Haffner's East!

Looking back on Haffner, he was so clear to himself – it was like he was made of the most transparent glass. He had always wanted to mean something: to reach the grandeur of the world-historical. Like all the characters in the grand novels: the American novels which Esther used to give as Christmas presents to Haffner, to further his education. But the problem wasn't Haffner, he was discovering: the problem was the world-historical. Not even the world-historical was world-historical. The instances of everything, Haffner thought, had turned out to be so much smaller than one expected. The magnificence was so much more minute than one expected.

He had gone to school with the man who later married the Prime Minister. He remembered her, from the days watching her son play cricket. Once, in the 1970s, before she became the party leader, he danced with her at a dinner at the Criterion. She was really very brilliant.

Haffner emptied his glass of its pale beer. He felt a little blurred, a little faded – a faded Haffner which dissolved even further as the tape in the restaurant came round to one of his favourite songs, in one of his favourite incarnations.

—You know this song? cried Haffner.

—No, said Benjamin.

—Then listen! said Haffner.

4

And Haffner floated away: forwards, into the past.

For when they began the beguine – according to Cole Porter, as sung by Ella Fitzgerald, as listened to by Haffner as he tried to educate his grandson – the sound of that beguine brought back the sound of music so tender; it brought back the night of tropical splendour; it brought back a memory evergreen. And then Ella's voice went higher. She was with him once more under the stars, and down by the shore an orchestra was playing, and even the palms seemed to be swaying when they began the beguine.

He had heard this song with Livia, sung by Ella, in Ronnie Scott's on Frith Street: and the shadow of the double bass's scroll on the white backing screen was a seahorse behind the Lady. She was in a gold lamé dress.

But you couldn't go back. This was the meaning of the song. But precisely because one couldn't go back, thought Haffner, was why one wanted to go back. Precisely because one had lost everything.

Yes, weakened, exhausted, melancholy, Haffner was beginning to revise his ideas of sin. It was so hard, he was finding, not to regret certain aspects of one's life, now that one considered one's life carefully.

And so the reason why Haffner so loved this song now, here in a Chinese and Slavic restaurant, was that it allowed you the romance of resurrection, of recuperation. It allowed you the dream.

For, against all expectation, the rhythm moved into a different beat; so that, as Ella's voice rose, she changed her rhythm against the beat – as she begged them not to begin the beguine; as she begged the orchestra to let the love which was once a fire remain an ember. And then again, in a contradiction which Haffner had always cherished (—Listen to this! he cried to Benji. Listen to this!), Ella with as much sad abandon contradicted herself, with the same push against the beat, the same refusal to give in to the obvious rhythm: that yes, let them begin the beguine, make them play till the stars that were there before return above them, till whoever it was who she loved might whisper to her once more, darling, that he loved her – and the song softened. And they would suddenly know, as she quietened down, what heaven they were in – she quietened to a becalmed softness – when they began the beguine.

5

—Yeah, it's cool, said Benjamin.

Haffner didn't know what to say. He was lost, in contemplation of his past.

Finally, Haffner spoke.

—You finished? he asked Benjamin. You full?

—I don't finish when I feel full, said Benjamin proudly. What kind of person finishes when they're full? Me, I finish when I hate myself. That's the treasured moment.

And as Benjamin said this, more dishes arrived: chicken in a black bean sauce; chicken with lemon. Then finally another porcelain plate, chased with fake Chinese scenes: on which cubes of beef were shivering. Then two more decanters of beer.

In a reverent silence, Benji's mind considered Haffner's ideas of loyalty. Oh Benji wanted so much to lose his loyalty! He wanted so much to leave his religion behind. He imagined himself in the backstreets of Paris, the docks of Marseilles, and it entranced him. But he found this subject difficult. The guilt distressed him. So, in defence against himself, Benji tried to talk himself out of his new temptations.

—I don't get this, said Benji.

—You don't get what? asked Haffner.

—I don't see why it's more cosmopolitan to be anti-Zionist, said Benji. It just means you feel more nationalist about Britain.

—Don't be clever, said Haffner.

Gluttonous, still perplexed by Haffner's ideas of loyalty, Benji continued to reach for the black bean chicken with his chopsticks: trembling in the air, like dowsers. Haffner continued too. On one thing were Haffner and Benjamin agreed: the absolute superiority of MSG – that glorious chemical. They adored its sweet and savoury slather – and there it was, unctuous, before them.

Through the prism of his newly sexual nature, Benjamin considered the problem of fidelity. Perhaps, he thought, there was something in what Haffner said. Maybe it was true that it was better to refuse one's own nation. And I think that I should repeat that Benji had inherited from Haffner the love of romance. So he liked the grander, political structure which Haffner's theory offered him when he considered his current predicament, more than the crudely sexual structure in which it was housed at the moment. It was nothing to do with the girl! Nothing to do with the smell of her, which Benji had caressed with his nostrils all the next day, and night, refusing to wash. Nothing to do with the wet warmth of her mouth on his penis. All of Benji's urges, he thought, were simply desires to be free. They were all about his new refusal to be faithful to irrelevant ideals.

It did seem possible.

—So then, said Haffner. Time to go.

—You can't, said Benjamin.

—I am, said Haffner. I'm meeting this man, and I'm meeting him now.

Had Benjamin, wondered Haffner, any better ideas? No, thought Benjamin. He didn't. He only knew that he had barely begun the conversation he wanted to have. He had barely begun at all.

If he wanted, said Haffner, if he was really worried, then Benjamin could call him. Haffner promised to keep his phone on. And then Haffner, replete with a final spring roll, having laid down his chopsticks on their concertina of wrapper, and given Benjamin a selection of banknotes to pay for the meal – a meal in which

Benjamin settled to the last dishes, as if to the last supper – ventured back out into the fading day.

And as he walked, he hummed. In the tropical night, the beguine washed over him.

Raphael Haffner was drunk.

Haffner Drunk

1

In the driveway of the hotel, Niko was in his car – now wearing a pair of outlandish tinted glasses – waiting for Haffner.

The sky was fading, elaborating its golden cloths. And all its other traditional effects.

—Yes we have it, he said. I have found your man.

Haffner peered into the car. There was a plastic bag full of Coke cans in the footwell behind the driver's seat. A packet of cigarettes was protruding from the open glove compartment. The radio, to Haffner's antiquarian delight, was only a radio – without even the empty slit for a cassette.

Niko's jacket had the word *death* stitched gothically at the back of its collar. He took it off, and threw it on to the back seat – so revealing a T-shirt which said *Godless Motherfucker*.

This was the company Haffner now kept. He decided that he rather liked it.

—You saw my girl, yes? said Niko chirpily, bending to slurp at the keyhole of a newly opened can of Coke.

—Yes, said Haffner, deciding that it would be best if he stopped the sentence there.

—Uhhuh, uhhuh, said Niko.

To this, Haffner maintained his politic silence.

—You like potato chips? said Niko: trying to begin a conversation as they drove off.

Niko, the athlete, was always snacking. He offered Haffner an angled tube.

—No, said Haffner: feeling drunk, and sick.

Their destination was a billiards and pool hall – on the opposite edge of the town to Benjamin's utopian Chinese restaurant, in an industrial complex – on the second floor of what appeared to have been intended as an office block. On the ground floor were a hairdresser supply shop – whose windows were hung with posters displaying the moustaches and side-partings of another era – and a shop selling carpet to the outfitters of mid-range business premises. Each window of the billiards hall was blacked out.

Their contact was already there. To Haffner's disturbed surprise, he discovered that he recognised this contact.

—I'm sorry, he said to Niko. I don't think I got his name.

—Viko, said Niko, pointing to his misprinted double.

—Ah yes, of course, said Haffner.

And Haffner gazed over at his masseur.

Haffner wondered if this would be awkward. All that was needed, he concluded, if the man could indeed do what he said he could do, was a brisk, businesslike demeanour.

He looked around: at the wall lamps, visored by green eyeshades; at a bar of chocolate on a table, its foil wrapper partially unwrapped, exposing its ridged segments – like a terrapin, or grenade.

He had hoped for something more; he had hoped for a man in a suit, with a briefcase and moustache. He had certainly hoped for a stranger. A powerful, authoritative stranger. If Haffner had ever had to imagine how this kind of business might be done, difficult as it may have been, he would have been able to be precise about the clothes. It most certainly would not have featured this man's obvious pleasure in contemporary sportswear.

As if, conceded Haffner, Haffner could talk: this man without a wardrobe.

2

Viko was a drifter; a man of travels. His career had taken him along the fabled European coasts: from Juan-les-Pins to San Remo, from Dubrovnik to Biarritz. His trade was that of the hotelier. Wherever he went, he found work in the spas of luxury retreats, the reception desks of grand hotels. In this trade, he had grown sleek. He had also become expert in the wiles of the world. Not for Viko, the moral life. He preferred corruption, blackmail: the free flow of information.

He kept himself to himself, this was how Viko put it. It was not quite how his colleagues put it. They knew him as rather more sinister: a fixer; a man who was protected, and who could, in his turn, offer protection to others. His ethics were those of the favour. He dispensed largesse. In return, he received the loyalty of chambermaids, office assistants, waiters, car-wash attendants. Often no one knew where Viko was: his movements were uncertain. His apartment was always blandly comfortable: on the walls, posters of Renaissance gods, and cubist still lifes.

Yes, out of his uniform – out of the shorts and cotton sports shirt, the tennis shoes – Viko was transformed. No longer the man who pampered the pampered rich. Now, he was in power.

Viko walked up to Haffner and Niko, nodded, then walked past them to the bar. But the barman was not there. He was taking the garbage out. Viko waited. He turned from the bar and reapproached them.

—How are you, my friend? said Viko to Niko. You are like Elton John, no?

Viko was wearing a T-shirt which did not conceal the fact that his forearms and upper arms were plaited with muscle, like challah bread. He put imaginary binoculars to his face. He grinned, behind his binoculars, scanning the limited horizon.

—In those glasses.

Niko smiled. He looked at Haffner. Haffner smiled at Viko, nervously.

The label of Viko's shirt, which lolled over the collar, was still pierced by its plastic hammerhead tag.

The billiards and pool hall in which they found themselves was reminiscent of an idealised gentlemen's club, from the nineteenth-century colonies. It was a vision of the past, where the players – dressed in waistcoats and bow ties – were meant to tend, like waiters, to the table. Portraits of forgotten stars, like imaginary aristocrats, were hung beneath lamps which bequeathed luminous rectangles to the aristocrats' foreheads, as if they were sweating. Each photograph was scribbled with an illegible imitation of a signature: as if the sign for a signature was its very illegibility.

Niko said that he would just go into the bathroom. Viko said he would be with them in one minute. First he had this little matter – they understood? He gestured over to a table, where an argument was taking place. They understood. So Viko wandered back over to the tables and took up his position, a little way off, on a bar stool; while Haffner waited on a banquette for Niko to return.

Haffner listened to the argument: like every argument, its intonations were universal.

He did not know the precise details: he did not know that a man was telling his teenage son that he was not showing any respect to Viko.

—When you were my age, he said. When you. When I was.

There was a pause.

—You're me, right, said the man.

On his bar stool, Viko lit a cigarette: aloof from the argument, in his ivory tower.

He was forty-two, said the anonymous father, and he had never said fuck in front of his mother. Never. Look, he loved him more than his bird loved him. He respected him. And he didn't need to go round saying things which weren't respectful. If he didn't show any respect.

—Him, if he wants to, said the man, pointing at Viko, he can have anyone killed.

And how was Haffner also to know, as he listened to this incomprehensible argument, that Niko was, at that moment, bending as if in solicitude over the tank of a toilet, inhaling a gram of cocaine which he had first neatly heaped in a thin straggling line? It wasn't Haffner's normal world. As he looked around, sipping the first of the vodkas which the barman brought him, he was simply trying to understand why there seemed to be such a lack of urgency; such a lack of businesslike flair. He wanted to be done with this. The urgent need to do what he had to do and secure this villa for Livia still possessed him, even in his drunken state. He wanted to be true to a domestic idyll. He wanted to be successful and in bed. But Haffner, in his finale, was fated so rarely to be in bed when he wanted, with whom he wanted.

He felt for the phone, bulging in his tracksuit top.

Niko propped himself on the patch of yellow foam under the ripped velour of the banquette, on which Haffner's hand had been resting.

—You want to play? said Niko. You like billiards? Why not? If we played a little game, for a bet?

—Really? said Haffner.

—Why not? said Niko. Why not?

Haffner was drunk. And he was good at billiards. After all, he had been Joe Davis's banker. Haffner, as the legend had often said, was a natural.

3

Along the walls of the billiards and snooker hall, a range of cues was propped – like an armoury. Haffner prised one out from its tight little omega, and rolled it on the empty and unlit surface of a dark unoccupied table. It drifted in an unprofessional curve. Haffner prised out another. The black butt of this cue was slightly sticky. He rolled this one also – noting its warp, its bias and slide.

He walked back to his table; asked if Niko wanted to break. Niko rested his cue, upright, against the table.

—You break, he said.

Haffner settled over the table, fervently. He jabbed the white, but somehow swerved his arm so the tip of the cue slid and tapped the white on top, then bounced beside it on the thin green baize.

—That's not a good shot no, said Niko.

—No, said Haffner.

—Listen, said Niko. You must keep your arm straight – no, yes, out, yes, better. Now try.

—But it's your turn, said Haffner.

—No no, said Niko. You go, you go.

Haffner recovered his form with an in-off red. He played gracefully, impressively. He relaxed into his talent. Intently – doing this for Livia, thinking of Livia, the tenderness he felt for the rashes she had been prone to, her skin weeping like honeycomb – he did not look at Niko during a series of fourteen in-offs. And then he missed.

—Come into my office, said Viko: he was standing beside their table, his arms wide, smiling.

Neatly, he sat down on a bench.

—So sorry, said Viko, nodding over in apology to the now becalmed and darkened table. A drink? he added.

A deal among men: this, at least, was a world which Haffner could understand. On his bench, as in the most masculine of steak houses, Haffner leaned forward, in the way that he had always done: the clasp of his palms dropped against his lap.

A genie, Niko returned with three bottles of beer – the flare of his nostrils, inside, was a glowing coral. He picked up his cue, scratched the turquoise block of chalk, with its shallow indentation, across its tip. He puffed the puff of chalk away. Then settled to his work.

And Viko outlined the situation. Haffner wanted the villa. The Committee was proving difficult. Haffner was interested in speeding the process up. This, so far, was what Viko understood. Haffner praised his grasp of the situation. And Viko, continued Viko: he was known as a man of honour. He liked to help his friends. And Haffner was a friend?

Haffner was a friend.

He thought he was, said Viko. So. Viko had done his research; he had asked various questions: he had made Haffner's situation known.

This was very kind, said Haffner.

4

Niko had been playing a monotonous series of in-off reds. He lifted his head from the table. What, he asked, did Haffner want the upper limit to be? Haffner wondered if 100 would be appropriate. Niko played another long in-off red.

And Viko therefore thought that, with the document he was now offering to Haffner, Haffner would find it ever so much easier to bring the matter to a close. He unfolded a square of paper from his pocket, and laid it in front of Haffner. Haffner tried to read it. As he expected, it was not in a language he knew.

This was what? he queried. It was the necessary authentication from the authorities, said Viko. It was the proof that the family of his wife were the rightful owners of the property.

—The deeds? asked Haffner.

—Not quite, said Viko. But this was all he needed.

Haffner had never imagined the world of corruption to work with such elegance, such dispatch. If only he had understood this sooner, in his career, he thought. He might have saved himself so many hours of work.

From the bar, they could hear a miniature ice-hockey match, on a miniature television, being brought to its conclusion. Niko paused: he strained to watch.

—You prefer which games? asked Niko, still straining.

—The game of cricket, said Haffner.

—Yes, the English game, said Niko, relaxing back into the real world.

From his cueing position, Niko wondered if Haffner could explain the game of cricket. Haffner thought this was unlikely. But it was true: he liked the higher games. The higher English games. Like cricket, and croquet. The games with intricate rulebooks.

—Or soccer, of course, said Haffner, in an effort to lower himself to the universal level, looking at his incomprehensible document with lavish pride.

— This is my game, said Niko. The penalties! This I love. The lottery. The goalkeeper's fear.

But no, Haffner said, putting his folded document down beside his beer, careful to avoid the ornamental water features on the scratched and sticky shelf. Not at all. The goalkeeper was never afraid of the penalty, said Haffner. The goalkeeper was in love with the penalty.

—You kill me, said Niko.

Hear him out, said Haffner. Hear a man out. What the goalkeeper didn't want was the difficult cross, the perfectly weighted through-ball. These were the tests of skill and psychology: the undramatic moments.

—Possible, said Niko. Possible.

The real dilemma for the goalkeeper, continued Haffner, was whether or not to leave his area. That was the moral crux of goalkeeping – to know when to curb one's courage. But the penalty was pure theatre. The goalkeeper, finished Haffner, in a penalty, could never be defeated.

—Interesting, said Niko, still watching the television. You like Barthez?

—Barthez? said Haffner. A showman. Just a showman. Never rated him. Now Banks, however, now there was a goalkeeper.

—Who? said Viko, bored.

5

With Niko's next shot, the red ball quivered against the angled upper jaw of a centre pocket, and settled there, unpotted. The white dribbled towards it and, miraculously, stopped – on the lower jaw of the same centre pocket.

—It's amazing what can happen, said Niko, meditatively, on this twelve-by-six-foot table. Then he smiled at Haffner, as if for appreciation.

There only remained, therefore, said Haffner, with decorum – trying to return the matter to his hoped-for conclusion – the matter of: and then he broke off, as he had always broken off before, when negotiating with clients. He understood?

Viko understood: he had consulted with Niko, he said. They were friends. Haffner nodded. They wanted to do this as friends. Haffner nodded again. They would therefore only charge him for the merest expenses. With a small extra compensation. For a third time Haffner solemnly nodded his assent, with gravitas. With gravitas, Viko named his price.

In this way these deals were done.

Haffner, in conclusion, nodded his agreement. In response, Viko stood to offer Haffner the manly theatrics of a less reserved hug.

Haffner looked at his phone, and considered calling Benji – to boast of his success.

—You want another drink? said Niko. Sure you do!

He decided that Benji could wait.

—So, said Niko.

They walked back to the bar, and sat down on the ripped banquette. There was also, he added, the question of his money too. Haffner looked at him, sad that matters should have turned so predictably filmic: with all the usual minor sins. He thought that had been taken care of, mentioned Haffner.

—For the bet? said Niko.

Had that been a real bet? asked Haffner. He had no idea that Niko had been serious.

Niko looked at the old man in front of him, and placed a paternal hand on Haffner's boyish shoulder. Could Niko talk about Haffner? Would he permit this? Haffner said he could. Sometimes, Niko worried, Haffner didn't seem to take things seriously which he should have taken seriously. Like, he pointed out, how Haffner had behaved in the club the night before. Whereas Niko, now Niko took things seriously. But then, Niko had been in a war. In fact, Niko had fought in two wars. Against the Muslims. And let him maybe tell this story. Once, Niko was on the border, in the mountains. They were laying an ambush. It was very cold in the mountains. And Niko's friend, he had been to America. In America, he had bought a special suit, with wiring inside. It was like an electric blanket? But there was no internal power supply to this suit. There was no battery. So they were at the front, in the mountains. And his friend did not bring so many of his clothes. Instead, he brought his suit, and also a car battery. So. They got to their position. He put his suit on, and then he wired it up to the battery.

—And what happened? asked Haffner.

He fell asleep, said Niko. It was freezing, all the enemy was there, close to them, and he fell asleep. He was snoring. And this, said Niko, was Haffner. The man asleep.

—I fought in two wars, said Niko. And I fired shots in anger, I can tell you.

6

In the difficult silence which followed Niko's portrait of Haffner, Viko proposed that they should go somewhere else to celebrate.

There was a place near here, agreed Niko: with such girls! Then he paused. He began to smile. In his lightness of spirit, Haffner said he would also, of course, pay for the drinks. First, however, Haffner downed a final vodka. He placed the glass back on the brittle bar towel. Then he drank another final vodka. His heart accelerated. And Haffner, searching for coins in his wallet, which emerged, scissored between two figures, leaned into the sense of flight – as into the exhilaration of a speeding curve.

He knew what Niko meant. The problem had always been to distinguish whether one was wasting one's life or truly living it. This was the conundrum inherited from Solomon, his father. But the anguish of Haffner's life had therefore been in identifying which was which: the two so often hid within each other.

Libertine man! This was all Haffner had ever wanted to be. Yet now, he was beginning to think, it had always been a mirage. Although it might have looked like waste – his life in the quiet suburbs – although it had so often seemed a waste to Haffner, in fact that life was everything. Renouncing a woman, after all, can be a form of heroism; this is famous. And winning her may be a form of discipline.

The war was everywhere.

And Haffner, thought Haffner, had finally proved equal to this war – as he contemplated his finale up here in the mountains, with Zinka in the foreground, Frau Tummel in the background, and Benjamin a shadow in the distance. This piece of paper in his pocket, thought Haffner, constituted an undeniable achievement. So Haffner rejected Niko's accusation. Haffner was exultant!

In recovering Livia's villa, Haffner saw his reconciliation.

A chorus of trumpeting putti, Viko and Niko and Haffner raised their ultimate vodkas, downed the glasses on the wet surface of the bar counter, then on they went, happy, to the next whisky bar.

Haffner had always liked the imaginary travel books: the voyages to the centre of the earth, the voyages under the sea. There were the Sciapods, one-footed, but whose one tremendous foot served as a sunshade in the desert; or the Cynocephali, with the heads of dogs and a language which resembled barking. His favourite, given to him by Livia as a Christmas present, was an illustrated edition of the adventures of Cyrano de Bergerac – the comical man with the grandiose nose, who imagined a trip to the moon. But all these mythical journeys could only lead their heroes home. And Haffner was moved to realise that this was also true of him – even now, when Livia was dead. The marriage was endless.

—It kind of baffles me, sometimes, how you sleep at night, Pfeffer once said, as they sat in the Overseas Bankers' Club in Lothbury: amazed how Haffner could lie beside the wronged form of Livia.

Haffner dropped a chunk of sugar into his coffee, observing the brief spawn of bubbles on the black surface.

With Pfeffer, the family man, when trying to defend his sexual record, Haffner had then developed a theory of the wife and the mistress. Really, said Haffner, people didn't understand: the wife was safe. The really vulnerable were the other women. Pfeffer queried this. Haffner was always good, he observed, at misplacing his tenderness. His sense of what was important and what was not had never been a thing of moral beauty.

Haffner's argument had never convinced Haffner, let alone Pfeffer. Now, however, Haffner was beginning to wonder if he had been right all along. He couldn't remember the other women. They meant nothing to him. It was sad to admit this, but it was true. Whatever Barbra was doing now, Haffner didn't care. Whereas Livia was different. Livia was everything.

And me, I might add something else.

It is still the same Promised Land, it is still the same story, whether we talk of Moses and his Promised Land, or Odysseus and his Ithaca; or Haffner and this villa in the centre of Europe. And in a version of the story of Odysseus, which I once read, when Odysseus finally arrived safely home in Ithaca, he found himself utterly disappointed. And yet, wrote the author, whose name I have forgotten, what did he want of Ithaca? What else did it really offer him, if not precisely that journey home?

Just as Haffner stepped out into the midsummer night – the longest night of the year, the longest night of Haffner's life – but did not see before him the deserted nocturnal retail village, but instead entered the noblest park, and stood there observing a spreading oak tree, under which a long-lost version of Haffner sat with his beloved wife. Around them, deer munched. They were in Gloucestershire, or Warwickshire: ensconced in England. A fox was a red blur in the dark of a blackberry bush. And this lost but momentarily recovered Haffner lay watching the yellow-green where the sun lit the leaves; the black-green where it didn't.

Haffner Defeated

1

The club which Haffner was speeding towards in Niko's car was located down a side street, pretending to be a milk bar. So went its name. It opened on to the street via a metal door. When this door was opened, the clubber walked down some steps to a checkpoint where a girl waited behind a table, branding you with an ink stamp, before letting you turn left, down a further flight of stairs, further underground, into the club itself.

In the first room, there was the bar, and a selection of chairs. In the second, there was a room where two girls were DJing. On the wall was projected a selection of childhood images: though from whose childhood, no one knew. In the final room, the kids were dancing; when the DJs finished, a live set began. Tonight, it was an electro band from Hungary who were pretending they were from New York: singing their lyrics in a filmic version of American. They screamed at their appreciative crowd, drinking vodka and Coke from plastic cups; drinking beer from bottles; drinking shots of absinthe from a cache of plastic espresso cups stolen from a hospital canteen.

Into this underground came Haffner: the back of his hand – freckled, brown-spotted – now stamped with an extra red stain, so prompting Haffner to the thought of all the major crimes he could have committed, but had not. Yes, Haffner descended into the night, as he contrived to answer his phone, into which he shouted to Benji that yes everything had gone smoothly, that yes it was very loud, he was in a club, called Milk Bar, or maybe it was a milk bar, he had no idea: and then he lost reception; and the collar on his shirt seeped with sweat, and his lungs filled with the smoke of 250 cigarettes, lit from each other by the manic youth of Europe.

It was an *inferno*. But to Haffner, triumphantly still reminding himself that Livia's villa was soon to be his, it seemed a blessed *paradiso*.

2

Inside, alone for a moment in the middle room, Haffner looked around. Behind Haffner, a boy was cycling along a mountain path. His path wobbled with the trembling grip of the super-8 camera which was working so hard to preserve his balance for eternity. A girl who was more real, in sunglasses and a bracelet made of pink plastic paperclips, was watching this film, intently, while shifting her feet to the beat from the DJs behind her. The boy continued pedalling, now observed by an ecstatic parent in mint-green sunglasses, encouraged by the severed hand of the camera operator.

Was this what the kids were up to? wondered Haffner. Their mania for nostalgia took them this far? This farrago of the sentimental. The kids observing the kids. Whereas all Haffner had wanted, as a boy, was the adult. He had wanted to wear a tie, to wear a suit. The two girls DJing were drinking from the same pink straw in the same glass of Coke. Although Haffner rightly doubted if it contained only Coke.

In this setting, his tracksuit, he thought, was more appropriate than he had imagined. Around him there seemed to be no dress code, no fashion which Haffner could recognise. The laws were gone.

So much posturing at the infantile! But now that he was old, Haffner rather applauded this resistance to the adult: the spirit of the flippant. The bare midriffs; the obvious bra straps; the visible panties. Everything in fluorescent colours. He warmed to this; as he warmed to everything which seemed unimpressed with the adult world. The nostalgia, perhaps not. But the infantile, this the older, less mature Haffner could admire.

Viko was offering to buy Haffner a drink. Haffner looked round. He suddenly realised that Niko was gone. With a depressed shrug, Haffner assented. He watched Viko lean against the bar, a man at ease. And Haffner tried to understand what was meant to happen next. He had hoped to avoid this, the time alone with his masseur. Their business relationship had been maintained with surprising ease, thought Haffner. This still did not resolve the question of where they stood more privately: what conclusion had been drawn after Haffner's curtailed massage. The problem was how seriously Viko thought that Haffner had taken it. Preferably, their relationship would have ended in the fog of its ambiguity – stranded, on a mountain top, with the night coming on, and only the cowbells for company.

Viko returned with the drinks. They chinked glasses, plasticly. Then Viko moved closer to him.

Viko, of course, didn't want Haffner. He only thought that Haffner wanted him. If there were more ways to make money from Haffner, then Viko was happy to explore those ways. He was a man of mode. The older men went for the younger men: this was the story of Viko's life. They offered you money to let them touch you; or watch you. So went the ways of the Riviera.

Haffner placed a palm on Viko's chest, girlishly: in a cute gesture of rebuff. Viko looked at it. He removed Haffner's palm, and held it tight.

He was drunk, Haffner. He was gone. He was there, at the crest of his ascent – in the glory of his absolute inspiration: just before it transformed itself, as if nothing had happened, into the absolute descent.

3

The descent of the grandfather, however, was being deftly matched by the ascent of the grandson. Even if, at the moment, this ballet was suffering from problems with timing. Oblivious to his future ascent, Benjamin was depressed. He was standing at a corner of the bar: trying to lean forward enough so that the deep folds of his T-shirt could hang down in a perpendicular line. For Benji's body in these clubs became a pastoral: the hillocks of his breasts, the trilling streamlets of sweat which ran between them.

This was not the kind of club in which Benjamin had ever felt happy. His grandfather's phone call, however, had disturbed him. So here he was, in his excited fear, and he felt alarmed. Packed as the club was with assured and sexual girls, it presented multiple temptations to Benji's soul. The temptation of lust, naturally, but also the darker temptations: of self-pity, and self-disgust.

His reaction to this state, before his Orthodox training, used to be a prolonged session at the bar, followed by a session of manic dancing. And it was to this practice, haunted by his recent erotic memories, worried for the safety of his grandfather, that Benjamin, against his moral code, returned.

His yarmulke was now stuffed, shyly, in the pocket of his jeans.

How many of his beliefs, considered Benji sadly, were really just romances? It seemed so very likely that his moral code was a romance too. It was all too possible. Benji wanted to be there in the Jewish East End: with Fatty the Yid, the fixer, handing out betting slips in Bethnal Green. Could he have told you why? Wasn't it obvious? These people had cool. On one street there would be

Jewish Friendly Societies, for Benjamin's relatives, newly emerged from Lithuania; and a house which concealed a miniature synagogue, whose ceiling would be azure with gold stars, and below which, on the walls, would be engraved in gilt the names of its benefactors – the Rothschilds, the Goldsmids, the Mocattas, the Montagues. Had Benjamin not been born too late, what a member he would have made of the Bilu Group, of Hovevei Zion! A group which he had once admired for the sarcastic praise they had bestowed on their nation for having woken from the false dream of Assimilation. *Now, thank God, thou art awakened from thy slothful slumber. The pogroms have awakened thee from thy slothful slumber.* No, thought Benjamin, this was the melancholy truth. In his identification with the marginalised, the bereft, he had been wowed by the romance of belonging to an elite. Because the persecuted could be an elite, of this he had no doubt.

Inside him lay Benjamin's grand emotions: envy, anxiety, self-hatred, self-contradiction. There they were, in their plush velvet case – snug, like a cherished heirloom; a polished silver piccolo.

They seemed unnecessary now.

Beside him, sitting on the plastic pod of a stool, a girl began to talk to him. She didn't want to talk to him about the state of his soul, nor the state of world politics: the endless problems of minority peoples. She only wanted to ask him what his plans were that evening, what his girlfriend's name was. Benji sadly admitted that he had none: no plans, no girlfriend. She offered him a cigarette. Her name was Anastasia, she said. And when somehow Benjamin inveigled into the conversation a mention of his Jewish origins, she looked at him. There was a pause. This was it, he thought: the moment when everything became obvious.

—Uhhuh, she said. So anyway.

He looked at Anastasia. She was the tallest girl he had ever met; and although he could not help remembering the distracting features of the girl to whom he had lost his virginity, he also could not help feeling that in Anastasia he had discovered something so much more refined. She was wearing a black shift dress, black tights: and red high heels. Her hair was cut in some sort of slick bob. There was a plastic butterfly visible on her left, diminutive breast.

—You are American? asked Anastasia.

—British, said Benjamin.

—Is better, said Anastasia.

And at that moment, as she shifted her weight, so accidentally placing her thigh in warm proximity to Benjamin's podgy hand, Benjamin finally noticed Haffner, talking to a man. He stalled in a trance of indecision. And although this was why he was here – to protect his wayward grandfather – Benjamin did nothing. He did not excuse himself and go to offer Haffner his protection. He simply looked into Anastasia's eyes, smiled, lit a cigarette which she had offered him, and desperately, feeling sick, hoping that he would not regret this, tried to take up smoking.

4

The smoke here was mythical. It was its own clouding exaggeration – not just in the usual secret places: one's nostrils, the creases of clothes. Here, it hurt the cornea, the tonsils, the ganglia of one's lungs.

Politely, Haffner wondered if Viko could perhaps put out his cigarette. It was terribly hurting his eyes. In fact, he said, he really did feel very tired. He really thought that he might sadly have to excuse himself and end his evening here.

But Viko, by now, was dictatorial in his drunkenness: a Tamerlane. Barbaric, he looked at his cigarette, and looked at Haffner, vanquished. He could not believe it, he said. It was a cigarette. And now this man in front of him wanted it to be put out. For why? It wasn't, he pointed out, as if he was the only person smoking.

And he gave out a staccato mirthless laugh – a studio audience of one.

Uneasily, Haffner looked around, into the crowd: the extraordinary overspill of beauty in this basement amazed him with its grace. It contrasted with Haffner. It contrasted less with Viko. He looked back at him.

Viko continued to stare – the cigarette hanging limply from his lower lip.

There was nothing else for it, thought Haffner. Any conversation which might restore some poise, some grace, seemed impossible to him now. And he had done what he needed to do. So he was leaving, said Haffner. He was very grateful, but now he really must go.

And Haffner turned – to discover Niko, bearing Zinka as a trophy. Gently, with distracted distance, she bestowed her smile on Viko, and then Haffner. And Haffner stood there, confident that if Zinka stayed here for ever, then so would he. With a gesture of European politesse, Haffner kissed the raised paw of Zinka's hand. He stood there, happily smiling.

And suddenly, Viko understood.

Viko believed in desire being rewarded. He believed in the myth of the kept man. No shame attached to money. The sudden way in which Haffner had left the massage table, having solicited Viko's attention, had not been forgotten. It irked him. Especially because he had heard the rumours of Haffner's friendship with Zinka. Why should Viko be spurned? It was the more galling for being the more unjust. This, after all, was the man whose property claims would be made easier by Viko: from Haffner, Viko had expected money in instalments, he had expected cash.

In this sad way, Viko talked to himself. His monologue took place before an unseeing audience of Zinka and Haffner.

Haffner was telling Zinka the story of his nightlife: how he had known the former Prime Minister of his country, and in a bar in

London he had danced with her and talked of world finance. And although the details of this conversation were inaudible to Viko, his rage was inventive enough to inflame itself just with its visionary gifts: observing Haffner's charmingly enfeebled touch on her arm, Zinka's dimpling smile.

It was incredible, said Viko. No one heard him. He said it again. It was utterly incredible. And he began to shout, in the language which Haffner did not understand. Spurned, Viko listed the million vices of Haffner. Ignoring Zinka's calming protestations, her anxious glances, Niko's confused scowl, he listed Haffner's lechery, his financial manoeuvres, his cowardice.

Haffner mildy asked what was happening. He seemed upset, observed Haffner. Zinka silenced him with an irritated flourish of her arm.

—You, said Viko, anxious to explain, jabbing at Haffner and Zinka and Niko in confused identification. You fuck her. His girl.

Haffner, full of justified smugness, tried to explain that this was not true, not at all. He really had to say that this was quite ridiculous. Viko refused his explanations. Everyone knew, he said. So Niko might as well know too. He glared at Zinka. Zinka lit a cigarette, and exhaled a plume of smoke in Viko's face, like the most classical of zephyrs.

The character of Niko was often inscrutable: so said his teachers, his mother; so said Zinka, the girl who tried to love him. It was difficult to predict. This difficulty was made more difficult by the various heaps of cocaine which Niko had inhaled that evening, the various drinks he had imbibed.

At first, he seemed only amused. He didn't care if Haffner had been trying to get more of his Zinka. Who wouldn't? said loyal Niko.

No, said Viko, doggedly, he didn't seem to understand.

While Haffner, as he listened to what he understood to be another attack on the soul of Haffner, realised that his feelings were oddly divided. It was true that he didn't want any violence; he didn't want a display of machismo. But on the other hand, he would have preferred Niko to be more worried, more ill at ease. At least violence would have demonstrated some form of sexual contest. Whereas Niko did not seem aware of any sexual contest.

So Haffner's pride debated with itself.

5

And, in this way, the ballet of Haffner and Benjamin began to find its synchronisation. For Benjamin was also considering the nature of his sexual pride. But not, however, with sadness. In the bathroom of this club – located in what seemed to be a makeshift plastic tunnel attached to the basement, reached through an emergency door – Benjamin was delirious with success.

—When you say obscenities in another language, it's only ever funny, said Benji. You can't do it. I mean, how do you say fuck me in your language?

She told him. He tried to repeat it. She started to giggle.

—You see? said Benji. I mean, say fuck me, in English.

—Fuck me, said Anastasia.

There was a pause.

—Oh no, said Benji, softly. Well maybe no. Maybe we could continue like that.

With no shiver of distaste, her hands were stroking the softness of his breasts; they were clasping the rings of fat which circled Benji, like a planet, and still she kissed him with abandon.

—Was that a practice sentence, or a real sentence? said Benjamin.

—Maybe both, said Anastasia.

And after they had kissed, Benji smiled at her.

—I haven't seen you smile that smile tonight. It is good, she said.

—I have a greater variety than that, said Benji, winningly.

Oh Benjamin's allegiances were all awry: they were jostled, irretrievably. He thought of the girl in Tel Aviv. Perhaps, he thought, he was not in love. Perhaps she was just a beginning. He didn't want to be what others made of him. Surely that was cool. No longer did he want to be defined by his loyalty: not to a race, and not even to his family. He wanted, thought Benjamin, to be himself.

—I want you so much, said Benjamin.

A sentence said with such ardent and charming sincerity, so in excess of Benji's pudgy demeanour, that Anastasia, helplessly, began to adoringly laugh.

6

It wasn't that Anastasia was cruel. She had simply become, by accident, the audience to an ordinary kind of comedy.

Himself! Benji wanted to be himself. So he exaggerated. And this is not so unusual. Maybe this is all the self is, really: whatever is most fervently displayed. It isn't difficult, to find this kind of story. It was, for instance, a theme in Benji's family itself.

In 1940, Cesare was interviewed by the British police – trying to ascertain his loyalty to Mussolini. In his defence, Cesare had not only proved to them in minute detail how he was a Marxist, a member of the Mazzini Garibaldi club; he had not only quoted to them the words of Garibaldi himself, imploring his acolytes to have faith in the immortal cause of liberty and humanity, because the history of the Italian working classes was a history of virtue and national glory – no, this was not enough for Cesare. To clinch his point he had stood on a chair and sung the Internationale, improvising an English translation. After the third verse, with three still to come, the British police allowed that perhaps they had been wrong in their suspicions concerning Cesare.

And when Cesare recounted this story, which was often, Haffner would riposte with the story of Bleichröder, Bismarck's Jewish banker, a hero of finance. An allegory for Haffner. For Bleichröder never managed to become Prussian, rather than Jewish. He tried, but he failed. He went for walks, Haffner would begin. And then Livia and Cesare would continue – in a ritual which they did not know was a ritual, since no one ever remembered that the precise same conversation happened at regular intervals which were not regular enough to prevent this amnesic repetition. So Cesare would tell his story of Cesare. Haffner would begin the riposte of Bleichröder. And Livia would finish, reminding Cesare, in case he didn't remember, how Bleichröder kept himself apart from the Jewish people, even in his weekend walks. On the promenades along the Siegesallee he walked on the western side: eschewing the east, with its Jewish crowds. And when asked why he walked on the other side, according to the police, added Haffner – yes yes, Livia would say, she knew this line: when asked why, Bleichröder answered that the eastern side smelled too much of garlic.

Benjamin, as he kissed Anastasia, and felt for her slim breasts, in the furore of his passion, was forming the final panel in this luminous family triptych. If his God could see him, he did not care. The neon light in this plastic cubicle did not disturb him, nor the seven empty beer bottles lined up, as if posed for some pop-art portrait, on a ledge. And Benji revelled in the sensation that in kissing Anastasia, on this night which he understood marked no high point in Benji's romantic life, no moment of deep conversion, still mindful of the girl whom he felt in love with, in Tel Aviv, he had made it impossible to return to the ways he used to think. In kissing Anastasia he had crossed over – through the looking glass, out the back of the wardrobe.

7

Haffner, however, found nothing new in this world. As Viko had elaborated the lays of Haffner, Zinka had led him out of the club.

At the door, a group of girls were waiting for a taxi. He turned to Zinka, anxious to enquire quite if he really needed to leave.

No, there was nothing new for Haffner. He knew this place. It was suburbia. Like everywhere Haffner lived. The clapboard pavilion on an artificial lake, with a landscaped golf course arranged around it; the hotel with souvenirs kept in a glass cabinet in the foyer; homes which once belonged to writers now preserved as monuments, complete with shops which sold tea towels on which were stitched, in italics, quotes from these great writers; or which were instead knocked down and replaced by an apartment block which bore the great hero's name; or restaurants which advertised a return to the ethos of the nineteenth century, or advertised the cuisine of Italy, or China, even though they were staffed by white and disillusioned teenagers: all this was suburbia. And so was this youthful display he could now see outside the club, where girls in thin dresses gathered together to whisper and giggle while sporadic boys lit avoidant cigarettes, affecting to ignore them.

And so was the manifest violence.

In the dark street Haffner stopped with Zinka, anxious to prove that he was scared of nothing, a speech which he had barely begun when Niko emerged from the crowded steps and stood there, in the doorway.

Even at this point, Haffner refused to believe in violence: he refused to believe it was possible – for Haffner was surely invulnerable. He still refused to believe that his story could really be serious. So Haffner was surprised when Niko moved to where he stood with Zinka and then pushed him, in a way which Niko imagined was only gentle, a tender threat: an amused gesture of gentle reproach. It was all the violence Niko would ever offer this aged man. But, unprepared, an unbalanced Haffner swayed backwards and then, in his effort to overcompensate, swayed forwards.

And Haffner fell.

He lay there on the street, but still refused to be downcast, beneath the chemical sky, its wash of cloud – like the most perfunctory of watercolours in the window of a fine-arts dealer behind the British Museum, on a Sunday in November, when everything is closed. No, opined Haffner, bleeding, wasn't it Cole Porter who used to say that, as he lay beneath the horse which was crushing his legs to a pulp, he worked on the lyrics of 'At Long Last Love'? Surely Haffner too could discover a *sprezzatura*?

Above him, like warring and disporting gods, Zinka and Niko were shouting. He was impossible, she said. What, she asked him, was he thinking – to attack an old and defenceless man? While Niko was shouting back, arguing with the facts as he now saw them, that he had never meant to hurt him, of course he had never meant to hurt him. And, then again, who was she to put the blame on Niko? Perhaps she should hear what Viko had to say about this man now lying there beside them. But Viko, suddenly, had disappeared.

And Haffner remembered with a sensual pang how he had once woken on Viko's massage table, surrounded by the scents of candles, the cries of whales, the tenderness of towels, in what now seemed to be a for ever lost vision of safety.

8

Defeated, bloodied, Haffner stumbled his way back inside, to find the bathroom. Against the basin, a girl was being roughly kissed, on her breast a man's splayed hand, a starfish: a hand which she was lightly coaxing away.

Into a stall stumbled Haffner.

Adjacent to Haffner, unknown, in another cubicle, Benjamin was gasping with abandon, as he touched the girl between the legs, his hand a little trapped by the elastic of her underwear. He was in a modern heaven. Through the bathroom's thin walls he could hear

257

the music, throbbing. The DJs had been replaced by the Hungarian band, featuring a girl who sang her American English songs in the highest voice Benji had ever heard: as if the world were house music.

While Haffner, oblivious, the end of all the modern, observed his ancient face, illuminated by one fluorescent tube. Behind him was a bucket with an indefinable mop drenched inside it. He should have known, he thought: this was how things tended to end up – with Haffner as a clown. He dabbled with the taps: they relinquished little water.

He had always wanted to be a libertine, but now he was something else. Just Haffner Silenus – a sidekick, so prone to fall over, so vulnerable to capture, so easy to wound: the same Haffner as he had become when Livia announced, two years before she died, that she was leaving him.

—Now? he said.

It didn't seem worth the effort. But yes, she said: she was finished. She was leaving him to live with Goldfaden. It was long enough after his wife's death. It was what they had always wanted to do.

And Haffner had looked at her amazed. He couldn't understand it. It was always Haffner who was the one to leave. No one else. But there she was, announcing that she would be going to live with Goldfaden. And although Haffner pleaded on behalf of his love for her, his family, Livia was unmoved. It was what she wanted, she said. And just as now Haffner stared into a mirror, hyperbolically lit, so Haffner had gone into the downstairs bathroom – the toilet with its pink fringed bib at its base, a china cow-creamer whose back overflowed with pot-pourri – and stared at the clown before him. There he tried to be precise about what he was feeling; he tried to be composed. But he was only possessed by a gigantic feeling that he missed Livia, that he had perhaps been missing her for many years: and Haffner wanted her back. He wanted to recover things. So he emerged, from the bathroom, ready to plead and beg – but found that Livia had gone.

Whereas this time he emerged, with wild wet hair, and discovered that, as in the puzzles of his youth – *Spot the difference, dear reader! Can you see it, kids?* – the picture had been doctored. Where Livia had been absent, there now stood Zinka, her arms folded, leaning against the bathroom's plastic walls. She unwrapped a wafer of chewing gum, and offered it to Haffner: its dusty granular surface.

She was taking him home, she said. She would spend tonight with him.

It seemed true, thought Haffner. She did not seem to be one of Haffner's visions. In the words of the very old song, the dream was real.

9

And yet, the dream life of Haffner was troubled.

It did seem all too possible that the brief moment of his triumph in relation to the villa was now over. The ordinary rules would soon reassert themselves. He doubted if the deal with Niko and Viko was still on. This seemed even less likely if he chose to allow Zinka to spend the night with him. Presumably, he could return to Viko and Niko and offer them the agreed sum. Presumably, he could try. But their goodwill might well be lacking.

Was Haffner to blame for this sudden fiasco? It seemed possible to plead that he was not – not responsible, in the end, for Niko's rages, for Viko's pride. He consulted the shade of Livia: would she really have wanted him to play the coquette with another man, simply to ensure her inheritance?

He could imagine the shade of Livia smiling.

Then Haffner was interrupted in this vision by a strong sense of nausea. A shiver took possession of his body, then relinquished it.

Yes, this, thought Haffner, was his return to the everyday. All his ingenuity had failed him. The Committee would have to be wooed all over again. So Haffner only felt a tired disappointment.

And yet, he thought, in compensation he seemed to have Zinka, in this party dress, beside him. But Haffner realised that even his joy in her was tempered. On arrival at this club he had felt so confident, so victorious. If he had been told he would leave with Zinka, it would have only made him a happy Haffner. Yet now here he was, still burdened with the problem of the villa, walking slowly through the dark streets of a spa town so marked with Livia's memory. And whether Zinka was a digression or in fact some covert route to Livia, Haffner did not know.

He still felt confident of his innocence. He had tried to remain faithful to Livia, and he would continue to try. But he was a connoisseur of Haffner's ability to be defeated. That Haffner had done his best, he was coming to realise, sadly, didn't mean he wasn't still guilty.

In this unaccustomed melancholy, Haffner followed after Zinka: his halting walk now embellished by the iambic rhythm of a limp.

But I am not so sure that Haffner should have felt so divided. Perhaps there is no such thing as a digression.

Zinka, it's true, was thinking in the same way as Haffner. She thought that it was an unusual event in Haffner's life – this dejected progress through the empty streets. She was moved by Haffner's comical plight. And it moved her more because she assumed that this comedy was all her fault. There was no way this man could have previously suffered the indignity from which he was suffering now. She didn't realise that in this story, as in all of Haffner's stories, there were certain patterns, certain repeats. She didn't know that farce was Haffner's constant mode.

This form was not new in the life of Raphael Haffner. Free from his ordinary customs, let loose in the wild East, Haffner was just allowed to become even more Haffnerian than ever – his own exaggeration.

So that every zenith was also a nadir, as usual, and all victory consisted of beatings. And, as usual, while illuminated with desire for Zinka, Haffner didn't know that a bruise was beginning to develop around his eye and on his cheek, like a Riviera sunset, the backdrop to a promenade bordered with palm trees, illuminating the night in green explosions, accompanied by the muzak of the rhyming cicadas.

Haffner Translated

1

So, said Zinka, as they entered Haffner's bedroom. Here they were.

It seemed undeniable. Here they were, at Haffner's finale. But Haffner was worried that his body was going to prove unequal to this finale. He was quite sure that he was getting ill. True, he was drunk. It could be just the drink. But Haffner knew about his body: its breakdowns and malfunctions. And this feeling was unusual: the dizzy sweating ague of it. He felt for his palms. They were sweating. He brushed the hair which still remained to him down with the Brylcreem of his sweating hand. As if to simultaneously produce a suavely dry palm and a suavely plumed forelock.

He offered Zinka a smile.

Tonight, Zinka explained to him, there was only one rule. Haffner asked what it was. The rule, said Zinka, was that everything came from her. Everything was her decision.

She liked Haffner, this was true, and she felt for his bruised pathos. But this did not mean that this was going to be Haffner's evening.

And Haffner said yes, absolutely.

He had never been one for the fantasies of permission: the allowed and the disallowed. But if rules were going to be a condition of this night with Zinka, then he didn't care. He revelled in them. He would content himself with the little which he was offered. Whatever the modern age would give him. At no point could Haffner touch himself, said Zinka; at no point could he touch her without permission. If at any time he broke these rules, the night was over.

Let Haffner submit! Let Haffner be debased!

All his life, the erotic for Haffner had been a matter of apertures: all the exits and entrances. And now he discovered that the apertures were something, but the rest was something else. There was so much else to play with.

Zinka pushed him gently to the bed, where he slumped down: his head raised, expectantly, like a yawning sea lion.

—You will do what I tell you, said Zinka. Yes?

—Yes, said Haffner, meekly.

Zinka stood between his legs, bent her head, and told him to open his mouth – which Haffner obediently did – then she let her spit dribble out: a thread slowly fastening with its own weight, then falling, gathered in by harmless Haffner.

2

Zinka went into the bathroom, crowded with the male accoutrements of Haffner, bought from a chemist in the town – a shaving brush, the tube of shaving cream, doubly creased in a sine curve which a parsimonious History had borrowed from the smudged blackboards of Haffner's prep school. With the door still open, she crouched on the toilet. She beckoned to Haffner. From below her crotch came the whispering sound of her pissing.

She told Haffner to come closer. He tried to sit down, like the men in Oriental street scenes exhibited at the Academy: a neat bobbing squat. It hurt too much. Instead, he therefore watched her on his hands and knees. Crawling, Haffner approached her closely. He could see her stream – braided, splurging.

—You like this? Zinka asked him.

—I do, yes, said Haffner.

As if there was nothing of the bodily about her, no smell emerged from Zinka. And Haffner, as he waited there, on all fours, only felt an overwhelming happiness. He was in the paradise of women; an island of intimacy, like Gulliver among the giants – whose travels Haffner had read when he was ever so young, so much younger than he would ever be again, in a miniature, octavo, red-leather edition. The eighteenth-century disgust remained with him now. It was there in his stomach, in his nervous system. But also the erotics. Gulliver astride a giant nurse's nipple! Even now, he felt himself rise up in applause. The rough pitted areolae which little Gulliver observed; by which Gulliver was entranced and perturbed. And when Gulliver – or did he? was this just a mistake of Haffner's imagination? – went on to describe the gaping maw of her crotch, Haffner, the delinquent eight-year-old, was not stricken by disgust at the human animal. Instead, he was overtaken by an acrid pleasure. The minuscule Haffner longed for this closeness to the women: the fur and softness. What was small was large, and what was large was small. The world was just a trick of perspective. It all depended, he supposed, on how good you were at magnifying, or diminishing.

Zinka came to an end. From his canine position, Haffner looked up at her, expectantly.

—Now you wipe, said Zinka.

Haffner tended to Zinka. He unrolled a small section of paper, then folded it into the most luxurious, downiest towel. He wanted to do the job with elegance: no one could ever accuse Haffner of not being a good sport.

—No. First with your mouth, she said. Your tongue.

It was for only a brief moment that Haffner paused in a qualm of indecision, before he bent his neck, uncomfortably, deliriously, and licked at Zinka's ferrous crotch. To his surprised disappointment, only a trace of her pale urine was detectable to Haffner's tongue: a sweetly sour herbaceous perfume.

—Now OK you stop, said Zinka.

Then he pushed the paper against her labia. He refolded. Pushed it again, a little harder. He dropped the paper between her legs, into the toilet bowl.

—So, said Zinka. We go through.

And Haffner followed her to the raised stage of his bed, where – earnest, dedicated – Zinka squatted over Haffner's face.

Zinka was hairless between the legs. Where the hair should have been, there was a brief tattoo: a mermaid easing herself against an invisible wave: sinuous, like Venus rising from her shell – a vision in dark green. And Haffner inhaled her.

Canine, Bacchic, Haffner thrived on the lower thrills: the women with their marine and sour aroma, the rotting rich smell of powdered roe, the ammonia rinds of cheeses. The spread of molecules in the still air was one of Haffner's most intense delights. They wafted and they drifted and they delighted him. He was undisgustable.

—You must not move, said Zinka. You move, I punish you.

Haffner wondered if this was serious. No one had ever said this to him before. Haffner had to admit that although he believed that Zinka possessed a charm he had never known in any other woman, it was true that he hardly knew her. He adored her, but she was unknown. He adored her because she was unknown. Unknown, and also young.

—Is this serious? asked Haffner, gaily.

In answer, Zinka pinched the twin wings of his nose together – their burst red cartilage poignant through the skin, like the surface of a butter bean – then pushed herself down on to his mouth. She was everywhere inside Haffner. His eyes goggled back at her, as she looked down, between her breasts.

—We do this how I like, no? said Zinka.

Haffner nodded. And she relaxed her grip on Haffner, flooding him with her delicate smell, a refined sweating bouquet.

Maybe it was better like this, thought Haffner. He began to

accustom himself to the absolute relinquishment of choice. Who needed to see Haffner holding in his stomach? Or his almost hollow shins – a veteran Roman legionary, the skin rubbed to a sheen? In this relinquishment, Haffner found his revolution.

3

His life had been shadowed by the counter-culture, the underground – and however much he disapproved of their childish politics, he admired the chutzpah of the protestors and the fighters, the uprisers and the deserters. Once, in New York, Haffner had helped a kid into the foyer of Chase Manhattan to extricate himself from the riot police, with their bright Lego helmets. Most orderly in his life, most savage in his imaginings, Haffner read with indulgence about the European anarchists, with their colourful cryptic names: the Black Bloc, the Tute Bianche. The Yippies in particular had gladdened Haffner's heart – especially the day they strode into the New York Stock Exchange, quietened the black security men into meek submission with raucous accusations of anti-Semitism, then stood in the public gallery and rained down dollar bills on the dealers in their braces, their visors, their pinstriped bespoke suits. He felt less attached to the Parisian revolutionaries, whom Haffner had watched on the BBC – the students in the lofts of the Ecole des Beaux Arts, attaching posters to washing lines with clothes pegs, so they could dry in time to be glued all over the city: the garish fonts and pointing hands – *Hypocrite reader! My double! My brother!* – proclaiming their escape from all the bourgeois normality, their new creation of an idyllic island, a utopia.

And now Haffner was stranded on this island, in this utopia.

Zinka, without explaining to Haffner, skipped off him and ordered him to undress. And this, thought Haffner happily, might be the moment, the reward for all his courage. In his exuberance he undressed, ignoring his habitual neatness, letting the bunched pair of his socks roll anywhere, his shirt remain in its pool on the floor.

He didn't care what form his utopia might take. Any revolution would do. If he had to be, Haffner would be the Saint-Just of the hypermarket, Guevara of the guava. And if in fact his utopia were here, in a hotel bedroom in a spa town, then Haffner would not resist. No, thought Haffner, if this was it, then he would take his place.

Leaning over the side of the bed, Zinka picked up the tracksuit trousers, and sloppily drew them up, like a snake charmer, along with the pool of his T-shirt. The trousers served to tie up one of Haffner's hands behind him, to the bedhead; the T-shirt served for his other. And Haffner was tied to the bed.

4

Stoical in his pursuit of pleasure, the true classical epicure, it wasn't the first time Haffner had been involved in the bedbound business of knots. It had been a habit of Barbra, his American secretary, to need to be tied to the bed, before being smacked with a book, struck with a cane, spanked until her buttocks turned a chaste and virginal pink. She liked to lose control, in the most controlled way possible. In her apartment in Chelsea, Haffner employed his ingenuity – even, in a moment of inspiration, lassoing a rope that had been stashed in a canvas bag left behind by her hearty and mountaineering brother over an exposed joist, so that Barbra could be tied there, standing naked, her arms above her head, her breasts raised with the tension – breasts which Haffner struck lightly but woundingly with the edge of his belt. When her breasts were raised like this you could see the mole which was usually a deft stowaway underneath the left. No, Haffner never minded these contrivances: but they were not for him. Not even medicinally. In the Russian Bath House in New

York, he never understood why Morton so enjoyed being whipped with switches, beaten with birch rods.

Here in Central Europe, however, the position was reversed. Haffner was the one who was tied. Lightly, it was true: with garish sportswear. But his power had still gone.

Haffner had abdicated.

Slowly, Zinka lowered her mouth to Haffner's chest. With her teeth she tugged at a nipple – its blunt miniature nub. To Haffner, this action still felt within the limits of the normal, or the possible. It hadn't yet gone beyond the border of the pleasurable. Then she continued to bite. And Haffner began to revise his definitions of pleasure. He wondered how far he could take this before she might draw blood. Nevertheless, he thought, nevertheless. His body took over – with its strange routes to enjoyment. Zinka began to bite the other nipple. As she did so, she dragged the sharp nails of her fingers over Haffner's delicate skin. Wildly, he felt his penis stir. She held his penis, tightly, painfully. It tried to stir some more.

Then Zinka began her game of teasing.

Stupendous, haughty, grand, the diminutive form of Zinka began its travails down the length of Haffner's body. She struck him; she bit him. Soon, he knew, his old body would become a palette of bruises – the yellows and browns of a landscape from the nineteenth-century French countryside, with cows, and sheep, and a misshapen cypress. She told him to close his eyes. He could feel her hover over him – her warmth and smell. With a calm hand, she rubbed her wetness on his eyelids, on his nose: a pensive Impressionist. And then she moved further down until she reached his penis, where she waited.

Oh Haffner was adrift! He was in a new ecstasy, confused beyond the obviousness of pain and pleasure. He began to whimper. As he made a sound, she hurt him. So that then Haffner lay still, silent, blinded: in the absolute perfection of his denuded state.

And this was it, he thought. It was the final liberation.

He had found a strange detachment – like the Zen-like kids in the sixties, on Wall Street, who used to tell him the world wasn't the way everyone said it was. Everything was perspective. The real object of the game, they told him, wasn't money: it was the playing of the game itself.

If Haffner had been a mystic, he could have found in this some kind of god. But Haffner was not given to the mystical. He preferred the reckless sensual. It seemed more rational.

5

In a fleeting, floating way, this reminded him.

Long ago, when Haffner was fitter and more beautiful, he had been having lunch with Livia, in Mayfair's Mirabelle. For reasons which were already obscure to them, they were arguing about the merits of the 1968 revolutions: the revolution in Prague, the riots in Paris, the protests in London, then the sit-ins in New York, which Haffner rather saw as pitiful imitations of the European originals.

But it wasn't just the Americans whom Haffner doubted. Even the Europeans, Haffner argued, couldn't be taken seriously. The kids with their posters! They were yearning for violence. And they hadn't seen what violence was. They couldn't understand it.

But Haffner had? asked Livia. Haffner had. Of course he had. She knew he had. And these kids wouldn't have been able to contemplate it. What about the one up the tree, the poet? Who on being asked to come down by a policeman replied that he wouldn't, and, on being asked by the policeman why, answered by saying that he would not come down because if he came down then the policeman would beat him. A pacifist revolutionary! But then: he was a poet. A master of theatricals. Like his friend, the theatre critic: who left the protests because his Berlutis were scuffed. No, Haffner, she had to concede, knew about violence. And so he was best placed to ask the following question. (At this point Livia, distractedly busy-ing herself with the tea, scalded herself on the stainless-steel tea-pot, where a teabag was in agony.) The following question. Could she honestly say that any of these students, these playwrights, these children, were motivated by anything except a desire to be seen in the newspapers? Could she? He didn't think she could. However much they might dress it up as something else, however much they might turn it into street theatre, or whatever, it was still the same old story: the ancient desire for glamour, for someone to notice you.

Livia asked when he would ever stop being flippant. At what point would he learn to take things seriously? Haffner considered his petits fours; the black water which was offering itself as coffee. He was, he assured her, taking it seriously.

She could put it this way, said Livia, spooning the teabag on to a saucer, bleeding its brown ichor on to the china. Haffner looked at her, and realised, with a small shock, that her hair was now white. So, said Livia, Haffner saw everything as selfishness. This was noth-ing new. A gangster, he thought that everyone else had the ethics of the gangster too: she knew this. But what revolution would sur-vive the accusation? What moment of human history? Everyone only cared about themselves. This was obvious! Less obvious was how much, said Livia, anyone should really care. So everyone – Robespierre, Brutus, Lenin, Mussolini – these were all men who wanted to be noticed. But maybe, said Livia, this wasn't the truth of Brutus. And Haffner had to concede – for he was a lover of the classics – that Livia wasn't absolutely wrong. He was always on Caesar's side, true. But even a Caesar was impeachable.

The revolutions happened – nourished by a healthy sense of melo-drama. Who was Haffner to judge the revolutionaries? asked Livia. Who was Haffner to judge the people who didn't care about all the irrelevant emotions – the self-consciousness, the self-pity: the people who didn't care what others thought of them?

So long ago, Livia had said this to Haffner. Now, when she

was dead, it occurred to him that perhaps he finally agreed. If she was right, then Haffner was finally behaving like a true revolutionary. Like the revolutionaries, he was untroubled by the usual emotions: the self-pity, the embarrassment. Here, in the East, in the remnants of Kakania, he no longer cared about social niceties. So a girl was treating him with absolute hauteur, and he was loving it? What did Haffner care? He was his only audience.

Solitary, realised Haffner, he was shameless.

6

Haffner's room still preserved the forms of the 1920s. As well as its view of the mountains, its Zarathustrian height, the room was also equipped with armchairs, an escritoire, and a marble fire surround, on which were two silver candlesticks, containing the unlit slim obelisks of two cream candles.

Haffner opened his eyes to see Zinka pluck a candle from its niche. This baffled him. Then she told him, lying there on his back, to raise his knees to his chest, so exposing himself to whatever Zinka might want to do to him.

It was a fantasy she had always had: to use a man as a woman.

Once, Zinka was talking to her friend, about love and its ramifications. Zinka's friend had explained how her husband's favourite thing was that she should perch there, behind him, and use a dildo on him, with its pink latex bobbles. Slavenka was happy to do this. She was a dutiful wife. But when Zinka asked her if she enjoyed it, if she found it sexy – because she thought it must be sexy, she envied Slavenka her exotic and fulfilling sex life – Slavenka sighed.

—Oh no, she said. It's so boring. I keep forgetting I'm doing it. It's like doing the ironing.

It wasn't how Zinka felt. The idea of it excited her. All her life, she had felt so managed, so in thrall. The idea of being the manager herself seemed so dense with possibility.

In an amazed trance of obedience, Haffner held his knees up. It felt so insubstantial, thought Haffner, that he could not rule out the possibility that this was all a dream. He rather hoped it might be. And as he raised his knees, Zinka noticed the creases which emerged on his stomach – as on a sofa, a clubman's Chesterfield. These creases, for Zinka, were tender with vulnerability. And this was what she wanted. To make the men unusual. To make them unprotected.

The unsure length of Haffner's penis was now being mimicked and outdone by the candle – slick with hand cream she had found in her handbag – grasped in Zinka's hand, like a light sabre.

There was no way, thought Haffner, that he could allow this indignity. But then again: why shouldn't he? It was his liberation. In it, he was prepared to entertain ideas for which he felt no natural wish to be an entertainer. It was not as if he hadn't done this to women himself. So why was it that he would blithely do to a woman – sure of their mutual pleasure, concerned to move with a more exaggerated tenderness – something he would not want a woman to do to him?

He had been content to let matters take their course when Zinka had entered his room that afternoon. In this way, Haffner meditated. Then, he had been moved by her pensive creativity. So why should he stop now?

The problems of philosophy were not, however, Haffner's primary concern. She let the thin candle, deftly coated in her hand cream, slip and settle slightly inside him. She watched him watch her. He could not see the oddity of it; he could not see this act's improbability – as it distended him, and enlarged him, beneath his tight testicles, as it made him wriggle and his stomach break out in sweat.

Then Zinka's other slippery hand became intricate around his penis, just as he had watched it elaborate itself on Niko's penis, two days ago: when his life, reflected Haffner, seemed so much simpler.

As she rested his rough, unpedicured feet on her soft shoulders, he felt moved to hazard the existence of a soul. Nothing else rendered his feelings explicable. And Haffner – Haffner cried out in his denuded, opened closeness to Zinka. They looked into each other's eyes and saw each other: illuminated.

Haffner's paradise! His translation to the supine, the passively cherubic!

She had begun by causing him pain. Now, gradually, she was gently moving the candle, back and forth, as she moved the skin on his penis, up and down, up and down, in front of her. She looked into his eyes and he looked back at her – comical, romantic. She didn't speak to him. Simply, they continued to look at each other, intently, while Zinka continued to make her motions inside Haffner. There was a blemish in one of her pupils.

And Haffner ascended.

With a burgeoning slow realisation, a shy astonishment, he could feel the slow progress of a climax he had not quite ever believed would be possible. Like the faintest music from a radio, playing in some car which pauses, behind an apartment block, as you lean out the window and enjoy a pensive cigarette, watching the unknown city below you, and then, when you think that no, you will never quite be able to make out the tune, that it will remain for ever just beyond you, the car turns a corner and with it you recognise with an unexpected glow of recollection the full volume of some hit made famous by the genius Django Reinhardt in the music halls of New York.

In this way, Haffner finally jolted his hips, and cried out.

Zinka scooped up Haffner's tepid liquid into an enticing paw. Then she told Haffner to open his mouth. Haffner opened. Then she tapped a fingertip on his tongue: a nymph tapping an aged demigod – asleep and drunk – with a finger stained with mulberry juice, to wake him and make him sing.

Haffner paused. Then Haffner swallowed.

And Zinka smiled at him. Plucking a tissue from beside the bed, she wiped the trickling semen from his belly – then flushed the heavy tissue discreetly away.

When Frau Tummel had left Haffner that afternoon, he had tried to argue that he was a libertine. Because he only cared about pleasure, he told her. This was why it would never work between them. And, furious, she had looked at him: her nostrils angrily flared.

—No, she said. No: you are too frightened.

The chutzpah of it had enraged him: because Haffner knew that it was true. For if Haffner were ever a libertine, it was never absolutely. He wasn't an absolute immoralist. He lacked the ruthlessness, the total selfishness.

But now, as he rested from Zinka's labours, he wanted to say that no, Frau Tummel was wrong. In some ways – the rhetorical ways – he wished that Frau Tummel could see him now. (He wished that Livia could see him now.) He wasn't too scared. He just hadn't wanted Frau Tummel enough. He just hadn't ever understood the ludicrous crazytalk of true desire.

Because, yes: desire is the ultimate in the improvised. This is the normal theory of desire. It was Zinka's – who was just about to explain to Haffner that now everything was over. But I am not so sure.

The difficult task is to improvise the seventeenth time. Or even, say, the second. It might have seemed so incandescent, one's impromptu smearing of chocolate mousse on the palpitating body of a woman – there where her flesh is most exposed. But if the next time one again moves doggedly to the refrigerator, then the prone and lovely woman will experience in her soul a tiny qualm.

The true libertines are the geniuses at repetition. Not the artists of the one-off, the improvised. Everyone can improvise. The true talent is in the persistence.

8

He woke up, to discover Zinka leaving.

He had drifted into what seemed like the deepest night of sleep, but which was in fact only a small moment; he had hardly closed his eyes. He looked down: his shrunken penis was sticky as an orchid bud.

—I have to go, she said.

—You could stay here with me, he said. Why not?

—I can't stay here, she said. I have to go home.

—But you can't let him make you, said Haffner.

—No one's making me, said Zinka.

Haffner looked woebegone. He felt worse than woebegone: he felt as if everything was over. Yet for a brief moment he had felt so utterly reborn. But then, who was Haffner kidding? How could a man be born, when he was old? What schlub was ever allowed the victory of a second chance?

—I mean, she said. Look at you. Look at me.

It was just a moment, she said. It wasn't love.

But, thought Haffner, he loved her. This seemed plausible. The speed of it was nothing for Haffner. It simply overwhelmed him with the evidence.

He knew, however, that he had thought that he had never thought like this before on previous occasions. The repetition, he had to admit, tended to produce a comical effect. So what was true? The feeling of uniqueness, or the feeling of a repeat?

And me, I do not know. Two answers seem possible, and only one can be true. Maybe Haffner was right to feel that he was always stuck in a repeat. He had always thought, every time he fell in love, that it had no precedent in the past. Just as a perplexed critic looks at a barbaric work of art, which seems to come from nowhere. And this was precisely why he repeated himself. He recognised nothing, because he forgot so much. And since he forgot so much, he always repeated himself. He always believed he was in love, when it was perhaps just another brief moment of desire. On the other hand, maybe the opposite was also possible. Every time he said he was in love, it was true. Every woman Haffner had loved had been unique. But he forgot so much, so lavishly. And the more he forgot, the more he tended to see each story as the same. Whereas, perhaps, no story was the same.

It is all a problem of perspective.

But whatever. Haffner, in however baffling a mess he found himself, was sure of this: the desire was nothing to do with Haffner. It wasn't a whim; it wasn't capricious. How could it be capricious if it was a compulsion? So maybe nothing was an imbroglio of one's own making. Maybe nothing was Haffner's fault. A new goddess appeared – that was all. And he surrendered.

9

Abandoned, Haffner began to argue with Zinka about the faithlessness of woman. He was aware that this was the opposite of what he had argued, a few hours earlier, to Frau Tummel: when he complained about the faithfulness of women. He was aware that he was beginning to resemble a character in the farces he had watched with Livia, in the 1960s, on Shaftesbury Avenue, the era when Haffner could still happily go to the theatre without being disappointed in the quality. But then, maybe this was fine. What else was farce but the way of understanding how quick one's ideas were, how soon their showers passed?

After all: this was why he liked Zinka. It was why he had loved Livia: he was always in search of the one who would leave him.

It had always been Haffner who was the one to leave. No one else. First Livia had destroyed this illusion of Haffner. But he had been able still to preserve one place of hope: that in the one-night stands, the brief affairs, it was always Haffner who left, cold-hearted.

Now even this was not true. Now that it was happening to him he was enraged by the injustice of it. Could a person simply choose whether or not they would have sex with someone else? Surely, if you had done it once, you had an obligation to continue for ever?

Although, as Zinka tenderly kissed him on the forehead, and left his room – not looking back at Haffner, naked on the bed – he could not conceal from himself the thought that this new incarnation did possess a certain logic. Maybe, thought Haffner, in a haze of contradiction, it was possible to love someone without wanting them: not to be tired with the need for possession. It didn't seem so unlikely. To want to inhabit the mind and body of someone else. For desire may involve possession. But also it might mean the opposite desire: to be possessed.

In his bedroom, Haffner was translated.

There was no reason, therefore, to be angry at Zinka. There was no reason to be proud. So what if she had left him? She entranced him precisely because she had never belonged to him at all.

Just as no one, thought Haffner, would belong to him again.

Or to put it in a way more familiar to Haffner, in the words of a great comedian . . . One day, this comedian, tired but happy, was walking down some street in Manhattan with his producer. The day's filming had gone well. Now they were off to some diner for a much needed salt beef sandwich, a much needed latke. Or whatever. As they sauntered down the street, two nuns, in wimples and solid shoes, walked towards them. And, solicitously, the great comedian took them aside, and very gently reminded them that he did apologise but they were in the wrong place. They had made a mistake. They weren't in this sketch.

In exactly the same way, what Haffner needed was the voice of a comedian, gently reminding him that now, regretfully, in the matter of Haffner, life was through.

Haffner, my hero, had outlived himself.

PART FIVE

Haffner Harmonic

1

The next morning – as the sun rose over the conifers, gilding the distant snows – Haffner woke up, raised his aching face and saw his battered suitcase: wrapped in creased and blotched cellophane, swaddled in blue adhesive tape, slashed by a diagonal tear which, according to the man who had delivered it – reception told him – could not be explained, and for which the airline admitted no responsibility.

In another era, perhaps Haffner would have instituted various legal battles. He would have written to the chairman and demanded compensation: donations to his designated charities. But not now. Haffner was no longer so proud of his property. He only felt a warm relief, as he abandoned his golfing trousers and tracksuits, and replaced the image in the mirror with a more familiar Haffner, in his brown tweed suit, his checked twill shirt, a muted tie: the handkerchief which Cesare had bought him in the Milan arcades stuffed with elegant negligence in his pocket.

Then he put on his glasses, and was fearful at his suddenly precise reflection. A livid stain was spreading across one cheek. A gummed splinter gelled in the tear duct of his right eye.

The reflection, however, perturbed him less than the pain within. His body seemed exhausted: he was shivering, worried Haffner, and his pulse was erratic. He felt for his clammy forehead: it seemed hot.

His first step, thought Haffner, in the life of this renovated, broken-down version of Haffner, should be breakfast. Then he should find Benjamin, and admit that perhaps Benji had been right all along. Though would he still believe that for a brief hour Haffner had been successful? Perhaps not, thought Haffner: perhaps not.

The dining room, by now, at this late stage of the morning, was empty. Haffner moved slowly along its buffet: with its sacks of grains and cereals, the contraption – which resembled no toaster Haffner had seen – for toasting bread, from which each slice emerged with its black insignia: a franking machine. All of these Haffner ignored. He took a croissant from some imitation of the rustic *panier*, and poured himself a coffee from the dregs of three silver Thermoses.

Haffner felt sick.

With flakes of croissant caught in the fibres of his tie, Haffner wandered out into the hotel's lounge: where the windows looked on to the mountains: their blues and greens and mauves. The absolute blue of the sky. It suddenly made sense to bespectacled Haffner now: this perfect view. He made for the bookshelves, but Haffner, whose flesh was sad, had read all the books he could. Humming to himself, he moved on to the miniature but eclectic collection of CDs – on a shelf, beside a book of mountain views, and a guidebook to the mountain walks, in French, from four years ago. And *Anne of Green Gables* in Spanish, and Volumes I and II of the *History of Nottingham* from the 1930s – but not the crowning Volume III.

Without expecting much, Haffner ejected someone else's CD featuring the classics of reggae from the 1970s, slid his own random choice into the waiting machine, and pressed play.

And Haffner discovered that he was in the orchestra stalls at the opera house.

2

As he gazed in the darkness, while fairies disported themselves on stage, Haffner was distracted by the surprise which had persisted, throughout the ballet's first half, at the smallness of Pfeffer's shilling tip to the cloakroom attendant in Rules, where they had eaten their theatre supper. In Haffner's opinion, no largesse was too much for the everyday retainers. So Pfeffer baffled him. But then Pfeffer often baffled him. Beside him, in the darkness, Pfeffer was holding opera glasses to his eyebrows like some marine instrument. They seemed to be directed at the mechanics of the flies.

Their respective wives were watching the ballet intently.

Haffner tried to settle into his velvet chair. He had accepted patiently this proposed outing, to celebrate Livia's birthday, to the Royal Ballet. It hadn't fit Haffner's idea of entertainment. But when he saw Bottom shrugging away his sorrow with a neat bend of his legs, Haffner began to enjoy himself. These people had humour, after all. While Livia watched beside him, on edge, transported – plucking at the plush velvet with her fingernails.

This theme recurred in Haffner's life. Twenty years later, in the living room of his daughter's house, he heard Benjamin trying to sight-read the same melodies: the cover of the score was worn like blotting paper. And in Benji's clumsy chords, Haffner rediscovered the sad emotion he had felt for the actor playing Bottom – the pirouettes, the tender holds! – in his massive ass's head. The sadness seemed to make sense to him now.

For what else was it as you lumbered across a room, towards the body of a woman, the prong of your penis straining to beat you in the race to touch her? It was farcical, always.

In the lounge of the hotel there was a curved bar made of vertical strips of pine, a collection of sofas, a box of board games. Into one sofa sank Haffner, as he played to himself, in the morning, the nocturne from Mendelssohn's ballet.

The horns, softly, their own echo, lay on the bed of the violins.

And as they did so, Haffner made a loop, descending from the childhood of Benji, back through Livia's birthday, to where this theme had first emerged. It was Haffner's theme tune. His first ever delicate kiss had occurred to this accompaniment, the music played with the film he had watched at the Ionic Picture Theatre, after which Hazel had allowed him to kiss her cheek.

In the window, outside, on the hotel veranda, he could see a woman emptying her rucksack – polyester in primary colours – of its crumbs, its lost cellophane wrappers from drinks straws, its crumpled tickets, its creased promotional leaflets to the most inauthentic restaurants.

Haffner contemplated the peaceful scene. There was no one in the lounge. Only Haffner. Everyone else was out walking, or swimming, or lying beside the pools. Or being cured of whatever they wanted to be cured of. But Haffner, instead, was lost in his persistent sense of floating, unattached.

Yes, checked Haffner, as if feeling in a pocket for his passport, the feeling was still there. Haffner was free.

3

As the soft nocturne continued, Haffner mooched among the CDs. He rejected showtunes from the movies; he rejected a selection of fados from the backstreets of Lisbon. And then, to his excitement, he found the Cole Porter songbook, as sung by Ella Fitzgerald.

If Haffner had an ideal musical form, it was the wordless harmonies of Duke Ellington's scat. But if there had to be words, then he wanted them to be Cole Porter's, with Ella's accent. She sang the songs so precisely, so simply. She confessed to her audience, as she had confessed to Haffner, that time in Ronnie Scott's, that ev'ry time they said goodbye, she died a little. And now, as he read the liner notes, he noticed the weird old-fashioned elision. Ev'ry! He'd only noticed the poetic quality of Cole Porter's title now, after – what was it? Sixty years? He rather liked it.

He was in the mood for preserving outmoded things.

—Benjamin! said Haffner, delighted.

Benjamin paused, and pointed a finger at his cheek, like a tearful harlequin.

—You've got a huge bruise on your cheek, said Benji.

Haffner asked him if he knew this one. Benjamin repeated his sentence; Haffner repeated his. Benjamin replied that no, not really. It was kind of not what he listened to, really. Then he should listen, said Haffner, raising a hand. As for the bruise – as for the bruise: the bruise was nothing, said Haffner.

Together they listened to Ella Fitzgerald explain to her silent audience how ev'ry time they said goodbye, she wondered why the gods above her thought so little of her that they allowed her lover to go. And then, once more, the strings came in, a trampoline for her voice.

—I'm not sure I like it, said Benji.

—How can you not like it, said Haffner, when it's true?

He had always loved this song for the frankness of its melancholy: its admission of being defeated by love. Perhaps this was the real America of Haffner – not so much the happy improvisation, as the stoic openness about pain. The acceptance of vulnerability was what moved Haffner now. He loved the Ella of this song, just as he had been charmed by his meetings with the innovative businessmen in the early seventies: the gunslingers, the white sharks. Sometimes, he had dealings with James Ling: the man who regarded the portfolio as a work of art, providing an escape from real life, and all its attendant risks. With his theory that one could diminish the risk of disaster by betting on everything. Patiently, over the years, Haffner had listened to their jargon – derivatives, risk arbitrage, hedge funds – all of them trying to pretend that these new ideas could diminish risk. And Haffner had listened to them, unconvinced – amazed by their ability to invent the idea of the rational bubble. So frank an oxymoron! So fragile a hope!

But Benjamin, this morning, was euphoric with optimism.

—Have you fixed things? Because I think I'm going to go back, said Benjamin.

—To bed? queried Haffner.

—Home, said Benjamin.

—To that summer school? said Haffner, looking down the song titles.

Benjamin said nothing.

—But this one, said Haffner to himself, is the real marvel.

—No, said Benjamin. I'm going back to her.

At this point, Haffner noticed something.

—You're in the same clothes as last night, said Haffner. You brought nothing else?

—I'm in the same clothes, said Benjamin. And then he grinned. To which Haffner offered a happily sceptical eyebrow.

—When did you arrive? said Haffner. Yesterday? I've hardly seen you.

Haffner had converted him. The legend of Haffner had now created the legend of Benji. For this would always be Benji's great story: the story of how he abandoned the practice of his religion, having slept with two girls in one week: in Tel Aviv, and then an Alpine spa town. Even if Haffner, in the mountains, had a finale all of his own. His story was all about the dismantling of his legend: the sudden zest for abandonment.

And, sultry in the mountainous morning, Ella began again to sing Cole Porter's classic: 'Begin the Beguine'.

—You're going to leave your school? asked Haffner.

—But have you fixed things? said Benji. I won't go if you still need me.

And Haffner considered this.

—No, he said.

—You haven't fixed things? said Benji.

—I don't need you, said Haffner.

—But no, began Benji.

—You ever heard of Artie Shaw? said Haffner, holding up the liner notes. Eight wives. Now let me tell you something, old boy.

But before he could continue Benjamin's education in the art of jazz, before he could continue to praise Benji for his liberation, before he could go on to explain that in fact uxorious panache wasn't what had made Artie Shaw remarkable – that in fact Artie Shaw's talent was his extension of the clarinet's upper range – there was an interruption.

4

Frau Tummel, clasping Herr Tummel's hand – like exhausted Olympic victors – appeared at the door of the hotel lounge. Like the overcrowded lounge at the end of a Parisian farce, an English murder mystery. Behind the Tummels, there was a man who was wearing his name pinned to his chest.

—He is here, announced Frau Tummel.

—Who? said Haffner.

—You, said Herr Tummel and Frau Tummel, in concert.

He had at least, thought Haffner, brought them back together. If this was the only good he had accomplished in this spa town, it wasn't nothing. Surely someone should acknowledge that?

The man with his name on his chest was the manager of the hotel. It was a pleasure to meet him, said Haffner, welcoming him with a handshake. This handshake was declined with a gentle cough, a gentle incline of the head.

Benjamin busied himself with the neat arrangement of a pile of magazines, dating from two years ago, concerning the niceties of couture.

Then the manager began his speech. He regretted to say it, he said, and he was sure that everything could be explained – just as, he added with what he imagined must seem an engaging twinkle, a teacher had once told him that everything, yes, must have an explanation, a rational explanation. So: he regretted the situation, but there it was.

Haffner watched him, silently.

Benjamin, in an attempt at disappearance, debated within himself the eternal oppositions: between the one-piece and the bikini; the bronzing or the elegance; the virgin or the whore.

So. There had been accusations. There had been comments raised to him of a personal nature, concerning Mr Haffner.

Haffner began to read the songbook's liner notes, with scholarly exactitude.

Yes, continued the manager, these allegations involved Haffner and a member of staff.

Haffner discovered with surprised satisfaction that the record – Haffner's vocabulary was not always modern – not only included Ella's renditions of Cole Porter, but also included a selection of live recordings: so that here, even here, in the least smoky and least cool environs of a spa town high in the backward Alps, Haffner could listen to Ella's improvisation of 'Mack the Knife' – an improvisation she delivered at the jazz festival in Juan-les-Pins on the French Riviera with Duke Ellington in 1966. Which Haffner himself had annoyingly missed. An improvisation, he then found out, which was in fact a staged version, since it went back to 1960 in Berlin, where Ella had first improvised these new lines to a song she couldn't remember.

Of course this could all be settled amicably, said the manager. He just needed to be aware of the facts. The facts as they had been made known to him by this lady here beside him. But he was sure that, perhaps, there had been a mistake.

—Present the evidence, said Haffner, simply.

Then he selected a new track, and pressed play. Because now he was truly bohemian: which is to say, he was bored.

Frau Tummel looked away, distressed.

—I'm sorry? said the manager.

He would of course have to determine the full facts, said the manager, raising his voice over the beginning big band. But naturally if this were true, he was afraid that naturally the young lady in question would have to be let go by the hotel.

—The evidence! shouted Haffner.

Furious, he turned away to the window, with his arms folded, and considered how he was going to save Zinka. It seemed unlikely. But Haffner wanted to try. For even if the world were a trap for Haffner, he saw no reason why it should be a trap for anyone else. Other people, he thought, could be done with being caught up in the farce of Haffner.

5

In other words, he no longer wanted to be Mack the Knife. It had always seemed to Haffner to be universal: this song which had begun in London, been rewritten in Berlin, then transatlantically re-rewritten by Louis Armstrong, Bobby Darin, and finally Ella and Duke. This universal ballad used to seem a statement of the universal facts as Haffner knew them.

But now, Haffner was less sure.

For Macheath was the perfect criminal. With Mack the Knife, anything was possible: on the Thames, a body was found; or there you were, in Soho, and a woman was discovered, raped;

or in the City of London, on a Sunday morning, there on the sidewalk was a body oozing life, and someone was sneaking round the corner.

This was how the song had gone, in Europe. Mack was the emperor of crime: the rewrite of a man like Tiberius, who made his guests drink lavish vats of wine, then tied a cord around their penises, so that their bladders burst. That was the usual story of how humans liked to be animals. But now that Ella sang it, something new occurred. Suddenly, realised Ella, the chorus had disappeared: and so that great singer, with her own bravado, had made up her own words.

Just like 'Begin the Beguine', the song had a way of extending itself. It went the distance. It possessed a final flourish of pure happiness.

For oh Bobby Darin, and Louis Armstrong, they made a record, ooh what a record, of this song, she sang. And now Ella, Ella and her fella, they were making a wreck, a wreck, such a wreck of the same old song. Oh yes yes yes yes they'd sung it, yes yes yes yes they'd swung it, they had swung Mack, they'd swung old Mack in town – for those people there, there, at the jazz festival, they were gonna sing, they were gonna swing, they were gonna add one more chorus.

And the Duke took over, with his big band.

Haffner, at the window, hummed along. And Benjamin, amazed at his grandfather's odd insouciance, amazed that one more time his grandfather was being accused of monstrous fidelity to pursuing love, went out on to the veranda. The prickly hair between Anastasia's legs returned to him, in the memory of his lips, his soft thick hands. It made him happy. While the manager, having been engaged in theatrical conversation, at this point left the hotel lounge with a final severe glance at Haffner: sweeping away in a flounce of Tummels.

It must, thought Haffner, have been Frau Tummel's doing: this catastrophe. And he could see why: always, the wives wanted to re-assert their dignity: the sanctity of their marriage. Betraying Zinka was simply Frau Tummel's way of doing this. He couldn't blame her. What else was Haffner doing himself – if not trying to reassert the sanctity of his marriage?

No, Haffner wasn't hurt by Frau Tummel's malice: the melo-drama of everyone's feelings. He was really done with all the theatre now. Because this was the point when Ella's scat began: the scat she had learned from Duke – the scat which Haffner admired. Twice she used it to push once more through, into a new repeat of the chorus. And then once more. And then finally again she sang: could they go with one, just one, one more? And oh they had swung it, yes they had swung it, they had swung old Mack, they'd swung old Mack for you. And once again they'd like to know, to let them know they were through.

And as the applause died down a voice said: You're the Lady – a voice which may well have come from the audience but which Haffner had always imagined, for Haffner liked his heroes to be friends, to be the voice of the admiring Duke himself.

6

Frau Tummel returned in the doorway. She called his name.

But Haffner was done with the romance of others. From the window, he walked across the room. As Frau Tummel motioned to speak, he held out a silencing palm. Instead, Haffner returned to the masterpieces of classical music.

Randomly, he chose a melody from the era of grand opera.

Oh but everyone knows the famous music where the music soars above the circumstances: like the beautiful aria sung by an unfaithful woman who is in love, without knowing it, with an unfaithful man. Or the song which is sung for a girl who is about to die beside her lover, immured in a tomb – music which somehow, as the master said, manages to leave behind the true circumstances of the singing, that two people were being buried alive; they would die together or (what was even worse) one after the other they would die from asphyxiation or hunger. Then the horrendous process of disintegration would set in until only two skeletons would remain, two inanimate objects quite un-affected by the presence or absence of the other. And yet, while all this was true, they continued to sing the most ethereal of melodies.

This is one version of music. It was the version which Frau Tummel believed in. Just as she believed in the eternal power of the feelings. But, for Haffner, music offered no lofty and ir-refutable soothing enhancement to life's unadorned and crude ugliness. He did not believe in music's triumphant power of transfiguration.

He stood and stared at Frau Tummel, who stared sadly back.

In this final meeting of Haffner and Frau Tummel, a gorgeous melody enveloped them. Unknown to both of them, a woman sang about her sad realisation, that the sincerity of passion is no argument against the corresponding truth of its comic portabil-ity. When a new god arrives – sang this woman, in a desert – we surrender.

Everyone moves from God to God.

But then, Haffner already knew this. He could have comforted Frau Tummel without the music. Think about it! Haffner could have said – if he had wanted to care for Frau Tummel in her romantic distress, sad at Haffner's betrayal, the speed of his feel-ings. Their liaison may have been brief, but it was still longer than many other more celebrated love stories. And the tempo of a love story's demise was no argument against it being a love story. The plot of *A Midsummer Night's Dream* takes just one night. In that night, so many couples swap over. The plot of *Romeo and Juliet* takes less than a week. Three days and three nights were all that was needed for a fairy tale. Three days and three nights were all that was needed for a fairy tale. In relative terms, the love of Frau Tummel and Haffner was endless.

And I think that it is possible to add one further comforting thought for Frau Tummel. There is a link, perhaps, between the transience of passion and the irony of the love songs. In the same way that a passion is always so much more fleeting than it believes itself to be, so a passion is always bestowed on an inappropriate object. But just because a passion might be bestowed on an inadequate object doesn't mean that the passion isn't real.

Everyone was on their desert island, waiting to be rescued by another god. It was true of Frau Tummel; it had been true of Haffner too.

Haffner auf Naxos!

Was Haffner laughable? Perhaps. But no more laughable than anyone else in love. To go for a young woman at seventy-eight was simply to add to the comedy of passion the comedy of the object.

7

The manager reappeared, with Viko.

—Yes, said Viko, looking bored.

That was the same man. Absolutely, improvised Viko. He had seen him kiss her too. Well then, said the manager. There seemed nothing more to say. He was sorry, but the matter seemed unambiguous.

Haffner had thought that a spa town would be a paradise of liberation. In his imagination, it was a bohemian idyll. And maybe it had been like this, for him, in some secret way. But the overt facts were disappointing. The morality of this place was so depressingly limited: a bourgeois, Communist morality – unoriginal even in its rules.

Haffner looked down, at his suit, at his shoes; at the tie which had been unaccountably crumpled by some customs official in Boston or Tehran. It seemed an adequate outfit for his own banishment.

There would be no need to let the girl go, he said. Instead, he would leave himself. He trusted that this would end the matter. The girl had done nothing wrong. He was sorry if he had behaved in an unbecoming manner.

This was really not what he had in mind, said the manager.

But no, Haffner halted him. It was the only just solution. He was sorry for the inconvenience.

And in the halo of his grandeur, Haffner nodded goodbye to Frau Tummel, to Viko, to the manager of his hotel, and strode out on to the veranda – where Benjamin was standing, looking out at the sky and its clouds, considering the phenomenon of Haffner.

—I am leaving in protest, said Haffner. This is a scandal. I will find another hotel.

—It's always like this, said Benjamin. It's kind of amazing. Everywhere you go, there's a crisis.

Haffner tried to protest. Once again, he had been the victim of an extraordinary set of circumstances. Benjamin said he had no idea.

Haffner changed the subject.

—So you're leaving as well, said Haffner.

—I'm really not sure now, said Benji.

—Come now, said Haffner.

—But Mama, said Benji.

—We will manage her, said Haffner.

And Benji, newly criminal, smiled.

—But you're sure you can handle this business? said Benji.

—It's paperwork, said Haffner.

He put his hand on Benji's shoulder, in his manly gesture of camaraderie.

—I always stick up for you, said Benjamin, looking out at the sun and the sky. Always.

And he broke off. He tried again.

--Even when she left, said Benjamin, – I still defended you.

And Haffner contemplated, for a moment, in an access of irritability at this kid's sincere demonstration of love, telling Benjamin the truth. For a moment, he imagined the conversation where he revealed, here, to Benjamin, and so to his family as well, the story of Livia with Goldfaden. How Livia had left Haffner not because she was enraged by Haffner's minor infidelities, not because of his refusal to take the art of ballet nor the religions of his forefathers seriously, but because she had been in love with another man. And then Haffner could have continued, and explained that the reason why Livia then lived for two years, the last two years of her life, on her own, in her flat in Golders Green, was not because she had so taken against the selfishness of Haffner that she had finally decided to abandon him, as her family believed, but because Goldfaden, when confronted by Livia's proposal that they could finally live together, now that his wife was gone, had gently but irreparably told her that this was a very bad idea. He was quite happy as he was. He couldn't understand what had come over her. There was no need for such theatrics, he had said.

This was why she had left, and not come back. She would not admit that she had been humiliated.

But Haffner would never tell Benji this. He would never tell anyone. No one would ever know about her defeat. He loved Livia with all the passion he was capable of; with an overwhelming care for her secrecy.

And maybe, I now think, as I watch Haffner stand there, that is how to truly be a libertine: to accept the libertinism of others.

For a final time, Haffner looked at the hotel's private landscape, the giant mountains, the infinite sky; then he patted Benji's shoulder again.

—You're a pal, he said.

And Haffner left the hotel.

Haffner Fugitive

1

Haffner stepped out into the midsummer afternoon, carrying his suitcase. It still trailed rags of cellophane.

The question was, thought Haffner, what he was to do next. Some form of shelter seemed imperative.

Wearily, Haffner made the long walk across the park, into the town, in search of a new hotel. The square was empty. The square was metaphysical. It was a Platonic form of sun. He passed a sports shop with a crate of plastic balls outside, printed with pictures of more leathery, more professional balls; he passed a patisserie with trays of greaseproof paper in the window. On a café terrace, a woman was pushing a folding chair flat with a pensive knee. On and on went Haffner, homeless in the heat. He was ancient. Everywhere was ancient: the imprinted gas vents were fossils in the pavements.

He couldn't stay just anywhere. He had his standards, his distastes. One hotel Haffner rejected because of the canaries kept behind the counter; another he rejected because of its incorporation of a nightclub.

So Haffner continued to walk, past the former medical institute, past the baths for men and the baths for women, and then, ahead of him, was the Metropole Cinema: its sign in handwritten squiggles of pink neon.

In general, if Haffner were forced to discuss the matter, he felt disappointed by the film industry. He did not feel the pictures had, as a rule, distinguished themselves. First the films were American. And these, Haffner had admired. Once, he had been Jayne Mansfield's banker: and she was a very handsome woman. Then there was a fashion for the French, which – as Haffner would inform the dinner party, the work colleague – left him cold. He never understood them: with their inexplicable cuts, their disdain for plot. Then Italian, then Japanese. Now they were God knows what. They were Mexican. But whatever their provenance, it really didn't matter, because one thing was sure: the new cinemas, with their speaker systems, were too loud for Haffner.

But Haffner, today, was tired. He wanted succour. At this point, Haffner would take anything.

He looked at the posters in front of the cinema. He recognised nothing; or no one. The language – as always, written in the language which for ease of reference Haffner was calling Bohemian – escaped him. The faces were foreign too. But Haffner didn't really want the film. He wanted the cinema instead: the rich festooned interior, the air conditioning and the darkness and the popcorn. He wanted peace.

So Haffner made his tentative way in.

In the foyer, a depressed salesgirl stood behind a stall which offered multicoloured packets of multicoloured chocolate. This combination tempted him. He bought two bars of chocolate. Then he approached the cloakroom. He lifted up his destroyed suitcase. The girl behind the counter looked at him.

—Is possible? asked Haffner, in his best imitation of foreign English.

She continued to look at him. Then she tore off a perforated ticket, and pushed it flat on the counter towards Haffner, letting it come to rest beside her magazine, which boasted of its proximity to the lives of the stars. Haffner heaved his suitcase up on to the counter, where a protruding plastic wheel caught the pages of her magazine, a circumstance which for a moment Haffner did not notice. As he pushed the suitcase across, he heard, to his alarm, a tearing sound, identical to the sound of glossy paper ripped.

She put the suitcase in a corner.

And Haffner turned round, to discover his interpreter from the Town Hall: Isabella.

—Is you, she said, pleased with this chance meeting.

—Is me, said Haffner.

—So how are things? she asked him. All good?

—Kind of, said Haffner.

— You will be glad to go home, stated Isabella.

Haffner considered this. He said nothing.

Isabella asked him where he was from, in Britain, and Haffner replied that he was from London. Isabella, she told him, had been to London herself. It was many years ago. She stayed at a hotel near Westminster. She told him its name.

—I don't know it, said Haffner.

—He knew it? asked Isabella.

He felt for his forehead. Now he was sweating profusely. He wasn't well: he wasn't himself.

—I don't know it, said Haffner.

And Isabella paused, lost in memories of bygone times.

Sweating, craving rest, Haffner excused himself, turned round, and – refusing the usher – entered the auditorium.

2

He realised that the reason for the usher's reluctance to let Haffner in – bearing though he did bars of chocolate and tickets, all the normal signifiers of an ordinary spectator – was that the film had started almost twenty minutes earlier. And perhaps, thought Haffner, if he had arrived at the beginning, then maybe he could have followed the plot. Now, it seemed unlikely.

Ahead of him, gigantic, loomed the dead.

He didn't really know, poor Haffner, why he was there. But then, the question of what he was doing anywhere had been posed so deeply to Haffner in the last few days that now he was tired of it. Happy, he settled into his bewilderment.

The film, it turned out, was in French, with subtitles; but Haffner no more understood the subtitles than he understood French.

One thing, at least, was clear. It was a war story. At first, he thought it took place in his war. Gradually he realised that it was taking place in his father's war: the Great War. Often wrongly called a World War. Whereas it was to be distinguished from Haffner's War, which was a truly World War. Though Haffner was increasingly unsure of both the greatness and the world.

Bereft of language, Haffner watched the slapstick. It seemed a reliable guide. Like so many war stories, this film was about escape. Happily, he watched as the prisoners propped a chair against the door, hooked a blanket over the blank window, prised up a floorboard. The alarm system was a tin can pierced by a string.

These escapes repeated themselves.

While, in the occasional background of an occasional shot, Haffner recognised what was left of his youth: sunlight, a horse passing by – its hooves and white ankles – watched by a slumped bored sentry.

How important could a man's life get? wondered Haffner. At what point would it ever become symbolic, or cosmic? Haffner was beginning to get a pretty shrewd idea. He was beginning to understand the abysmal length of the odds.

On the screen, the boredom continued. The prisoners tried to amuse themselves with amateur theatricals. They dressed up as girls, in stockings and heels. And Haffner with approving assent noted the silence, the deep hollowed silence as the prettiest kid emerged on stage in his chemise and stockings and hairband. The parody of the wife you hadn't seen for the last three years. The parody which broke the obvious rule: you couldn't think about sex, not in a war. But you only thought about sex. The last thing you needed was the reminder. And then a singing comedian came up on stage, who could neither sing nor make his audience laugh: a vampire, backlit, in white tie and tails.

And this was Haffner's past. He knew it intimately. The boredom was Haffner's domain – an infinite suspension. One had always lived, during the war, under the illusion that everything would be over very soon. Whereas now Haffner wondered whether both victory and defeat were for ever deferred. Although Haffner could not have said why – because one was endlessly defeated, or simply because the war was never over.

In the life of Raphael Haffner, maybe a truth became obvious. the great illusion – the true schmaltz – was always the illusion of victory.

3

Above him glowed the tired and blissful face of a French actor, licking his way along the rim of a cigarette paper: a harmonica. And although Haffner was almost happy here, in this cinema, after the initial coolness, the initial comfort of the velvet and the choco-late, he was still finding it difficult to focus.

He looked at the audience instead. It was sparse. The usual collection of misfits, the bedraggled loners: the geeks, the aca-demics.

Then Haffner noticed a tall lean angular neck, with a crest of hair, and seemed to recognise it. Was that Pawel? He couldn't tell. Pawel from the Committee waiting room: Haffner's exposed twin.

Haffner tried to get his attention – coughing, leaning forward – but Pawel simply sat there, entranced in the picture. And then, in Haffner's bored scan of the audience, his heart jolted.

Was that Zinka sitting a few rows ahead of him, diagonally across? He could not be sure. But before he could try to look closer, there sat down, late, a woman whose face was darkly hidden from Haffner, but whose scent clouded towards him: the delicious mixture of perfume and sweat. He had a thing for the imperfectly adorned, did Haffner. For the sorrow and the pity. But not now. Now he only wanted her to move.

He was going mad, he knew this. As if suddenly, in this backstreet backwater cinema, everyone he knew would have gathered, for Haffner's finale.

Concentrate! Concentrate!

And Haffner settled back into his seat, begrudging the cheapness of the velveteen, the dead springs inside.

He was oddly adrift from everything he knew. Haffner, now, had no one. Not even the troubles of his heart. No, not even the women troubled Haffner's thoughts.

On their holidays, Livia always had her little ritual. Happy at their escape, she used to ask him how far they were from the West End – the bright theatres – snug in her couchette above him, as they sped through the mountains of Italy to Venice, or Lake Como. Their daughter, with her husband and their son, was in the adjacent compartment. And the rain fell, wriggling in jerky zigzags down the pane. Against the wall was pinned a bulging net for Haffner's book and glasses. Yes, thought Haffner. She was always intent on putting distance between them and the rest of their known world. So how far was he now from London? He tried to imagine the distances. And in this way, making this calculation, in the full emergence from his chrysalis, Haffner fell asleep.

But maybe, to understand the full happiness of Haffner, I should contrast it with another metamorphosis: for Benjamin had undergone his own metamorphosis, his conversion to a world of pleasure. But this conversion had not led to a happiness impervious to fear.

In his room, the twin buds of his earphones in his ear, he was once more listening to his favourite hip-hop song of the moment, called 'Darkness'. And as he listened, he brooded, darkly.

The song called 'Darkness' was by Saïan Supa Crew, rappers from Marseilles. It opened with a sample from the most romantic song: 'Anyone Who Had a Heart' – with an abrupt drum roll and first faint orchestrated crackle, like the oldest radio in the world. And then, almost simultaneously, began the wistful violins. But the words – oh the words – Benji could not understand them. The rap, apart from one moment which he was sure mentioned the metro, eluded him. All he could recite, without understanding, was the chorus.

Ho, c'est le darkness, recited Benji, grandly: *adieu à l'allégresse, c'est le darkness, c'est Loch Ness, c'est le madness, la lumière se baisse.*

The first time he heard the song was in Tel Aviv, in the apartment of the girl whom he once hoped would become his girlfriend. Or, more precisely, whom he once hoped would let him see her naked. He wasn't ambitious. She shrugged a nonchalant record from its sleeve and made it frantic. On the cover was a black-and-white photo of a cream block of flats in the most modern version of Paris, with a patchy sky and burnt-out cars.

Since then, he had listened to this song called 'Darkness' over and over. And he still did not know precisely what it meant. But to him it was so beautiful – with its plush American romantic violins, crackling with nostalgia, and sarcastic clever French rhymes (rhymes whose meaning he did not understand). It seemed so poignant with poise, so world-weary with sadness.

Luxuriously, therefore, romantic, Benji contemplated his fears.

It wasn't the first time. Three years earlier, Benji had been stricken by a vision of his death, in some club in an industrial part of north-west London: for the first time in his life he had not only taken a tab of LSD but had added, recklessly, a pill as well. So Benji could soon be found sitting on his own, carefully near the accident and emergency room, feeling sick, and terrified, as hippies with matted dreadlocks bent forward to leeringly if kindly ask about his health. He had decided that he would not go into the emergency room until it was absolutely necessary. He was mortified by appearances. This tendency to be mortified was adding to his panic, since all too easily he could imagine the headlines in the newspapers the next morning: the school photo, the tearful parents, the charity estab-lished in his memory. It would have to be him, the amateur who died after taking a pointless and accidental overdose: the bourgeois boy adrift in the world of cool.

The great screw-up: this was Benji's constant anxiety. He always went in fear of doing or saying the minute thing which would place everything in the greatest danger.

Really, thought Benji, there was no need to understand the words of this, his favourite song. He knew what it was about. True, the moments of incomprehension were everywhere. He was not convinced, for instance, that in the chorus of one of their songs, a hip group of French hip-hoppers, whether from the graffiti'd *banlieue* of Paris or the graffiti'd suburbs of Marseilles, could really be saying *c'est Loch Ness*. Maybe Loch Ness, with its monstrous Scottish depths, connoted darkness to a group of French hip-hoppers, but this seemed hopeful and unconvincing. This seemed his provincial, unlikely mishearing. But then, what did this mistake really matter?

He knew what this song was about. The song was about the fear.

The voices were all he needed, because the voices were grave, and delicate: they were, for him, the meaning. The meaning of this song was in the collage of serious, careful voices, trying to resist the melancholy romantic violins.

Because they couldn't. No one could resist the romance, he thought: as he contemplated the screwed-up mess which was the life of Benjamin.

5

When Haffner woke up in his uncomfortable velvet seat, he discovered the black-and-white outlines of a new prison for the characters on the silver screen: a grander, more feudal kind of prison. It was some kind of schloss – with pines and stones, and Gothically written signs warning against escape. The scene took place by night. And this time a man with a French accent and a man with a German accent were talking to each other in English: a fact which led Haffner to wonder if he was still dreaming.

—Have you really gone insane? said the man speaking with a German accent.

—I am perfectly sane, said the man speaking with a French accent.

He really couldn't be sure, thought Haffner, at what point any of this had been a dream. From the moment he met Zinka until now. From the moment he met Livia until now. With depressed accuracy, however, he felt compelled to admit that no moment of his life could really be excused or explained by a theory of unreality.

The German and the Frenchman continued their elegant debate in English.

—It's damn nice of you, Raffenstein, but it's impossible, said the Frenchman.

And with that, he began to climb, while the Germans trained a searchlight on him, like a music hall artiste: the famous actor in his follow spot. As, presumed Haffner, he was. In another version of the world entirely. And when Haffner then saw the man halt, arch his back, and stumble; when he saw the Frenchman on his deathbed, tended to by the German who had shot him, he wished he could believe it. He wished he could be moved. But partly there was the problem that he could hardly be moved by a film he had barely seen, and barely understood; and also there was a deeper reason.

Haffner didn't care about nobility. He didn't care about the soul. Just the beauty of escape.

All of Haffner's dreams of escape were suddenly incandescent. He sat there. And when the house lights came up – revealing to Haffner's placid eye the empty drinks cartons, packets of sweets, the crisp cellophane from cigarettes – and the credits rolled, he sat there while the small audience filed out, checking the footwells for coats, for wallets, for all the human belongings. The man he thought was Pawel was just conceivably Pawel: he could not be sure.

The girl he thought was Zinka turned out to be a teenage boy.

6

And Haffner, left behind in the cinema, considered how, on the one hand, there was the myth of the escape. Everyone understood the need for this myth. But maybe the need was explained by another wish: the safety of a refuge.

He had always assumed that he would go back home, to London, when the paperwork on the villa was completed. It wasn't as if he was here as an exile. But then, anything could become an exile, if it became impossible to go back.

And Haffner considered this spa town.

In Haffner's mind, his vision of Livia's villa was now merging with his vision of the cottage in the film, a cottage where the Frenchman had conducted some form of love affair with a lonely woman on her farm. The husband, presumed Haffner, must have been away, at the war. This cottage represented some kind of idyll. And now Haffner was wondering if he was beginning to understand the need for this cottage, he understood the need for a refuge. It was the deeper meaning of every escape. Just as he now understood how deeply he missed the girl who had stayed with them, in 1939: the girl whom none of them could understand, who took her own life. She was looking for a refuge, and she had not found it. And just as how – if one discovered the most minute version of Haffner, the slimmest, most concentrated fraction of Haffner – in some way, he thought, he understood what their marriage had represented to Livia. It might have seemed inconceivable to the outside observer, but to her it was a place of safety. For she knew he would never leave her. Haffner mimed the act of leaving, but he never would.

He had always believed that there would always be another girl; just as he had always believed that he would always have another city. However much he might have made mistakes, however unsure he may have been that he had made the right decision, he could always start over again. But now, he thought, he didn't.

And me, I might put it more sadly. I might use the words of the poet – the poet of a disappeared empire · who once said that in the way a man destroys his life here, in this little corner, so he has destroyed it everywhere else. But Haffner's pessimism was more euphoric. The problem had always been in finding the right elopee. But surely the elopee was obvious. It was always only Livia. If he added up his women, he decided, he had only ever had two: Livia, and then everyone else. Yes, thought Haffner. He had always seen everything in terms of repetition. And now it turned out that there was such a thing as a singularity. And love proved it.

The *trompe l'oeil* of the ending! The false bottom of the ending!

Could he manage one more? wondered Haffner. He thought he could. Let him swing it one last time.

His century was over, and all Haffner wanted to take from it was the memory of Livia. He only wanted, now, to assert his constant fidelity.

Why did he need to go back, when the paperwork was completed? Why couldn't he, thought Haffner, live there in the villa – surrounded by the history of Livia? And in the excitement of his decision, Haffner wanted to see the villa, now – the villa which he had not thought he ever wanted to visit. He wanted to pay homage to Cesare's famous ceiling – executed in the dining room when he was sixteen, when he still believed in his destiny as a great European painter. Homeless, he wanted to observe what would be Haffner's final home.

7

Haffner marched out into the foyer. The window to the cloakroom was shut. At the ticket booth, he pointed to the cloakroom. The woman in the ticket booth shrugged, helplessly. Haffner mimed, like a monkey, the heaviness of twin suitcases, invisibly weighing down his arms.

—No no, said the girl.

—No? said Haffner.

The girl said a word which Haffner did not understand. She turned to the calendar behind her on the wall, one half of which was a series of mountain views, underwritten by romantic poetry; the other half of which was a grid with numbers. She pointed to one square, containing one number.

And finally Haffner understood that he would only be able to recapture his belongings the next day.

With a renewed sense of triumph, therefore – since what more could he now lose? – the untold story of Haffner reached its conclusion. He would go to look at the villa, unencumbered by his possessions. And eventually he would live up here, in this spa, in this place of his escape: in the solitude of their infinite marriage: its absolute irrelevant immortal secrets.

For this, thought Haffner, was the true version of Haffner – a husband.

In a bar out on North Beach once, in San Francisco, he had talked to the barman about DiMaggio. DiMaggio, said the guy behind the bar, had been a regular. And the barman confided in him that when Joe was dying, he used to say that it was no sadness to him. At least, he said, it would maybe give him another chance with Marilyn.

It had shocked Haffner then. Now, however, it seemed bleakly accurate. It seemed adequate to the facts.

Always, he had wanted out, thought Haffner. And now he didn't.

Haffner Mortal

1

As the twilight began, the subtlest twilight, Haffner walked up the long road towards the villa. He tended to his memories of Livia. It was his triumph, his procession through the city's streets: with his conquered slaves before him – and his personal freedman behind him, whispering that Haffner was mortal.

And that former slave, for now, is me.

Yes, the conjuring with tenses was now all over. For Haffner had indeed caught a cold two mornings ago, when he swam in the lake with Frau Tummel: finally, the symptoms were for real. And in two weeks' time this cold would develop into a virulent form of pneumonia, which would be imperfectly treated, here, in the Alps, by a junior doctor whose concentration was distracted by his concern to keep calling his girlfriend and assure her that he loved her, stricken as he was by his lone moment of infidelity, an impulsive regretted kiss at a soirée after a conference; so that by the time Haffner was flown home to London – successful, true, in his legal pursuit of the villa – he would have already suffered a stroke. And in that weakened, muted state, began the long dying of Haffner.

It wasn't the defeat he had intended, or predicted: like everyone's defeat. It was just the one that Haffner got.

But at this moment, Haffner was still happy in the bliss of his escape. Up the hill he walked, out of the town, into the depleted suburbs: his natural habitat.

On reaching the drive which led to the house, however, he was struck by a problem. What Haffner had not considered, in his moment of emotion, was the legal problem. He did not own this property, obviously. He knew this. The company who used it as a holiday home still owned it. It now struck him that he had no idea how he might explain why it was that he was here: a bedraggled ancient madman with a bruise above his eye and around his cheek.

For a moment, his bravado disappeared. A homesickness over-took him. In Benjamin's bedroom, which had already not existed for years, he began to describe to Benjamin, in his bunk bed, how easy it was for Santa Claus to fly: he was buoyant, said Haffner. He simply floated.

In this cloud, Haffner stopped at the gate of the house. Perhaps, thought Haffner, no one was there. It could be standing empty.

Haffner paused.

He was here, thought Haffner, so he would brave it. And Haffner walked across the grass, and opened a door.

2

Haffner found himself in the kitchen: bare, lined with white tiles. A spiral iron staircase seemed to lead to all the other floors. Haffner stood at the base of the stairs, listening. He could hear nothing. So Haffner ascended and found himself in a corridor – covered in grey wallpaper, with brown stains, like stock market graphs, rising from the skirting – which led to the roofed veranda. Haffner knew about this veranda. On this veranda, Livia's father used to sit, watching each Alpine sunset. It used to have wooden floors, with zigzagging parquet. Now, the floor was lino; and the view had been glassed in.

It seemed to be a dining room: two Formica tables were lined up against each other. On one of them, there was a plate with a slick of butter flattened on its rim.

Haffner stood there. He looked down. Just like Uncle Eli, who – so Goldfaden told him – at one point in his late escape from Warsaw reached a wall: and there below him was a courting couple. They were sitting on a bench. A plane tree was growing in its wire netting beside them. The man was begging his girl to come inside with him, up to his apartment. It was just up there, he said. Her mother would never know. The girl was not so sure. And Eli had perched there, looking down on them, begging this girl silently to ignore her moral scruples, to go into the room. This resistance fighter, said Goldfaden, his slight jowls shaking with laughter – imploring her to give up her resistance!

Even now, Haffner found this amusing.

From the veranda, another door led into an empty room, containing just a photo of the President, and a plastic sign advertising the various ice creams to be found in a miniature freezer, there in the corner, humming to itself. So Haffner did not know that this, in fact, was the room which had once contained the grand brick fireplace beloved by Livia's mother, which had now been blocked up and plastered over. Nor did he know that Cesare's treasured ceiling, on which he had depicted The Dream of Europa, being squabbled over by two women who represented two continents, had been boarded over by another dropped ceiling, twenty years ago.

Everything was missing.

Upstairs, the bedrooms were filled with bunk beds; and more grey wallpaper. The bathroom which had been Livia's mother's personal project, obsessed as she was by all the conveniences of modern hygiene, with bidet, toilet, mirrors, handshower – all the delightful gadgets – had been replaced by a stone floor and three doleful showerheads, hanging their heads from the ceiling.

And when Haffner ascended, finally, into what had been the eaves, where Cesare kept his painting things and Livia kept her costumes from all the plays she had ever been in, there were now four small mansard rooms. Above each door there was a sign demanding that no one should smoke.

Haffner pushed one door open. Again, there was a bunk bed. A bra was resting on a chair. He turned to go, and as he turned he saw the notice which was on the back of every door, extending a most cordial welcome to this vacation home. Haffner was wished a wonderful stay. To guarantee order in the home, however, he was asked to observe some simple house rules. Sadly, Haffner read the times for meals, and the pickup of picnic lunches; the time for the afternoon rest period. During this time, Haffner was asked to refrain from playing the radio: instead, he should walk quietly on the stairs, and close doors quietly. In the immediate vicinity of the house, children were also required to play quietly. Lying on the beds in day clothes was not permitted. Requests and complaints should be addressed to the house manager.

All the ornament, all the marginalia and doodling were gone.

Unlike Solomon Haffner, his son believed in inheritance. The European museums always left Haffner sad. He saw no reason why a home should be given to the state. If Haffner had his way, if Haffner were a president, or a mayor, he would restore these ancestral homes to their rightful families. The pleasure of the chateau tour always eluded him. He could not help thinking of the dispossessed. This sensation returned to him now.

Yes, Haffner wished that he could bring everything back. He wished everything could be revised. In this, Haffner's last judgement, everything he had once consumed would be made whole again: the cigarettes would ravel themselves back into neat cylinders, the wines would loop back into their bottles; all the newspapers he had ever thrown away, all the detritus, would be restored in Haffner's sight. And finally the women. Everyone would be returned to him – resurrected: all the people he had loved. Because the problem with Haffner, really, was that he loved too many people. Thought Haffner.

He tugged at a venetian blind's toggle. It snapped up, like an aperture.

And Haffner, ignoring the landscape, remembered how, ten years earlier, when Morton was dying, he had gone to see him in Brooklyn. And because he couldn't think of anything which seemed in any way adequate to the monstrous fact of Morton's death, he tried, as he had so often tried to explain to Morton, the nature of a draw in cricket. It wasn't the simple matter of the scores being level. As always, this was where the foreigner became confused. But this time Haffner didn't bother with the detail. He didn't try to explain the technicalities: he just tried to explain its beauty. What it meant, he said, was that in cricket you could never be sure of victory or defeat: you could snatch defeat from the jaws of victory and victory from the jaws of defeat. And this was wonderful. It meant, Haffner tried to explain, that there was no reason for the strong to win.

Morton's contribution to this had been to tell him a story.

Was it like this? said Morton.

Man, said Morton, Haffner didn't know what the British had missed, sitting outside Rome, waiting on the Americans. When they had gone into Rome, said Morton, it was crazy. And Morton then told him a secret. So there Morton was, in Rome, in bed with two girls. One of them was his girlfriend, the other one was not. They were simply trying to sleep. Because everything was a mess. He had no idea why they'd ended up in the same bed. And in the middle of the night, he turned to the girl who was not his girlfriend. For she undid him. She was so beautiful. And they kissed. He shivered with the memory of it. They kissed and kissed. He put his hand down her skirt. He felt her, there where her legs became so intricate with flesh. The soft cleft with the strong bone above it. And this was the great moment of his life, said Morton. Beyond anything he had ever felt with his adored wife. It was the moment of absolute excitement.

—And? said Haffner.

—And nothing, Morton said. Nothing happened. My girl woke up. So we both pretended to be asleep.

3

No doubt about it: Morton understood.

In the end, you had to get over the victories and the defeats.

—You know, said the celebrated movie star Hugh 'Tam' Williams, on the way to Aldershot in 1939 for their training, you're going to make it. You've got it in you. You have star quality. I can tell these things.

And Haffner had never forgotten this. Slick compliment it may have been, to pass the time in some station café more pleasantly, but Haffner believed he meant it.

He didn't need his wallet and its mute photograph album now. Haffner was quite happily his own mausoleum. The pictures came back to him so easily.

What had been Haffner's victories? The Athletics Cup in 1934. The Divisional Cricket Championship in Jerusalem in 1946. The presidency of the City branch of the Institute of Bankers in 1982.

But the real victory, thought Haffner, was elsewhere. It could take place anywhere: not just in the eternal cities, with the Colosseum for backdrop, or disporting in the Roman swimming pool, watched over by a Fascist eagle. And Haffner, remembering that night, when Rome was liberated, then thought of another swimming pool – in LA, where Goldfaden's Uncle Eli lived. He was having some kind of pool party. And Eli had begun to reminisce about the Ghetto in Warsaw. Of course, said Eli, after the third year people started reminiscing. It wasn't like this in the beginning, they used to say: then things were so much better.

With a bottle of beer in his hands, tipped with a crescent of lime, Haffner had guffawed.

In this humour, in this privacy, Haffner reckoned the true triumph might be found.

And then Cesare – who had wandered over, dressed neatly in his European and academic suit, refusing all West Coast dress codes – entered the conversation and reminded Haffner and Eli of a resistance fighter's great interview, twenty-five years after it was over, when he pointed out that the history of the Warsaw revolt wasn't going to be one for the military historians. The outcome had never been in doubt. It wasn't notable for its strategy. But if there was a school to study the human spirit, then it should be a major subject. The importance was the force shown by the Jewish kids, after years of degradation, to rise up against their destroyers: and choose their own death. Was there, asked this hero, a standard which could measure that?

This man here, said Cesare, pointing at Haffner, he didn't want to be Jewish. He would never acknowledge, said Cesare, how much the Jews were hated. How much strength they had to be capable of. And Haffner, only wanting to locate Livia and go with her to the edge of the garden, to look out over the city, disagreed. It was true that he loved the image of the Jews as musclemen, the men of steel. But really what he admired was something else entirely. It wasn't Jewish – the revolt. This was Haffner's theory. It was a triumph of something much more universal.

Such confusion! said Cesare. But it was only to be expected. This was the constant problem. You try to assimilate, and in fact you just lose everything: you lose your family, but you also can't make friends. You can neither go forwards nor backwards. Wasn't this right, Raphael?

Oh he had loved Cesare so much, thought Haffner. Cesare had courage. But even Cesare was not as courageous, thought Haffner, as he should have been. The deepest courage belonged to those who chose to withdraw. To be doubly rejected, encircled by rejections – by the Jews and the non-Jews – allowed you an absolute freedom.

Haffner didn't care if he was a contradiction, an impossible hybrid. After all, he liked the hybrids. The greatest piece of music in the world was Mozart's Clarinet Concerto, as improvised by the great Benny Goodman. Haffner went for such impossible beings: the sphinxes, the centaurs.

And maybe, I think, Haffner was right – as he stands there at the window of a dismal bedroom, which had once belonged to Livia. His century had been a century of metamorphoses. And at its centre was his greatest invention of all: the strange winged beast of Haffner's marriage.

4

In the darkening sky, the reticulate constellations were nets, hauling in Haffner.

He had left Frau Tummel behind. Zinka, it is true, troubled Haffner's thoughts: but gently, tenderly. She still eluded him. He could only think of her obscured: taking off her T-shirt, an arm making shadows of her face.

So, for one last time, I want to go in search of Zinka.

She was in her apartment, in front of her television: in the living room decorated with prints of haystacks, a cathedral facade disintegrating in the twilight. She sat there until the light went, then went to sleep. And then that night, as usual, Niko came home, and made for Zinka's bed, where Zinka was doing her best to form the letter S. Her bed was in fact a sofa. It disguised itself as a bed in the darkness of the night. Its covering was ribbed polyester, dyed grey. Niko tried to follow the breathing which made her chest ascend and descend, cleanly silhouetted in a sheet. He tried to synchronise his breathing to hers. In the same way, in the dark mornings, before school, when he was eight, and it was snowing, he had crept into bed beside his mother, and tried to match his breathing to hers. Someone once had told him that men's respiration was quicker than women's, which was why women lived longer. So he tried to calm his breathing down.

Very slowly, Niko then began to move.

He felt his usual combination of the erotic and the uncomfortably sad. As he laboured inside Zinka – as she lay on her stomach, her legs cramped in angles which he could not alter, which would not let him extend himself in the way which Niko might have liked – he tried to tell himself that although it was not the life of desire he had imagined, perhaps it was enough. Perhaps Niko was happy.

But he could not.

No, long after he had finished with Zinka, who was pretending to pretend to be asleep, Niko lay awake, watching the shapes of the books melt and blur against the wall, in the dark, in dawn's twilight   yes, long after his bleated, blurted defeat as he reared over her, stabbed in the back by his soft orgasm. While Zinka lay there, imagining all the other lives she could be living.

And then they fell asleep.

5

Haffner walked downstairs, and went on to the villa's enclosed veranda. He looked out into the landscape: where the colours were. Yes, there they were: pure, like the colours Haffner had seen in the museum in New York – more neatly arranged there, true, more vibrant, but with the same lightness, the same absence of any human mistake. They obeyed their own mute logic.

Haffner was horticultural. He knew about the breeds of roses: how they formed an ideal order, invisible to the human brain. His life had often led him to gardens. Like the gardens of Ninfa, near

Rome. Or Haffner's own rose garden, where Solomon had taught him the two possibilities for a life: to live it, or to waste it. As if the choice were Haffner's.

The forest was a smudge of greens and blacks: a giant discarded palette. Through the trees, the sun was a precise gold disc pressed on to the horizon.

It was an industrial pastoral, with the sounds of the sibilant freeways in the distance: the twentieth century's automobiles and dryads, its fauns and chemical plants. He tried to hear the tune which had been playing at his first ever dance with Livia in Southwark. Naturally, he could not. He was not romantic enough for that. There was now just the sound of the wind in the trees, and the sound somewhere of the cattle bells – those bells, thought Haffner, which must so irritate the proud cow, reminded with every move of their ownership by others. Or maybe, thought Haffner, it was no more irritating to them than the weather. Maybe the bell was part of the bovine condition.

But before he could continue his meditation on the limits of a cow's perception, he was distracted by a bumble bee, hovering against the glass. And then another. And Haffner, in his exasperation and fever, began to wave the bees away: so that from a distance, from the position of the imaginary spectator, all that could be seen was Haffner, standing at the window, beating time to the grandest and most transparent orchestra.

6

And maybe, as he stands there, I should balance Haffner's faults and virtues. Perhaps this is the point to decide whether Haffner was a hero or a monster. But even if I could truly describe him now, as he looks out of the window, in his wife's villa, would that portrait equally apply to the soldier in Palestine, the husband in New York, the romantic in London?

He always saw himself in poses. And this series of receding Haffners could continue diminishing, into infinitely vanishing fractions.

I wanted to preserve the real Haffner. I wanted to resurrect him. The Haffner I actually knew was a man of reticent privacy. I only had the stories to work with. I only had my inventions. But whether they were true or not, Haffner was inescapable, in all the stories he gave rise to . . .

And this was, perhaps, how history worked.

As an admirer of the classics, Haffner wanted to understand what caused the great empires' decline. I was more modern. I wanted to know how the emperors had turned into legends. But maybe both these questions possessed the same solution. The law of unintended consequence – the law which governs every empire's decline – was so definitive that every emperor became a legend: enveloped by their own defeat. No historian, after all, could ever know all the causes. So they had to write a legend. A legend is just a story which is missing most of its causes; a legend is just a feat of retrospective editing.

The more I knew of Haffner, the more real he became. this was true. And, simultaneously, Haffner disappeared.

7

Haffner walked away, down the steep road back into town, towards the spa, to find a hotel. In the same way as that classical king who, as the poet says, when deserted by the Macedonians did not behave like a king. Instead he threw away his golden robes, borrowed someone's everyday outfit, then left – like an actor who, once the play is over, changes back into his clothes and wanders away.

As he walked, he remembered Livia's funeral: how from the window he had seen the undertakers waiting outside, like paparazzi, for the body; and the organist, playing the funeral march as everyone shuffled away, finished with a comic trill, a final flourish, when he thought that everyone had gone – a squiggle of pure flippancy. Just as Haffner would have told her, afterwards, in the refuge of their bedroom, if it hadn't been Livia who had died.

Think about it, thought Haffner.

Exiled on St Helena, Napoleon continued to be chic. He cared about his waistcoats, the gold stitching of his shoes. Yes, it was unbelievable, but it was true. All the victors were masters of retreat. They cultivated retreat. Even Tiberius, the ruler of the world – a god with his giant pied-à-terre in Rome – preferred the quiet island of Capri.

But me, I might put it like this: there you are, dear reader, at the pool party, by the sea, in the sunlight, with the pine forest sighing behind you, and the blue sea sighing in front of you, ceaselessly bringing you tribute, while in the distance the dolphins show off the sheen of their backs; and then, from somewhere invisible, out of your field of vision, you hear a deep splash, a forsaken cry, and when you turn to look – there it is, the surface, settling in circular ripples, which enlarge, and then enlarge some more: until they enlarge into nothing.

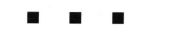

Postscript

This book contains quotations, some of them slightly adapted, from works by W. H. Auden, Saul Bellow, Bertolt Brecht, Mel Brooks, Constantine Cavafy, Blaise Cendrars, George Eliot, Ella Fitzgerald, F. Scott Fitzgerald, Gustave Flaubert, Edward Gibbon, Alfred Goldman, Robert Graves, Alfred Hitchcock, Courtney Hodell, Hugo von Hofmannsthal, Christophe Honoré, Horace, Bohumil Hrabal, Peter Stephan Junk, Franz Kafka, Velimir Khlebnikov, Ladislav Klíma, Stéphane Mallarmé, Thomas Mann, Groucho Marx, Thomas Middleton, Vladimir Nabokov, Marcel Ophuls, Georges Perec, Petronius, Alfred Polgar, Alexander Pope, Cole Porter, Alexander Pushkin, François Rabelais, Saïan Supa Crew, Viscount Samuel, William Shakespeare, Tupac Shakur, Stendhal, Laurence Sterne, Alexander Stille, Suetonius, Tacitus, Junichiro Tanizaki, Leo Tolstoy, Paul Valéry and Virgil.